Healing
and Restoring

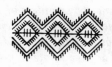

Coordinating Editors
Martin E. Marty   James P. Wind

Also available from Macmillan Publishing Company is Caring and Curing: Health and Medicine in the Western Religious Traditions, *eds. Ronald L. Numbers and Darrel W. Amundsen (1986).*

The Park Ridge Center, which sponsers the series, is an interdisciplinary, multireligious research institute founded on the premise that studies in health and medical ethics cannot be complete or satisfying unless they take into account basic human belief systems. The Center was established in 1985 to fill a perceived international need for the study of religious aspects of human well-being, especially as they relate to prevention and treatment of disease, interpretation of illness and health, and ethical issues connected with these matters.

Through its Associate membership program, the Center brings together thousands of representatives from religion, health care, history, science, and the humanities who reach across traditional disciplinary boundaries to relate their own fields of interest to many others. The Park Ridge Center disseminates its research and discoveries through numerous publications which are sent to all Associates or made available at a discount. The Center welcomes contributions from its Associates in the form of letters, research suggestions, and articles for review and possible publication in Second Opinion *or in the Center* Bulletin.

Additional information may be obtained by writing to The Park Ridge Center, 676 North St. Clair, Suite 450, Chicago, IL   60611.

Healing
and Restoring

Health and Medicine
in the World's
Religious Traditions

EDITED BY
Lawrence E. Sullivan

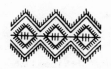

MACMILLAN PUBLISHING COMPANY
A Division of Macmillan, Inc.
NEW YORK
Collier Macmillan Publishers
LONDON

The chapter opening decoration in this book is a medicine-man sand painting design from *Navajo Medicine Man Sandpaintings* by Gladys A. Reichard © 1977 and is reproduced by permission of Dover Publications, Inc.

Macmillan Publishing Company
866 Third Avenue, New York, N.Y. 10022

Collier Macmillan Canada, Inc.

Library of Congress Catalog Card Number: 89-30298

Printed in the United States of America

printing number
1 2 3 4 5 6 7 8 9 10

Library of Congress Cataloging-in-Publication Data

Healing and restoring : health and medicine in the world's religious
  traditions / edited by Lawrence E. Sullivan.
    p.   cm.
  Bibliography: p.
  Includes index.
  ISBN 0-02-923791-2
  1. Health—Religious aspects.   2. Medicine—Religious aspects.
I. Sullivan, Lawrence Eugene, 1949–
BL65.M4H43   1989
291.1′75—dc 19   89-30298
                                                            CIP

For my parents,
Lawrence and Bertha

Contents

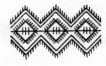

Foreword

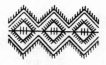

An earlier and companion work to this one dealt with the subject of caring and curing "down the block," as it were—with issues of health and medicine as they relate to religions in that part of the world we call the West. In that volume scholars informed and served professionals and laypeople alike in the fields of medicine, religion, and ethics.

This second volume, which stands independently, moves us figuratively beyond the block on which most of the readers live to the neighborhood "across the street"—to cultures, in both the East and the West, that few of us have until now encountered. The readership for this volume expands in equal measure with the scope of its subject matter to include those who enjoy the study of culture and the history of religions. While there are good reasons for this book to find its way to libraries around the world, most readers will probably be in the Western world. Mentally and metaphorically they will find themselves opening a large road map that charts the world of health, medicine, and religion.

These case studies take readers from native American communities and Haitian devotees of Vodou (who may be down the block more than across the street) through sub-Saharan Africa or Latin America, to the widespread religious traditions of Islam, Hinduism, and Buddhism.

Among the peoples studied here are Bantu-speaking peoples of Africa. Several Bantu languages possess a proverb I have long cherished, one that applies to readers of a book like this: "He who never visits thinks mother is the only cook." This book will help us enlarge the repertory of options and learn our way around other figurative kitchens, not just in order to sample à la carte but to come to a more profound understanding of the world.

If we take the offerings in this book as insights into the thinking of large populations, we are looking at a majority of the world's people: Buddhists, Muslims, Hindus, Taoists, Confucians, and those following the traditions of local ancestors in Asia, Africa, Oceania, South Asia, the Caribbean, and the Americas. What do we make of them all?

Before we try to make something of them, let me issue a guarantee. Having attended the conferences at which these essays were first presented and then having read them, I can warrant that if you begin reading almost anywhere, you will read on, with fascination, sometimes delight, at times shock—but you will read on. For example, start with the essay on Haitian Vodou or with an insider's view of practices in Ghana. You will, I repeat, read on.

This book has something to say about our ever-smaller world, a world of citizens whose life and destiny are increasingly bound together. What it says is important on several levels that I want, right off, to point out.

These essays have intrinsic worth, inner quality, and character that impel attention. A Beethoven string quartet, a beautiful person or poem, a rose, a well-crafted short story, the lark's song: these exist and attract us by their inner aspect. We cannot avoid dealing with them. So it is with these well-wrought scholarly essays. We have made every effort to bring together some of the world's foremost scholars, and we are pleased by their efforts.

These essays address our humanity. They tell life-and-death stories and give historical, theological, and scientific accountings of how people cope with suffering, how they care, how they cure. They lead to expansion of human awareness and cut across the disciplines of the humanities, that zone in which, through imagination, we confront other people. These disciplines include history, literature, philosophy, religion, linguistics, law, anthropology, and more. Through them we enlarge our own distinctive possibilities by encountering notions about what it might be to be someone else, somewhere else.

These essays bring self-knowledge. Again and again in reading these chapters I not only glimpsed through a window the lives of others but saw myself, as in a mirror, and saw my world in new lights.

These essays probe the interactions among the diverse centers of culture in our contemporary world. The so-called "West" does not exist in isolation. It interacts daily, in countless ways, with the people and products of the "East," the "South," and very many other cultural and geographic spheres of influence. Such interaction has *not* led to an integration, a convergence. Thomas Mann said that the world has many centers and will not likely see them disappear as a single Center emerges. Whatever the long-range view, for the lifetimes of all who read this, the West will be interacting with other worlds, worlds that survive, endure, transform, and prosper. These worlds will make their mark and act upon the West, a West that they once viewed as always and only imperial. The study of health, medicine, and religion improves understanding of the interactions.

These essays about unfamiliar places and sometimes exotic experiences teach lessons. Reading them would be a creative experience if one were to jot down clues for improving care and cure in one's own world. My notebook would refer to the environmental understandings, the webs of relations—the larger contexts that are easy to forget in our own society where, sealed off in intensive-care wards, we are likely to die "alone." What do suffering and death mean in places where they are social experiences, undergone with a variety of emotions? Can we learn from such approaches? We can. Are there views of nature, of time and space, that are somehow transportable and importable *here?* There are.

These essays tease the imagination and stretch the mind. They are useful to the professional and the layperson alike in fields of health, religion, and the academy, for professionalization, sooner or later, leads to a focus on an ever-smaller set of issues. The inventory of problems and possibilities from elsewhere enriches one's mental account books.

These essays provide grounds for critical and constructive self-judgment. One of the telling features of this book of antiromantic essays—essays that educate us to the real conditions of real people with ambiguities and flaws—is its possibility for contributing to a valid critique of Western ways. The missionaries, the medical agents, the manufacturers, the ideologues of the West have often in their ventures trampled upon what was valuable. Here one will read about how the West brought alcohol and alcoholism to places like Hawaii and how it brought other distinctively Western blights to other lands. We do not all feel or have to feel collective guilt for ancestral sins or mistakes, but here we have the opportunity to deduce from our new insight, strategies and instruments that will not add to the export of suffering.

These essays make possible the reform that comes after judgment. They offer clues about how and what one exports and how one reforms practices and attitudes at home. Not all changes wrought elsewhere because of Western contact were wrong; there were creative reforms as well. In like manner, the importation of insight from elsewhere can lead to new concepts of health care and cure in the West.

These essays can spur us on to personal transformation. We have come back to themes provoked above: one is changed by travel. Medical doctors learn much from visiting clinics that serve the poor and from health facilities that use uncommon technologies. Religious people are changed by their experience of worship in other settings. Anthropologists are transformed by their experiences during fieldwork. The Bantu saying about mother's being the only cook to the untraveled does not imply that those who have traveled reject home cooking. Not at all. I, for one, figuratively run home from elsewhere to be near the modern hospitals, the anesthesia, the societal security of the world I know, and I am ready to pay a price for these even if part of the cost is that I lose something of value that people elsewhere preserve, depend upon, and cherish. But I, this figurative runner—I hope I represent most readers—will enjoy home in new ways, as a person with enlarged imagination, a stock of new information, and fresh empathy.

Finally, for all the light this book casts on cultures far from the West, there remains what we might call a bonus question. Having partly satisfied a curiosity about how faraway peoples think of health, having come closer to becoming world citizens through the experience, will readers who stay at home find anything practical for up-close existence, for life with their neighbors, for understanding and contributing to medical care?

The answer is an emphatic *yes*, a *yes* that will resound more loudly and in ever-widening circles as America continues to grow more pluralist. Of course, such pluralism is already palpable in many places. In Dearborn, Michigan, one had better understand Islamic Shī'ism if one is to make sense of the people next door. In many parts of Harlem in New York City, talk of healing procedures in terms of Vodou, Santería, or devotion to Shango is as common as the high-tech vocabulary of the hospital. In Los Angeles, Catholic Mass is said in scores of Asian languages each week. Still, such concentrations seem remote to most Americans.

To counter such notions and seemings, let me take you next door, or next county, from the Cook County, Chicago, center in which I am writing this. West of us is DuPage County, an expanding, prosperous-to-plush area where industries and commercial centers abut luxury homes and apartments—which in turn border the middle-class residences of Middle America. DuPage County is a Republican stronghold, one that carries images of rectitude and refuge from the pluralist mélange and malaise of the city of Chicago to its east.

DuPage County, however, like so many other straight and square-seeming places, is changing, and already it embodies evidences of such change. Of course, being near Chicago, its population is predominantly Catholic. Again, of course, having long been suburban or exurban, it has a good mainstream Protestant representation. For a variety of reasons, it is also an evangelical bastion, even to the extent that one of its towns, Wheaton, has received the playful designation "The Evangelical Vatican." There is Wheaton College, an evangelical flagship school. In that county Billy Graham had his first church and radio program, and thence issues the magazine *Christianity Today*. Christians built fine and prosperous hospitals there. Any number of evangelistic organizations bear DuPage County letterheads. Safe territory for Western religion it decidedly seems to be.

Then one opens the yellow pages of any of the local phone books in the county. If I collected all such phone books, I am told, there would be evidence of several dozen non-Western groups, non-Judeo-Christian worshipers, to say nothing of living-room gatherings of groups that do *not* advertise in the yellow pages. The people who attend are not leftover hippies, aging, long-haired relics of the sixties, who once upset the culture. No, these are Iranian engineers, Pakistani physicians, Indonesian nurses, Japanese computer experts, and other permanent settlers who brought their faiths with them and quietly spread them. They give and need medical care; their children are in the public schools, representing alternative ways in faith and life and care and cure.

So my eye falls, in the present case, on the Nichiren Shoshu Temple in West Chicago, deriving from the name the pleasing image of a Japanese Buddhist community. And there is an SVS Temple in Aurora and a Shri Venkateswara Temple of the same faith in the same town. I have a choice of being part of Glen Ellyn's Ahmadiyya Movement in Islam or Villa Park's Islamic Foundation. Culturally oriented somewhere between West and non-West is the DuPage Religious Science Center in Lisle. I also note the Bochasanwasi Swaminarayan Sanstha group in Glen Ellyn. I expect that Baha'i is somewhere in the county. Not in the yellow pages before me, but well known, is a Zoroastrian group in well-off Hinsdale. While planning for a meeting of the American Academy of Religion in Chicago I was surprised to learn of the Academy members who could overlook the lures of the metropolis of Chicago in order to get their chance at seeing the lighting of the fire by Hinsdalean Zoroastrians. And all this is only a sample of what is actually out there.

Of course, one would not meet such an exotic array in a Tennessee village or on a Nebraska plain—yet options are springing up in ever more communities. These groups of citizens may remain minorities, but they signal a phenomenon of great importance. Many chapters of this book will enlighten those who would care for and be cared for by, and who would cure or be cured by, the once faraway people now so close to home—all of whom have their own practices and ideas about well-being.

Martin E. Marty

Acknowledgments

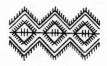

This volume is the work of many hands whose labors merit thanks.

The directors of the Park Ridge Center supported this project with generosity and patience: Martin E. Marty, President; James P. Wind, Director of Research and Publications; and, especially, George B. Caldwell, President of Lutheran General Health Care System, who encouraged the Park Ridge Center to pursue historical research into the cultural background of medical systems.

Clair J. Carty edited the manuscript in preparation for publication.

Readers combed through the first draft of this volume and delivered their suggestions to authors at a plenary working session in Chicago: David Carrasco, Director of the Mesoamerican Archive and Professor of Religious Studies at the University of Colorado, Boulder; Jean Comaroff, Professor of Anthropology at the University of Chicago; Winston Davis, Professor of Religious Studies at Southwestern University, Georgetown, TX; Frank E. Reynolds, Professor of Buddhist Studies and the History of Religions at the University of Chicago; Marilyn Waldman, Professor of Islamic Studies and Comparative History at the University of Ohio, Columbus; and James P. Wind, Director of Research and Publications at the Park Ridge Center. David T. Stein arranged our international conference. Kathleen A. Cahalan, Program Coordinator at the Park Ridge Center, proposed improvements in the final copy.

Lawrence E. Sullivan

Contributors

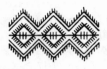

PETER ANTES (Th.D., University of Freiburg/Breisgau, 1970; Ph.D., University of Freiburg/Breisgau, 1971) is Professor and Chairman of the Department for the History of Religions at the University of Hanover (West Germany). He has published studies on Islamic theology and ethics as well as on methodological problems concerning the phenomenology of religion. Since 1974 he has coedited the *Zeitschrift für Missionswissenschaft und Religionswissenschaft*.

KOFI APPIAH-KUBI (B.Litt., Oxford, 1973; Doctor of Public Health, Dr.P.H., Columbia University, 1982) is a free-lance consultant and part-time Lecturer at the Ghana Institute of Management and Public Administration. He is a social scientist, theologian, and public health specialist. He is the author of several books and articles; principal among them are *Man Cures, God Heals: Religion and Medical Practices among the Akans of Ghana* (1981) and *African Theology Enroute* (1979).

RAOUL BIRNBAUM (Ph.D., Columbia University, 1976) is a member of the Department of Religion at Princeton University. He pursued post-doctoral research for two years at the Metropolitan Museum of Art. His research has centered on the world of Buddhist practice in medieval China, and his principal works include *The Healing Buddha* (1979) and *Studies on the Mysteries of Mañjuśrī* (1983). He currently is completing an extended study of sacred geography in medieval China, with special focus on the history and lore of an international center for Buddhist pilgrimage located in northern China, Mount Wu-t'ai.

ÅKE HULTKRANTZ (Ph.D., University of Stockholm, 1953), Professor of the History of Religions and head of the Institute of Comparative Religion from 1958 to 1986, is a specialist on North American Indian religions. He is the author of many books, of which the latest concerning North American Indians are *The Religions of the American Indians* (1979), *Belief and Worship in Native North America* (1981), *The Study of American Indian Religions* (1983), and *Native Religions of North America* (1987).

JOHN M. JANZEN (Ph.D., University of Chicago, 1967) is Professor of Anthropology at the University of Kansas, Lawrence, and Director of Kauffman Museum at Bethel College, North Newton, Kansas. He has carried out extensive research on health and healing issues and on the medical anthropology of Central Africa. His publications include *An Anthology of Kongo Religion* (1974), with Wyatt MacGaffey; *The Quest for Therapy: Medical Pluralism in Lower Zaire* (1978), with William Arkinstall, M.D.; and *Lemba 1650–1930: A Drum of Affliction in Africa and the New World* (1982). Since 1985 he has been editor of the monograph series Comparative Studies in Health Systems and Medical Care for the University of California Press.

SUDHIR KAKAR (Ph.D., Vienna, 1967) is Senior Fellow at the Centre for the Study of Developing Societies, Delhi. A psychoanalyst, he is the author of several books including *Frederick Taylor* (1971), *The Inner World* (1978), and *Shamans, Mystics and Doctors* (1982), and he is the coauthor of *Tales of Love, Sex and Danger* (1986).

JOSEPH MITSUO KITAGAWA (Ph.D., University of Chicago) taught the History of Religions at the University of Chicago from 1951 to 1984, both in the Divinity School and in the Department of Far Eastern Languages and Civilizations. He is also a former Dean of the Divinity School. He has lectured in many European, North American, Asian, and Australian universities, and his books have been translated into various languages. His major works include *Religion in Japanese History* (1966), *On Understanding Japanese Religion* (1987), and *The History of Religions: Understanding Human Experience* (1988), as well as various volumes that he edited on the history of religions, Eastern religions, and the writings of his mentor, Joachim Wach.

DAVID M. KNIPE (Ph.D., University of Chicago, 1971) is currently Chair of the South Asian Studies Department, Director of the South Asian Center, and Chair of Religious Studies at the University of Wisconsin. He is a historian of religions specializing in the religions of South Asia, in particular Vedic studies and contemporary Hinduism. His book *Hinduism: Experiments with the Sacred* was published in 1989.

KATHARINE LUOMALA (Ph.D., University of California, Berkeley, 1936) is Professor Emeritus of Anthropology, University of Hawaii. She is an

Honorary Associate of Bishop Museum, Honolulu, and of the Association for Social Anthropology of Oceania. She is a Fellow of the American Anthropological Association and the American Folklore Society, a Vice President of the International Society for Folk-Narrative Research, and a former editor of the *Journal of American Folklore*. Her anthropological fieldwork has been in the Pacific area and among the American Indians. Her numerous articles and books relate principally to Polynesian and Micronesian cultural and social anthropology, but she has also written on Navajo and Diegueño Indian life. In 1987, the Bishop Museum in Honolulu reprinted her best-known book, *Voices on the Wind: Polynesian Myths and Chants*.

KAREN MCCARTHY BROWN (Ph.D., Temple University, 1976) is Professor of the Sociology and Anthropology of Religion at the Graduate and Theological schools of Drew University. She has published numerous articles on Vodou as practiced both in Haiti and among Haitian immigrants in New York. Her book *Mama Lola: A Vodou Priestess in Brooklyn*, a multigenerational study of the healing arts in Haitian traditional religion, is forthcoming from University of California Press.

GANANATH OBEYESEKERE (Ph.D., University of Washington, 1964) is Professor and Chairman of the Department of Anthropology at Princeton University. He has written extensively on South Asian medicine and religion; his most recent books are *Medusa's Hair: An Essay on Personal Symbols and Religious Experience* (1981) and *The Cult of the Goddess Pattini* (1984). His book *Buddhism Transformed*, coauthored with Richard Gombrich, was published by Princeton University Press in 1989.

EMIKO OHNUKI-TIERNEY (Ph.D., University of Wisconsin, Madison, 1968), a native of Japan, is the William F. Vilas Professor, Department of Anthropology, at the University of Wisconsin, Madison. She has published extensively on the Ainu, the Japanese, and theoretical issues in symbolic and historical anthropology, including *Sakhalin Ainu Folklore* (1969), *The Ainu of the Northwest Coast of Southern Sakhalin* (1974), *Illness and Healing among the Sakhalin Ainu* (1981), *Illness and Culture in Contemporary Japan* (1984), and *The Monkey as Mirror* (1987). Her honors include a Guggenheim fellowship (1985–86), appointment as a member of the Institute for Advanced Study, Princeton (1986–87), and a Santori scholarly book award (1986).

BERNARD R. ORTIZ DE MONTELLANO (Ph.D., University of Texas, Austin, 1965) is Professor of Anthropology at Wayne State University in Detroit. From 1980 to 1985 he was Director of the Center for Chicano Boricua Studies at Wayne State. He has published extensively on medical anthropology, folk medicine, and the Aztecs. These publications include "Empirical Aztec Medicine," *Science* (1975); "Aztec Cannibalism: An Ecological Necessity?" *Science* (1978); and *"Caida de Mollera:* Aztec Sources for a Mesoamerican Disease of Alleged Spanish Origin," *Ethnohistory* (1987).

FAZLUR RAHMAN (1919–1988, D.Phil., Oxford, 1950) was Harold Swift Distinguished Service Professor of Islamic Thought at the University of Chicago. Prior to coming to Chicago in 1969, he taught in England and at McGill University and was Director of the Islamic Research Institute of Pakistan. He has published numerous articles, and his books include *Islam* (1966; second edition 1979), *Major Themes of the Qur'an* (1980), and *Islam and Modernity* (1982).

LAWRENCE E. SULLIVAN (Ph.D., University of Chicago, 1981) is Professor of the History of Religions and Acting Director of the Institute for the Advanced Study of Religion at the University of Chicago. Before coming to Chicago he helped establish the Department of Religious Studies at the University of Missouri, Columbia. He has carried out special research in Latin America, Central Africa, and Japan. He is Editor of *History of Religions: An International Journal for Comparative Historical Studies* and of *The Journal of Religion,* and he is Associate Editor of the sixteen-volume *Encyclopedia of Religion* (1987). His book *Icanchu's Drum* (1988) was selected as the most outstanding book in philosophy and religion by the Association of American Publishers. It probes the nature of religion by examining the native cultures of South America since the Spanish conquest.

Introduction:
The Quest for
Well-Being and
the Questioning
of Medicine

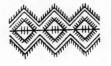

LAWRENCE E. SULLIVAN

If illness is part of the human condition, so is the questioning that accompanies it. Why am I sick? What makes me suffer? Who or what can help? In any human community, these questions require answers.

1

Could the peculiar way in which humans experience illness have sparked their very capacity to inquire? Who can say? One thing is certain. Every culture responds creatively to these queries, and, curiously, the responses open new lines of questioning. Probing the mysteries of suffering and death, which no explanations finally dissolve, each culture furnishes itself a vocabulary for critical inquiry in the form of myth, meditation, philosophical speculation, and scientific hypothesis.

The questioning of medicine can never be restrained, because the sickbed is a maelstrom of forces that are historical as well as organic. History has not yet ended, and startlingly different tales reveal the first appearance of historical existence and the unfolding of subsequent historical forces. Medicine treats as questionable the forces that intrude upon the sick body or mind and it probes their origin, nature, and effects.

From puzzles about the body, even about any one of its cells, it is a short ride to riddles concerning the ultimate causes of the universe and enigmas about the meaning of existing in time. Lewis Thomas, the biology watcher, wonders whether we can any longer think of our bodies as entities in themselves, made up only of "successively enriched packets of our own parts." Instead,

> [we may be] shared, rented, occupied. At the interior of our cells, driving them, providing the oxidative energy that sends us out for the improvement of each shining day, are the mitochondria, and in a strict sense they are not ours. They turn out to be little separate creatures, the colonial posterity of migrant prokaryocytes, probably primitive bacteria that swam into ancestral precursors of our eukaryotic cells and stayed there. Ever since, they have maintained themselves and their ways, replicating in their own fashion, privately, with their own DNA and RNA quite different from ours. . . . Without them, we would not move a muscle, drum a finger, think a thought. . . . They feel like strangers, but the thought comes that the same creatures, precisely the same, are out there in the cells of sea gulls, and whales, and dune grass. . . . Through them, I am connected; I have close relatives, once removed, all over the place. This is a new kind of information, for me, and I regret somehow that I cannot be in closer touch with my mitochondria.[1]

Cultures throughout the world have noticed such similarities in form or function between processes of the human body and structures of the universe. The shape of these homologies varies widely, from the image of the physical body as a microcosm or the cell as an ecosystem as complex as Jamaica Bay to that of the human mind as an archive of coded information, universal categories, or ideal forms of reality that exist elsewhere.

The sick lie at the intersection of histories that are genetic, social, individual, microbial, and spiritual. Who defines the differences among the kinds of history that afflict the ill? Sickness is not just an event wherein microbes, after threading their way through the germ and genetic pools of space and time, converge on the afflicted body of the patient. Around the sickbed swarm conflicting interpretations of disease and competing prescriptions for cure. The medical arena turns adversarial forum. Curers not only battle disease there. They confront one another's opposing views of sickness or health—beliefs molded in personal development, social events, and cultural history.

Medical lore warehouses these human evaluations of self, history, and cosmos. That is why Oliver Wendell Holmes, a physician and the father of the American jurist, pushed scholars to undertake the study of old medical books. "The debris of broken systems and exploded dogmas," Holmes argued, "form a great mount, a Monte Testaccio of the shards and remnants of old vessels which once held human beliefs. If you take the trouble to climb to the top of it, you will widen your horizon, and in these days of specialised knowledge your horizon is not likely to be any too wide."[2]

Medical knowledge has always included weighing alternative explanations, a symptom of the curer's willingness to become familiar with what is new or strange in the repertoire of cultural wisdom. By comparing ideas about illness and well-being, medical questioning becomes an exercise in cultural history and not only an experiment in anatomy or biochemistry. Practiced as a cultural science, medicine can view sickness as a human problem as well as a material disorder. What social circumstances engender illness? What powers render disease devastating and cure effective? Which cultural images express the meaning of afflicting and recuperative powers? The historical and social forces converging in the sick patient are physical and ideological. Thus, "medicine is a social science in its very bone and marrow."[3]

Allowed its full social extension, the study of health and sickness conditions the moral climate of action. What is my neighbor's suffering to me? How shall I understand a friend's death? How should I face my own? What meaning does life hold in the presence of tragedy? What value sustains medical care in the teeth of death—whether the patient's death appears imminent or remote? What ties bind public health to the public good?

If sickness provokes innumerable questions, the quest for well-being spawns fantastic schemes for cure. The impulse to experience ultimate well-being looses the imagination, which begets utopian visions, nostalgic longings, physical urges, and political movements. Medicine and religion reveal their kinship here. In the pursuit of well-being that undergirds some world religions, physical cure signifies the coming of the paradisal state of salvation. In the beginning of the first millennium BCE, for example, Zarathushtra (Zoroaster) taught humanity divinely given techniques of cure. These medical practices would vanquish evil manifest as illness and return the world to its original perfection. *Frashokereti*, which means both healing and salvation, is still the Zoroastrian goal of the entire story of creation, from its fall from light to its final redemption. At the end of time (a time beyond death), the saved will enjoy an everlasting existence in a new body. Similarly, in the Pali canon of Buddhist texts, Śā-kyamuni Buddha (sixth or fifth century BCE) heals through instructions on impermanence and prescribes meditation as an exercise for curing illnesses that, from the Buddhist view, reflect psychic states that have gone awry. The Buddha's cures deepen the spectators' insight into the nature of existence and can thereby occasion even complete liberation. Half a millennium later, Jesus of Nazareth performed miraculous cures as distinctive signs that the Messiah dwelt among humans and that the new age of the kingdom of God was at hand.[4]

Strange reversals occur. Taking paradisal bliss as its goal, the quest for well-being, which often arises out of medical inquiry, effects a critical bent of mind and turns on medicine by questioning it back. Thus, the questions of medicine become a questioning of medicine, a religious and moral interrogation of its resources, purposes, accomplishments, and limits. Having made the human condition questionable, medicine falls subject to question. The imminent prospect of more perfect and more abundant life prompts reevaluation of explanations of illness, rejection of outmoded concepts of the body, and demand for new standards of care. All cultures are the outcome of such complicated histories of critical quest and requestioning. Emil Cioran, the Romanian philosopher, observes that a society incapable of giving birth to and calling upon a utopian notion of well-being is menaced with ruin, for the desire for wholeness and health transforms the social universe in accordance with its wishes.[5]

Regard for alternative cultural concepts of well-being inspires the critical questioning of medicine. What visions of health have filliped human freedom in cultures across the globe? A truly critical medical knowledge considers, compares, and familiarizes itself with their strangeness.

Cultural Responses and the Responsibility of Modernity

Medical inquiry and its critical counterpoint, the interrogation of medicine, breed quandaries that lurk in the heart of any culture. This volume of essays does not expose them all to the light of day. The Park Ridge Center gathered a panel of men and women from all corners of the curative setting within North America. They were patients, critical care staff, psychiatrists, pediatricians, hospital lawyers, internists, pastors, patient advocates, and medical ethicists. This panel listed ten topics it most wished an assembly of historians and anthropologists to address in writing, through an exploration of the relationship between religion and medicine: well-being, sexuality, passages, morality, dignity, madness, healing, caring, suffering, and dying. The panel asked the writers to address a wide, general readership that was not specialized in their fields of scholarship.

With this assignment, the Park Ridge Center picked an investigative team whose members not only study the cultures beyond the margins of North America (and the emarginated cultures within it) but in many instances had been born into those cultures; they came from West Africa, Sri Lanka, India, Japan, Pakistan, Mexico, and the Pacific Basin, as well as from Europe. At a meeting in Chicago, the contributors to this volume plotted the ten topics across the human life cycle and explored them under the paired headings of wellness and illness, care and cure, and ethics and justice, as these concepts appear in the cultures under study. Contributors were encouraged to diverge creatively from one another by reshaping questions to suit the communities they describe. In this way, the distinctiveness of each medical and religious tradition has come to sparkle through the diverse content and style of the essays. In some chapters, the texture is broadly historical or comparative, and in others the focus falls on particular cases.

In view of the simplistic way medical beliefs of the world are still often cataloged on a single time line, ranging from "outdated," on the one end, to "modern," on the other,[6] one must underscore that the cultures presented in this volume are not antiquarian curiosities. The peoples described are the contemporaries of so-called "modern" medical practice. The ancient system of Āyurveda (described by David Knipe), the historical outlook of Buddhism (chronicled by Joseph Kitagawa), and the classical tradition of Islamic medicine (portrayed by the late Fazlur Rahman) are presented because they vibrantly color the estimations of health and sickness for large numbers of patients and practitioners in today's world. Most of the people sketched in this volume struggle under the signs of the same modernity that empowers the research and industry of modern medicine. Far from being modern history's agents or the beneficiaries of its wonders, however, they more often suffer its ravages. Such has been the fate of the many Native American communities surveyed by Åke Hultkrantz. In her inventory of the Polynesian materia medica employed in the Hawaiian islands, Katharine Luomala points out that, within forty-five years of first contact with the English in 1778, the population of the islands was cut in half by new diseases, displacement, and warfare conducted with more lethal imported weapons. Disease and conquest exterminated the population of South American peoples compared in my article, and reduced them to a fraction of their full strength. In the first 150 years of colonial contact in Latin America, it is estimated, one-quarter of the world's inhabitants were exterminated, taking into account only the number of native South Americans who died. The Aztec empire of Mesoamerica was sacked and leveled by the first wave of Spanish conquerors.

Bernard Ortiz de Montellano reconstructs the Aztec medical system and argues that, in spite of the ravages of history, its theories have survived to undergird contemporary Mexican folk medicine. The process of medical questioning needs the medical ideas of these communities, for they are participant observers of the modern world. They complement or challenge Western perspectives and furnish critical commentary on modernity, seen as a historical movement, a social experiment, a medical crossroads, and a way of knowing reality.

No fifteen essays could cover all the medical systems in the world that bear on the ten topics assembled by the panel at the Park Ridge Center. Nor does any single essay treat all the medical practices current in the area it presents. Raoul Birnbaum's coverage of Chinese medicine concentrates on Buddhism and explores the importance of the *Scripture on the Master of Healing* and the meditation manuals of Chih-i (b. 538), a master of T'ien-t'ai (a line of Buddhist thought and practice). For fourteen centuries East Asian medical specialists have pondered Chih-i's syntheses. Birnbaum now asks us to do the same. Adequate coverage of these rich materials requires setting aside other Chinese medical traditions, such as the influential one based on the systematic descriptions recorded in the *Inner Classic of the Yellow Sovereign (Huang-ti nei-ching su-wen; Ling-shu)*. Similarly, Emiko Ohnuki-Tierney delineates the principles underlying general concepts of health and illness in contemporary Japan and instantiates them with a close look at popular devotions at public shrines. Of course, there are other kinds of Japanese religious medicine not detailed in her essay: practices associated with the history of Shingon (esoteric Buddhism) and with the formal rites performed by Shinto priests, New Religionists, and free-lance curers.

Rather than impose uniform, exhaustive coverage of a checklist—an unimaginative way of dulling readers' senses—each essay presents an exemplary case in its own way. Sudhir Kakar, a Delhi psychiatrist, uses an individual case to analyze the broader cultural background of his Hindu patient's anxiety. Gananath Obeyesekere begins with several interviews with the sick in Sri Lanka in order to evaluate the distinctions that separate existence from illness and meditation from trance (possession by a spirit).

Each essay samples the richness one can expect to find in the wider world of religious medicine. Together they represent large areas and populations of today's world: the Pacific, South Asia, Africa, the Americas, East Asia, and the Islamic, Hindu, and Buddhist spheres of influence. Readers are welcome to wade into the volume at any point. Each essay contributes to the volume's larger purpose: to show how cultural medicines differ, just as religious expressions do, from one tradition to another and how knowledge of these distinctions enriches our understanding of the human desire for health and capacity for freedom. Each tradition of religious medicine roots itself in the creative soil of its culture and its history. By sampling an assortment of influential worldviews, the collection entices, encourages, and enables readers to encounter others.

Taking diverse approaches to these materials has proven a fruitful tack. Indeed, they teach a lesson: encourage the development of different approaches in order to uncover the diverse facets of religious medicine in any single culture. In regard to Islamic medicine, for instance, whether one begins with the piece by Fazlur Rahman on classical Islamic medicine or Peter Antes on the contemporary Islamic medical scene, one's picture of medicine and health in the Islamic world will be enlarged by reading the other article. The complexity of Islamic history calls for both kinds of treatment. Indeed, one could imagine still other presentations. The same could be said of any culture treated in this volume.

The different styles, interests, and capacities of each author disclose something new. This phenomenon is apparent in the treatment of African materials. Kofi Appiah-Kubi's impassioned presentation of religious medicine among the West African Akan people of Ghana pushes him toward the poetic end of prose when he praises the virtues of life-giving Earth and berates biotechnical images of the body that arrived with industrial colonialism. John Janzen's discussion of Central African history, on the other hand, broadly compares medical terms used by a large number of ethnic groups. Janzen's article lucidly illustrates the value of the science of comparative linguistics and the fact that fascinating medical ideas are systematically transmitted from one group to another over time. The tendency of medical systems to travel with the social systems in which they are embedded enables Karen McCarthy Brown to provide a vivid picture of Haitian Vodou, which develops from traditions of the Fon people of Benin, the Yoruba of Nigeria, and the Kongo people of Zaire. Brown's approach to African spirituality in the Caribbean focuses on the family and the view of the person within it.

Lest delving into these alternative systems of cultural medicine appear an exotic exercise, it is well to picture any large North American clinical setting. Given the diverse heritages of patients and staff, it is a whirlwind of cultural views on medicine. Religious experience helps shape these perspectives. In any urban hospital, the attitudes and values of both patients and healers are fundamentally shaped by their background in Christianity, Judaism, Islam, Hinduism, Buddhism, the folk medical systems of Asia, Africa, Hispanic culture, or native American belief.* The religious and medical situation is no less complex in the hospitals of Uvira, in Kivu Province, Zaire, than in Los Angeles or Beijing or Stockholm. In all large

---

*An earlier volume, designed by the Park Ridge Center, has presented the medical impact of Judaism, Afro-American religious life, and various Christian denominations. See Ronald L. Numbers and Darrel W. Amundsen, eds., *Caring and Curing: Health and Medicine in the Western Religious Traditions* (New York: Macmillan Publishing, 1986).

medical centers one finds patients and staff, as well as beliefs and medical techniques or curative substances, summoned from many parts of the globe and issuing from distinct historical consciousnesses. Never before have the broad cultural reach of medical questions and the religious responses to the human condition imposed themselves so perceptibly.

Cognizance of the plural beliefs at work in any medical setting effaces, in some measure, the specious dichotomy between "home" and "away," or between "Western" and "non-Western," or "us" and "them."[7] The distinctively human reality is a richer and more confused tangle. The contributors to this volume illustrate the point. Speaking on behalf of the foreign communities that they know intimately and are perhaps a part of, they also are at home in North America, through their experience as students or working professionals. By rendering more permeable the lines drawn by culture and language to keep categories apart (West/East; religion/medicine; tradition/modernity), their lives and their essays help us regard the diversity of cultural creations as evidence of a single history of human striving, and, full of questions, they make us wonder about the place we are assuming in it.

Notes

1. Lewis Thomas, *The Lives of a Cell* (New York, 1974), pp. 4, 73.
2. Cited without attribution in Edward Theodore Withington, *Medical History from the Earliest Times* (London, 1964), p. 1.
3. Rudolph Virchow, *Einheitsbestrebungen* (Berlin, 1849), p. 40.
4. See Lawrence E. Sullivan, "Healing," *Encyclopedia of Religion* (New York, 1987).
5. Emil M. Cioran, *Histoire et utopie* (Paris, 1960), pp. 70–80.
6. Johannes Fabian, *Time and the Other: How Anthropology Makes Its Object* (New York, 1983).
7. Regarding the way in which cultural practice contrasts with the dichotomous categories used in the study of cultures, see Catherine Bell, "Discourse and Dichotomies: The Structure of Ritual Theory," *Religion* 17 (1987): 95–118.

CHAPTER 1

Buddhist Medical

History

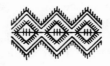

JOSEPH MITSUO KITAGAWA

Buddhism arose in the sixth century BCE in northeastern India, where the indigenous culture and the Indo-Aryan, Brahmanic tradition converged. It was an ascetic movement (*śramaṇa; samaṇa* in Pali), based on the enlightenment experience of its founder, Śākyamuni, or Gautama Buddha. Like the ascetic movements of Jainism and Ājīvikas, Buddhism did not develop out of the Brahmanic-Hindu tradition. Consequently, it was regarded as a rival heterodoxy.

From the time of the Buddha, early Buddhism attracted lay followers, for it was patronized by the rising mercantile families in northeastern India. King Aśoka (274–232 BCE) advocated Buddhism not only as the religion of his vast Mauryan empire but also as a missionary movement to other parts of the world. Buddhism was enthusiastically promoted again during the second century CE by King Kaniṣka, who ruled northern India and Central Asia. Following the route of Hinduization, it expanded into various parts of South and Southeast Asia. It came to Central Asia and China along the so-called Silk Road, and China then became the center of Buddhist expansion into other parts of East Asia. Another route of expansion brought Buddhism into Tibet and eventually to the Mongolian steppe. Since the latter nineteenth century Buddhism has also penetrated various parts of the West.

E. J. Thomas astutely pointed out that the Buddhist movement began "not with a body of doctrine, but with the formation of a society bound by certain rules."[1] The early Buddhist community had four components: monks *(bhikṣu, bhikkhu)*, nuns *(bhikṣunī, bhikkhunī)*, male lay followers *(upāsaka)*, and female lay followers *(upāsikā)*. The monastic path, however, was acknowledged to be more central.

A century after the demise of the Buddha his community began to develop many informal factions. In the course of time, the community split into three major traditions, each with many subdivisions: (1) Hīnayāna ("small vehicle") or Theravāda ("way of the elders"), a monastic-centered tradition adhering to the Pali canon, became established in South and Southeast Asia; (2) Mahāyāna ("great vehicle"), which follows Sanskrit and/or Chinese scriptures and recognizes both the monastic and the lay paths, became established in East Asia; and (3) the Esoteric or Tantric tradition, the latest form of Buddhism, became established primarily in Tibet and Mongolia but also in Japan. In Tibet this tradition developed a *de facto* theocracy. Unlike Christianity and Islam, Buddhism accommodated many local religious features and thus developed a series of culturally oriented religious forms such as Thai Buddhism, Mongolian Buddhism, and Korean Buddhism.

All Buddhist traditions affirm the centrality and interrelatedness of the *tri-ratana* (or *tri-ratna*, "three jewels")—Buddha, *dharma* (or *dhamma*, law or teaching), and *saṃgha* (or *saṅgha*, Buddhist community)—although each tradition interprets them differently. Buddhist teaching is traced to the Buddha, who, as a supreme physician, diagnosed and presented the remedy for the spiritual health of humankind in Four Noble Truths: (1) the fact of suffering as the basic feature of existence; (2) the cause of suffering; (3) the cessation of the cause; and (4) the eightfold path that leads to cessation—right understanding, right thought, right speech, right action, right livelihood, right effort, right mindfulness, and right concentration. Other notions central to Buddhist beliefs are *anatta* (nonself), "dependent cooriginition" (which explains how all physical and psychical phenomena, from ignorance of the true nature of existence to old age and death, are conditionally related to each other), and *karma* (action with inevitable results, the moral law of cause and effect). From the time of King Aśoka, *dharma* came to be understood as the foundation and guide to empirical social and political order as well as to cultural life.

Characteristically, the Mahāyāna tradition stresses the way of the bodhisattva or Buddha-to-be and the mutuality between saving wisdom *(prajñā)* and compassion *(karuṇā)*. The Esoteric tradition acknowledges the importance of superhuman knowledge and power *(abhijñā)*.

In 1957, Benson Y. Landis estimated the number of Buddhists as roughly 350 million.[2] But since many of those listed by him as adherents of other religions—Confucianists (300 million), Taoists (50 million), and Shintoists (25 million)—may consider themselves Buddhists at the same time, the total number may be much larger. Buddhism is now one of the most widely diffused religions, scattered over every continent with the probable exception of Africa. There is a sizable Buddhist community in the USSR and in the West as well, where the number of Buddhists has been increasing steadily since World War II.

Wellness and Illness

HEALTH

According to the canonical tradition, the Buddha was concerned with the health of monks and took a keen interest in medicine. Once he and his trusted disciple, Ānanda, found a monk suffering from dysentery and lying fallen in his own excrement. They washed the body of the sick man themselves and then the Buddha told the assembled monks: "Monks, you have not a mother, you have not a father who might tend you. If you, monks, do not tend one another, then who is there who will tend you? Whoever, monks, would tend me, he should tend the sick."[3] Then, after giving rules for the care of the sick, he proclaimed:

> Endowed with five qualities, monks, is one who tends the sick fit to tend the sick: he comes to be competent to provide the medicine; he knows what is beneficial and what is not beneficial; he takes away what is not beneficial, he brings forward what is beneficial; he tends the sick (from) amity of mind, not in the hope of gain; he does not become one who loathes to remove excrement or urine or sweat or vomit; he comes to be competent to gladden . . . delight the sick from time to time with *dhamma*-talk. Endowed with these five qualities, monks, is one who tends the sick fit to tend the sick.[4]

As far as we can ascertain, Buddhism did not develop its own medical tradition. The Buddha himself was attended to by Jīvaka Komārabhacca, who had studied surgery and medicine at Taxila and was in service at the court of King Bimbisāra. According to A. L. Basham, the science of medicine in India became known as Āyurveda, "the science of living (to a ripe) age."

> The term is significant from the semantic point of view, since its first component *(ayur)* implies that the ancient Indian doctor was concerned not only with curing disease but also with promoting positive health and longevity, while the second *(veda)* has religious overtones.[5]

Health was believed to be conditioned by the balance of three primary fluids in the body (wind, gall, and mucus), and five separate breaths or winds were supposed to control bodily functions. The harmonious operation of these factors was thought to maintain good health, while discord was thought to result in disease.

Buddhism was concerned with physical health as an important condition for striving after spiritual health, as told in *Anguttara-Nikaya* (III, 16): "The monk wisely reflecting partakes of his alms food . . . merely to maintain and support this body, to avoid harm and to assist the holy life."[6] Following this principle the early Theravāda tradition tried to confine the monks' medical activities to the monastic orders, without much success. But Basham reminds us that "with the Mahāyāna, medicine became one of the five secular sciences that the monk might study, and Indian medical knowledge was taken by Buddhist monks wherever they went."[7]

The Buddhist view of health and illness has basic ambiguities. According to the doctrine of *karma*, one's existence is the result of one's past actions; yet one can improve the physical and mental state of his or her future by the right mental attitude and by careful attention to measured food, proper digestion, and a regulated living style. On the whole, the laity were less concerned with doctrinal matters. They simply rejoiced when they were blessed with good health, which to them was an essential condition of happiness, as the *Dhammapada* (The path of virtue) teaches: "We live happily indeed, free from ailments among the ailing! Among men who are ailing let us dwell free from ailments!"[8]

SUFFERING

Because Buddhism is a nontheistic religion, it does not ask why God allows suffering. No outside agent, divine or demonic, causes suffering. Nevertheless, suffering is an all-important issue for Buddhism because suffering *(dukkha)*, impermanency *(anicca)*, and nonself *(anatta)* are considered to be the three basic characteristics of existence. According to the canonical tradition, in his First Sermon the Buddha explicated suffering as the first of the Four Noble *(ariyan)* Truths: "Birth is suffering; decay is suffering; illness is suffering; death is suffering; presence of objects we hate is suffering; separation from objects we love is suffering; not to obtain what we desire is suffering."[9] Walpola Rahula reminds us that the Pali word *dukkha* (*duḥkha* in Sanskrit) carries the idea of suffering, pain, sorrow, or misery, as opposed to the word *sukha* (happiness, comfort, or ease), but that in the First Noble Truth the term referred not only to suffering in ordinary usage but also to deeper philosophical notions such as imperfection, impermanence, emptiness, and insubstantiality. In short, "whatever is impermanent is *dukkha*."[10]

Understandably, such a radical understanding of the nature of existence results in a uniquely Buddhist approach to the meaning of suffering. Above all else, suffering is edificatory. From the Buddhist perspective, recognizing the fact of suffering means understanding the truth of impermanency *(anicca)*: everything is in a constant state of changing, disappearing, and dissolving from moment to moment. Understanding this leads to understanding the truth of nonego or nonself: there is no abiding ego entity, no ontological substance within these bodily and mental phenomena of existence that are usually mistaken as a self or a person. Indeed, without a realistic understanding of the universal fact of suffering as taught in the First Noble Truth, no one can enter the path of the Buddha, who alone discovered the way of emancipation from the universal predicament of suffering.

SICKNESS OR INJURY

It is well nigh impossible to make generalized statements about Buddhist views of sickness or injury. For brevity's sake we may delineate three different approaches practiced by Buddhists, namely, medical, doctrinal, and magical, provided we remember that in reality these three approaches are often interfused.

For the most part, Buddhist communities in India, as well as those in Southeast Asia, followed the Āyurveda, the pan-Indian science of medicine mentioned above, and its deviations, while Buddhists in China depended heavily on Chinese medical science as exemplified by the *Yellow Emperor's Classic of Internal Medicine* and *Shen Nung's Classic on Herbs*. According to these medical views, the functioning of the human body, thought of as a microcosm, is controlled by natural laws, just as the universe is regulated by the laws of cause and effect. Disease results when the constituent elements of the human body malfunction. Thus, as Obeyesekere points out, Sinhala Buddhists accept on one level the Āyurveda's notion that "disease is caused by the upsetting or excitement of any one or more of the three humors basic to the human organism: *vāta* or *vāyu* (wind), *pitta* (bile), *slēshma* or *kapha* (phlegm). Collectively these are known as the *tri-dōsa*, 'the three troubles'"[11] Chinese medical science interprets the natural cause of disease in similar fashion. Evidently, everywhere in Buddhist communities monks and laity alike have always accepted such naturalistic medical views of disease, at least on one level.

On another level, however, the Buddhist view of disease and/or injury cannot be divorced altogether from the doctrine of *karma (kamma)*, which refers to "the wholesome and unwholesome volitions and their concomitant mental factors, causing rebirths and shaping the destiny of beings."[12] Thus, whether or not and to what extent disease and injury are caused by one's karmic volitions have remained serious questions in the Buddhist community, questions without clear-cut resolutions. As early as the second century BCE a Greek king in Bactria, Menander (Milinda), asked the Buddhist master Nāgasena concerning the relationship between *karma* and the Buddha's own injury and disease. In his answer Nāgasena insisted that although the Buddha had burnt all evil (all consequences of *karma*), a splinter of rock had pierced his foot at one time and he had suffered from dysentery at another but that his injury and disease were not caused by *karma*. Nāgasena explained that not all suffering has its root in *karma*:

> There are several causes by which sufferings arise, by which many beings suffer pain. And what are they? Superabundance of wind, and of bile, and of phlegm, the union of these humours, variations in temperature, the avoiding of dissimilarities, and Karma. From each of these there are some sufferings that arise, and these are the eight causes by which many beings suffer pain.[13]

Nāgasena admitted, of course, that "there is the act that has Karma as its fruit, and the pain so brought about arising from the act done." He also recognized that the Buddha, who was "above all gods" and in whom there was no evil left, was a very special case and that "no one without a Buddha's insight can fix the extent of the action of Karma" vis à vis diseases and injuries that cause pain.[14] The difficulties involved in the question as to which diseases and injuries are caused by the action of *karma* have haunted generations of Buddhists in many lands.

As stated earlier, Buddhism has always been conciliatory to local cultural and religious traditions and has accommodated many non-Buddhist beliefs and practices such as spirit worship in various parts of Asia. Invariably many forms of magical beliefs concerning disease and injury developed, especially in the folk-religious traditions. Obeyesekere, for example, depicts the popular beliefs concerning diseases presumably caused by external (supernatural) agencies (for example, demons and gods)—beliefs that are held by the Sinhala Buddhists in Sri Lanka. "Ultimately," according to his observation, "all misfortunes caused by external agencies are due to unfavorable planetary movements *(graha dōsa)*: astrology in turn however simply indicates a person's *karma*, in this case bad *karma* or *karma dōsa*." He goes on to describe the interesting manner in which the demonic theory of disease causation is linked to the classical medical theory. Moreover, the Sinhala hold that "the identical disease may be caused by either naturalistic (Ayurvedic) or demonological factors. For example, *lē māle* (menorraghia) can be caused by a natural excitement of heat *(uṣna)* or bile *(pitta)* in the body, or by the demon *Sanni Yaka,* or *Riri Yaka* (blood demon)."[15] Similar observations may be made about folk Buddhist traditions elsewhere.

MENTAL ILLNESS

Among other characteristics, early Buddhism was known for its tendency toward absolute idealism as exemplified by the opening sentence of the *Dhammapada:* "All that we are is the result of what we have thought: it is founded on our thoughts, it is made up of our thoughts."[16] Related to this idealism were psychological and mental analyses of the human condition so sophisticated that Heinrich Zimmer calls the Four Noble Truths "psycho-dietics."[17] In fact, these characteristics run through all aspects of Buddhist doctrine, ethics, and soteriology. The canonical tradition stresses the importance of equilibrium, harmony, and balance in relation to mental faculties (faith, energy, mindfulness, concentration, and wisdom). Yet the canonical tradition rarely deals with what we now call mental illness as such, because trance and vision experience, divine hearing, and stupefaction, psychogenesis, obsessional neurosis, and paranoia are difficult to evaluate.

The popular or folk Buddhist tradition, on the other hand, has inclined to the view that a variety of nonhuman agents, spirits, or demons cause mental illness. As a consequence, it has practiced many forms of healing cults, exorcism, pacification of spirits, and divination, side by side or in collaboration with established Buddhist institutions. Fortunately, we now have a large number of books and articles by scholars on these eclectic beliefs and practices concerning what we regard as mental illness. Evidently, the religious universe of many lay Buddhists is inhabited by many spirits and demons of non-Buddhist origins, and lay Buddhists today, as in the past, depend on a variety of cultic specialists in addition to Buddhist clergy and physicians in dealing with irregular mental conditions caused by these nonhuman agents.

ALCOHOL AND DRUG ABUSE

One of the five moral rules in the canonical tradition forbids the use of intoxicants and drugs such as wine and liquor because they lead to moral carelessness. This precept was observed more or less faithfully within monastic orders, but it often broke down in village temples where monks served as *de facto* parish priests. Moreover, many lay Buddhists indulged in intoxicants and drugs for medicinal purposes, among others. In the modern period, Buddhist reform movements have advocated strict prohibition of alcoholic beverages, but they have not met with significant success.

Caring and Curing

IMPULSE TO CARE

There are many facets and meanings to caring in Buddhism. At the risk of oversimplification, we might discuss the Pali canonical tradition (the tradition inherited by Theravāda Buddhism in South and Southeast Asia), including both its monastic and its lay orientations, and the Mahā-yāna orientation.

Although in principle Buddhism affirms that its truth (dharma) can be known and actualized only within the corporate life of the Buddhist community (saṃgha), the monastic-centered canonical tradition quickly developed according to an elitist model. It encouraged monks to strive spiritually toward the states of the Stream Winner (the lowest stage of the path of the noble disciples), the Once-Returner (the state of the noble individual who, after returning to this world once, can overcome suffering), the Never-Returner (the state of being born in a higher world from which one may reach nirvāṇa without having to return to this world), and the Holy One (arahat, the state of the saint who has been freed from all craving and rebirth and has attained enlightenment). For the sake of this spiritual striving, monks are urged to cultivate four kinds of emotions: loving-kindness (mettā) that eliminates the boundary between oneself and others, compassion (karuṇā) that enables one to share the suffering of others, sympathetic or altruistic joy (muditā) that enables one to rejoice over others' happiness, and equanimity or evenmindedness (upekkhā), the feeling of total identification of oneself with others. Thus we read:

> Therefore, O Brothers, the monk with a mind full of loving-kindness pervading first one direction, then a second one, then a third one, then the fourth one, just so above, below and all around; and everywhere identifying himself with all, he is pervading the whole world with mind full of loving-kindness, with mind wide, developed, unbounded, free from hate and ill-will.[18]

As Winston King reminds us, however, such ethically good emotions and deeds as loving-kindness, compassion, and equanimity do not bring a man to sainthood or enlightenment (nirvāṇa). The perfect deed, according to the canonical tradition, "is the detached thought, word, or deed which has no kammic [karmic] consequence. Hence the highest life seems to be a complete escape from, or transcendence of, the ethical sphere."[19] Thus, caring, as an expression of loving-kindness and compassion, is not an unquestionable virtue. Unless compassion is guarded by a perfected state of equanimity rarely attained, it tends to push the path-seeker to enter again and again the sensuous sphere of this world.[20] The following verses of the Dhammapada may be read in this light:

By oneself the evil is done, by oneself one suffers; by oneself evil is left undone, by oneself one is purified. The pure and the impure (stand and fall) by themselves, no one can purify another.

Let no one forget his own duty for the sake of another's, . . . let a man, after he has discerned his duty, be always attentive to his duty.[21]

It is clear that in the canonical tradition caring involves ambiguities. Monks are urged to strive toward their own enlightenment, an enlightenment that transcends all ethical and human considerations. Although we may be a bit surprised, we can certainly understand why a sick monk was left unattended in the famous incident when the Buddha and Ānanda were touring the monks' quarter. "Lord," said the other monks, "this monk is of no use to the monks, therefore the monks do not attend that monk."[22] Helping the sick monk would not really help other monks in their spiritual striving. It would only interfere with their main religious task. Confronted by this difficult situation, the Buddha advocates a sort of middle way: "He becomes one who does what is beneficial; he knows moderation in what is beneficial; he becomes one who takes medicine; he makes clear the disease just as it comes to be to one who tends the sick and who wishes him well."[23] But it is easier to say what the Buddha advocates than to do it. The history of the canonical tradition reveals that monks were inclined either to strive for their spiritual growth at the expense of compassion (caring for others) or to give themselves to the work of caring for others at the expense of their own spiritual vocation.

Lay Buddhists in the Pali canonical tradition do not aspire to attain *nirvāṇa*, for it is the prerogative of the monks. Their life is based on (1) piety toward the Buddha, his image and pagoda, and toward the monastic order; (2) ethical conduct following the Five Precepts against killing (human or animal), stealing, lying, sexual aggression, and intoxication; and (3) charity (almsgiving) and generosity toward the monks, other human beings, and animals. Following all of these precepts enables them to accumulate good *karma* and thereby to gain rebirth among the gods in heaven. Consequently, the lay Buddhist's impulse for caring is motivated and conditioned by the notion of merit, which governs all aspects of his or her life. Acquiring merit for the next world is so important that, according to Rahula, some laymen in Sri Lanka (Ceylon) had a so-called "Merit-book" in which they recorded their meritorious deeds: "This was usually intended to be read at the death-bed, so that the dying man might gladden his heart and purify his last thoughts to ensure a good birth [in heaven]."[24] S. J. Tambiah found that lay Buddhists in northeast Thailand ranked meritorious deeds according to their importance, as follows: (1) financing the building of a *wat* (monastery), (2) becoming a monk oneself or having a son become a monk, and (3) giving food daily to the monks.[25] Curiously, this ranking does not include any act of charity or service toward fellow human beings or animals, even though such deeds have been considered meritorious in the history of Buddhism.

The attitude of the Mahāyāna tradition toward caring is conditioned by its "social emotions," as Edward Conze rightly emphasizes.[26] These were inspired by the Mahāyānist ideal of the all-compassionate bodhisattva or Buddha-to-be who postpones his own attainment of Buddhahood because of his vow to save all beings. The complexities of Mahāyāna doctrine are not important here, but we should at least mention its fundamental conviction that all sentient beings are endowed with and share the same Buddha-nature. Also significant is its notion of the field of merit or the field of compassion. The early and/or Theravāda Buddhists regarded the Buddha and the monastic orders as the fields of merit for the laity. The Mahāyāna tradition, however, expects the monks and monasteries to offer gifts to both people and animals, especially to the poor and the needy, the orphaned, the aged—even to the ant. Now these are considered the field of merit or compassion.[27] Furthermore, many Mahāyāna schools regard the paths of the monastics and the laity as two different but equally legitimate options of religious vocation, urging both monks and laity to cultivate a compassionate heart and to participate in the saving enterprise of the bodhisattvas by practicing the perfection (pāramitā) of charity.

Buddhist opinion varies as to whether the impulse to care should extend to those outside the Buddhist fold. For early Buddhist monks and those in the Theravāda tradition, the dividing line did not separate Buddhists and non-Buddhists but monastics and nonmonastics. The latter included Buddhists as well as non-Buddhists. There was no question that the canonical tradition expected monks to care for fellow monks. But whether monks extended their caring deeds to nonmonastics—thereby interfering in effect with the karma of other beings and diverting energy from their own spiritual striving—is another matter. The evidence points both ways.

The primary field of merit for the laity in early Buddhism and the Theravāda tradition has always been the Buddha and the monastics, while other human beings and animals have taken second place. Here one finds an intricate mixture of altruism and merit-making for one's own spiritual welfare.

For the Mahāyānists—monks and laity alike—compassion (karuṇā) is inseparable from saving knowledge (prajñā). Therefore, deeds of caring must be extended, at least in principle, not only to persons outside the Buddhist fold but to all sentient beings.

MEDICAL MISSIONS

Even before the time of the Buddha, Indian medicine had been well established. Consequently, Buddhist medical missions in our sense of the term did not exist in the early period of Buddhism. There were, to be sure, some monks who had medical knowledge, but they were cautioned against having too many contacts with householders. The first significant public association of medicine and Buddhism took place during the reign of the newly converted Buddhist King Aśoka. In one of his Rock Edicts, dated circa 257 BCE, we read:

> Everywhere in the dominion of the Beloved of the gods [Aśoka himself] . . . (provision) has been made . . . (for) two (kinds of) medical treatment, (viz.) medical treatment for men and medical treatment for animals.
>
> And wherever there are no (medicinal) herbs that are suitable for men and suitable for animals, everywhere (such) have been caused to be brought and caused to be planted.
>
> And wherever there are no (medical) roots and fruits, everywhere (such) have been caused to be brought and caused to be planted.[28]

Aśoka makes it clear that he is doing all this as an expression of his commitment to the cause of *dharma* and for the sake of merit in the next world.[29] It is difficult to ascertain how extensive or how effective the medical service he initiated was. Nevertheless, his example inspired many later Buddhist rulers in other parts of Asia. For example, the famous king of Ceylon, Duṭṭha-gāmaṇī (101–77 BCE), is credited with providing extensive social welfare services, including eighteen centers at which medical treatment and medicines were made available.[30]

With the rise of the Mahāyāna tradition, medical service became an important act of compassion and charity. Hindu physicians had been restrained by ritual purity from cutting the body of the deceased, whereas the less inhibited Buddhist physicians made great contributions to the knowledge of anatomy. Earlier, pious kings and queens or the state had established medical services, but increasingly monasteries came to offer such services. In addition Mahāyāna Buddhism popularized the cult of the Buddha of Healing *(Bhaiṣajya-guru)* and the practice of reciting certain scriptures for the prevention of and recovery from sickness.[31]

CURING: FAITH AND MEDICINE

Buddhism has many contradictory strands, from rationalistic nontheism to a pietistic wing that borders on theism. All recognize the importance of faith *(saddhā)* over against faithlessness—together with energy over against laziness, mindfulness over against forgetfulness, concentration over against distractedness, and wisdom over against ignorance—as essential ingredients for the striving toward purity. But in Buddhism, faith in the sense of religious affirmation is directed toward the Three Jewels, which are the Buddha (the Enlightened One who discovered and taught the law of deliverance), the *dharma* (the law of deliverance), and the *saṃgha* (the Buddhist community). Since medicine deals with natural laws governing the physical condition of human beings, it is thought to belong to a different sphere from faith. But inasmuch as the same human beings are involved in both religious and psychological-physiological life, questions have been raised ever since the time of early Buddhism as to how or whether religious faith and ritual aid the process of curing one's illness. For example, a question is raised in *The Questions of King Milinda* regarding the validity of the Pirit service, a ritual used for the sick. The service has been widely used to the present day, and many Buddhists have believed it was created by the Buddha. The canonical texts do not state this, but Milinda believed that the Pirit had the Buddha's authorization.

Milinda's Buddhist mentor, Nāgasena, also accepted the view that the Buddha sanctioned the service, but he gave a classical Buddhist interpretation of the relation between religious ritual and medicine. He states:

> [The Pirit service] is only meant for those who have some portion of their life yet to run, who are of full age, and restrain themselves from the evils of Karma. And there is no ceremony or artificial means for prolonging the life of one whose allotted span of existence has come to an end. . . . no medicine and no Pirit . . . can prolong the life of one whose allotted period has come to an end. All the medicines in the world are useless . . . to such a one, but Pirit is protection and assistance to those who have a period yet to live, who are full of life, and restrain themselves from the evil of Karma. And it is for that use that Pirit was appointed by the Blessed One.[32]

Nāgasena states further that just as a disease can be turned back by medicine, the power of the Pirit is such that diseases are allayed and calamities depart from the sick person. He was careful to add the qualification, however, that Pirit is a protection to some and not to others:

> And there are three reasons for its failure—the obstruction of Karma, and of sin, and of unbelief. That Pirit which is a protection to beings loses its protecting power by acts done by those beings themselves.[33]

Early Buddhism tried to maintain a balance between religious belief/rite and medicine by giving a qualified approval to both. The Mahāyāna tradition, by contrast, influenced as it was by the Hindu Bhakti movement, gave greater emphasis to faith, while the Esoteric tradition, which appropriated many features of Hindu Tantrism, stressed the magical power of the Buddhist divinities. The folk Buddhist tradition, which allied itself with spirit cults of all sorts in various parts of Asia, developed various cults of faith healing and various forms of magical incantation, some of which have been studied by Tambiah, Obeyesekere, and Yalman.[34] It is important to add that many Buddhists do not depend on faith healing exclusively. They go to medical doctors simultaneously or they resort to faith healing only when they are not cured by medicine. There are also cases in which Buddhist clergy act as faith healers. To give one example, Joel M. Halpern cites an account given by a French-educated Lao official about a friend who was a supervisor of road crews. One day the man evidently fired a laborer who was idle on the job, not knowing that the laborer was an evil spirit. When the supervisor went home, he developed body pains. His wife did not know that his sickness was caused by an evil spirit, so she took her husband to a Western-educated doctor who found nothing wrong with him. But when the illness persisted the sick man "went to see a wise old bonze who told him that his malady was an evil phi [i.e., an evil spirit] at work. This particular bonze had stronger spiritual power than the evil spirit and was thus able to force it to leave [the sick person's] body. After this he immediately felt better."[35] The account represents the attitude of many folk Buddhists toward faith healing and/or the relations between faith and medicine in general.

MEDICAL TREATMENT

Before the time of King Aśoka in the third century BCE little is known about the nature of Buddhist medical institutions, if there were any. All we know about Aśoka's medical provision is what we read in the Rock Edict previously mentioned: that he was making medical treatments as well as medical herbs, roots, and fruits available for men and animals. His purpose (the welfare of all people) is in keeping with Buddhist principles. He also adds: "Whatever efforts I am making are in order that I may discharge (my) debts to (all) beings, that I may make them happy here (in this life) and that they may attain heaven in the next (life)."[36] Undoubtedly medical institutions established by Duṭṭha-gāmaṇī in Ceylon and Buddhist kings elsewhere had the same purpose.

What medical treatment was given in those institutions is largely a matter of conjecture. The canonical text contains legendary accounts of the physician, Jīvaka Komārabhacca, who once attended the Buddha. An illegitimate son of a courtesan, Jīvaka was brought up by the royal family. When he had completed seven years of medical training, his teacher told him to tour the vicinity of Taxilā and to bring back any plant that was not medicinal. When he returned empty-handed, his teacher told him he was ready to practice medicine on his own. From the legends about Jīvaka we learn how physicians treated patients in the early days of Buddhism. With a handful of ghee mixed with medicine Jīvaka cured a woman of a severe headache. He removed King Bimbisāra's fistula with ointment. He cut open the skin on the head of a merchant who suffered from a head disease and drew out two living creatures. He cut open a man's stomach in order to correct a twisted bowel, and he cured a neighboring king of jaundice.[37]

From the medical text of the physician of Caraka, a contemporary of another Buddhist king, Kaniṣka, we learn some of the major components of the Indian medical science, Āyurveda, that the Indian Buddhists accepted: pathology, diagnostics, physiology and anatomy, prognosis, therapeutics, and pharmaceutics.[38] In the main, Indian physicians sought to restore the primal state of health (restitutio in integum) by means of a "regimen of preliminary purgatives, enemas, and emetics, followed by a light and wholesome, restorative, sāttvic diet."[39] With the rise of Mahā-yāna, medical study (chikitsā-vidyā) became one of the five disciplines basic to understanding Buddhism itself.[40] This encouraged the prolifera-tion of priest-physicians who aspired to follow the path of the compas-sionate bodhisattvas. Many Mahāyāna monasteries and nunneries in East Asia operated clinics and dispensed medicine for the sick.[41] The Esoteric tradition, too, stressed medical activities as central to Buddhism. Indeed, Buddhist medical institutions, including a Buddhist medical college (in a strict, literal sense), have remained intact in Tibet until our own time.[42] What has happened to them since the departure of the Dalai Lama from Tibet cannot be verified.

Buddhist medical institutions vary greatly in regard to personnel. For the most part, institutions in the Theravāda tradition depend heavily on professional physicians. In institutions of the Mahāyāna tradition, lay physicians, chiropractors, and others assist priest-physicians, while insti-tutions of the Esoteric tradition are generally staffed by priest-physicians. Most Buddhists have no hesitations about seeking medical advice from non-Buddhist physicians.

Ethics and Justice

ETHICAL DECISIONS REGARDING BIOETHICAL CONCERNS

In sharp contrast to many ethical systems in the West, the ethical prin-ciples that one may derive from Buddhism, like the ethics of other Indian religious-philosophical traditions, are more biological and cosmic in ori-entation. The term dharma usually refers to the fixed position of duty and right. It also designates religious observance, secular law, and the law of nature. In a more basic sense, dharma implies universal justice based on immanent necessity, for "all that has ever come into existence produces its specific reaction or effect—the law of action and reaction as laid down by the principle of Karma [activity]."[43] According to this biologically ori-ented view, the deed itself, or the psychic disposition to do it, is trans-mitted by psychical inheritance from one karma-bearer to another because of the inviolable and ethically indifferent law of cause and effect. The uniqueness of the Buddhist stance may be clarified by comparing it with the Brahmanic-Hindu tradition's substance-view of reality (ātma-vāda), which conceives reality "on the pattern of an inner core or soul (*ātman*), immutable and identical amidst an outer region of impermanence and change."[44] As Murti succinctly points out:

> Buddha came to deny the soul, a permanent substantial entity, precisely because *he took his stand on the reality of moral consciousness* and the efficacy of Karma. An unchanging eternal soul, as impervious to change, would render spiritual life lose [*sic*] all meaning. . . . The ātman is the root-cause of all attachment, desire, aversion and pain.[45]

The Brahmanic-Hindu tradition affirms further that every person is destined to be born into a fixed place (*sva-dharma*), a place that mediates the eternal *dharma* and the person. Buddhism, however, rejects the notion of personal *dharma* and affirms that the *dharma*, the liberating law discovered by the Buddha, can be fulfilled only in the Buddhist community (*saṃgha*) (cf. the threefold affirmation of Buddha, *dharma*, and *saṃgha*). Consequently, early Buddhism conceived ethics primarily in terms of a personal morality prerequisite for an individual's salvation, that is, the achievement of *nirvāṇa* for the monks and of better rebirth in the next life for the laity.

As far as we can ascertain, early Buddhism did not attempt to combine ethical and medical concerns in a unified category of bioethics. To be sure, early Buddhists knew a great deal about the constituents of the body—the hair of the head, hair of the body, nail, skin, teeth, flesh, nerves, bones, marrow, kidneys, heart, liver, pleura, spleen, lungs, intestines, bowels, stomach, feces, bile, phlegm, pus, blood, sweat, fat, tears, serum, spittle, mucus, nose mucus, synovial fluid, and urine[47]—and they knew the processes of the formation of the fetus and of the birth and growth of human bodies. They also had access to rather advanced surgical and medical arts. But they considered prevention and treatment of diseases to belong to the sphere of life that had no direct relevance to moral and spiritual striving. They accepted religious life and medical treatment as two separate spheres without articulating a system of ethics that might mediate between them and provide guidance to physicians. As a result, physicians were compelled to make medical judgments in specific cases solely on medical and surgical grounds. Of course, even if early Buddhists had wanted to develop a positive system of bioethics, the fundamental doctrine of no-self (*anātman*) did not encourage the systematic reflection needed. In addition the doctrine of *karma*, the law of cause and effect, would have presented a real dilemma to any would-be Buddhist bioethicist. Consider a physician confronted by a situation in which he could save either a mother or a baby but not both. What principle, according to his best medical judgment, could he invoke to determine how he should act according to Buddhist ethics? How would he know whether it was the mother's *karma* to die or the child's? If the mother should beg him, should the physician save the child, or should he save the mother at the request of her family on the grounds that the mother could bear another child? Either way, the physician might interfere with the law of karmic justice.

Yet another important factor was not conducive to the development of a system of bioethics: early Buddhism was not inclined to develop any coherent system of social ethics in general, even after King Aśoka affirmed *dharma* as the guiding principle of his vast empire. We have already seen that Aśoka, motivated by his compassion and by his desire to gain merit, provided medical treatment and planted medical herbs for the benefit of people and animals. Suppose a contagious disease had broken out in a crowded community and the families of the sick had begged a physician not to disclose the nature of the disease. What would the physician have done? There were no carefully worked out ethical principles to guide either the physician involved or the Minister of Dharma, whose duty it was to enforce *dharma* according to Aśoka's scheme.

Winston King astutely observed the inherent difficulties Buddhist ethics faces in balancing the issues of intention and result. It is taken for granted that a good intention does not produce an evil deed; conversely, a good intention or a good result cannot compensate for an evil deed. But, King asks, what should one do if one sees a snake ready to attack a child? If one kills the snake, will the act of killing—a sin with evil consequences—be compensated by the act of saving a child? A Buddhist might question our commonsense judgment that the intention and the deed of saving a child might compensate for the sin of killing an animal. The child, one might reason, might not have been killed or might have been saved by other means. Yet King correctly asks whether a person who killed a snake and saved a child would interfere with karmic processes, or would that person simply be the agent of *karma* "and hence guiltless"?[48] It is easy to see that Buddhists would confront similar ethical ambiguities in dealing with many medical cases. Should one take the course of nonaction in order not to interfere with karmic processes? Should one act, assuming that one is just an agent of *karma*? Or does one have a karmic duty to perform a specific act even if one's acting inevitably involves the possibility of other evil consequences?

RESOURCES AND EXPEDIENTS USED IN DEALING WITH BIOETHICAL PROBLEMS

Although Buddhists have as a matter of course faced many bioethical problems, the Buddhist tradition has not acknowledged them as bioethical issues until quite recently. The assembly of the monastic orders was the form closest to a "resource" in the Buddhist tradition. It dealt, however, only with the activities of the monks. To judge from the *Vinaya* texts, the assembly placed high priority on "intention" in evaluating the monks' deeds. We read, for example:

> Whatever monk should intentionally deprive a human being of life or should look about so as to be his knife-bringer . . . or should incite (anyone) to death: he also is one who is defeated, he is not in communion.[49]

The *Vinaya* texts cite numerous case histories:

> At one time while a certain monk was eating, some meat stuck in his throat. A certain monk gave a blow to that monk's neck; the meat fell out with blood, and that monk died. He was remorseful . . . "There is no offence, monk, as you did not mean to cause his death."[50]

> At one time a certain monk had a headache. The monks gave him medical treatment through the nose. The monk died. . . . "There is no offence involving defeat."[51]

But other acts were condemned, as when one monk was asked by a pregnant woman to give her an abortive preparation, which resulted in her child's death, or when another monk, at the request of a barren woman, gave her fertility medicine that caused her to die.[52] Despite recording individual medical cases, however, the *Vinaya* does not seem to provide positive principles for dealing with the difficult ethical issues involved.

The Buddhist tradition provided no resource or guidance to the laity except general moral principles, such as those found in the eightfold path: "right understanding" regarding the characteristics of existence (impermanence, suffering, and no-self or no-soul) and the nature of moral law regarding "right thought," "right effort," "right mindfulness," and "right action" ("(1) Not to kill, but to practice love and harmlessness to all; (2) Not to take that which is not given, but to practice charity and generosity; (3) Not to commit sexual misconduct, but to practice purity and self-control; (4) Not to indulge in false speech; . . . (5) Not to partake of intoxicating drinks or drugs").[53] Beyond these, the laity usually consulted the clergy and medical experts on a case-by-case basis for help in dealing with medical-ethical problems. The consulting of practitioners of fortune-telling, divination, palmistry, and related magical arts has also been rather widespread.

GUIDING AUTHORITIES

The most significant Buddhist medical institution developed in Tibet, where religion and medicine achieved a high degree of integration. Under the thirteenth Dalai Lama (1895–1933), the College or House of Medicine and Astronomy was established in Lhasa, equipped with lecture halls, a hospital, living quarters for teachers and students, and laboratories. Until the flight of the current Dalai Lama to India, the college received one student from each provincial monastery in addition to able private students.[54] Outside Tibet, the Buddhist community did not develop anything like a Buddhist medical academy or college. Historically, however, large Buddhist monasteries, especially in Mahāyāna countries, had clinics attached to them, and the people turned to these institutions for authoritative advice. Moreover, physicians of Buddhist persuasion served in such government institutions as the Great Medical Bureau (T'ai-i-shu) in China during the T'ang dynasty.

Since the introduction of modern Western medicine during the past two centuries, many medical colleges, hospitals, and clinics have been established in various parts of Asia. Most operate under secular auspices, but Buddhist groups have founded some. Side by side with westernized modern medicine, herb medicine and other traditional forms of medical practice continue to be in demand. As a result, it is difficult to generalize about authorities to which Buddhist adherents turn for guidance. It is probably safe to assume that the religious universe of contemporary Buddhists is spacious enough to embrace westernized modern medicine, traditional medicine, and a host of diviners, sorcerers, and fortune-tellers. All maintain varying degrees of authority in guiding those faithful who encounter difficult bioethical problems, whether they recognize them as such or not.

Passages

A few words may help explain why there is such a bewildering variety of notions and practices concerning passages of life in the Buddhist world. The Buddha had forsaken the world; and mendicant disciples, following his example, left home to lead the religious life. At the same time, he attracted many lay disciples, male and female. It was taken for granted that monastics were the core of the Buddhist community. After the demise of the Buddha, they took upon themselves the role of guardians and transmitters of the founder's teaching. But Caroline A. F. Rhys Davids astutely reminds us that although the Pali canon was "compiled by members of a religious order and largely concerned with the mental experiences and ideas of recluses, and with their outlook on the world," it included a discourse on domestic and social matters based on the Buddha's doctrines of love and goodwill. The discourse was entitled the "Sigala Homily," and it testified to the continued importance of the lay components in the early Buddhist community.[55]

Even so, in contrast to many religious traditions in India and elsewhere, early Buddhism said virtually nothing, positive or negative, about the religious and social significance of the various stages of the house-holder's life. As Eliot points out, "the Buddha prescribed no ceremonies for births, deaths, and marriages, and apparently expected the laity to continue in the observance of such rites as were in use."[56] Thus, unlike the monks, whose stages of life were guided by the code of discipline (Vinaya), early lay Buddhists in India followed the non-Buddhist mores and observances familiar to them in dealing with the major events in their lives. Since the Indian Buddhist community did not develop Buddhist forms to celebrate life-passages, the same pattern was followed later by lay Buddhists in other parts of Asia. Each group appropriated the non-Buddhist customs in its own locality. This practice accounts for the wide variety of interpretations and customs concerning life-passages in the different Buddhist nations of Asia. There are accounts of Buddhist traditions in South and Southeast Asia, the Himalayan border area, Tibet and Mongolia, China, Korea, and Japan. In the limited space available here we cannot cover all local variations; we can discuss only those bare essentials that are shared, more or less, by Buddhists in various parts of Asia.

BEGINNING OF LIFE

At the expense of oversimplification, we might distinguish three layers of meaning in the Buddhist tradition for the "beginning" as well as for the "end" of "life": religious, empirical (physiological), and cultural. In religious terms, the all-important doctrine of anattā (nonego, no-self, or no-soul) states that what is known as a person is a temporary combination of bodily and mental elements that lacks any self-reliant substance, such as an ego or a self. What is called life, marked by birth and death, is only an insignificant part of an unbroken chain, the continuous combination, dissolution, and recombination of physical and mental elements known as saṃsāra (round of rebirth or transmigration). Saṃsāra implies a constant repetition of birth and death in the three worlds and the six realms of existence according to the law of karma. Thus a single lifetime and its beginning have no religious significance except as they testify to the doctrine of impermanence of life and the world. It should be stressed that in this cosmic scheme, human beings share equal status with other beings.

On the empirical level, birth or the beginning of life is accepted as a natural consequence of conception, which is instrumental in bringing into existence the temporary combination of corporeality, feeling, perception, mental formation, and consciousness, as well as sensitive organs, with all the identifiable physical and mental marks.[57] Even on the empirical, physiological level, however, there is no unanimity concerning what constitutes the beginning of life. One canonical text leads us to believe that "from the mind's first arising, from (the time of) consciousness becoming first manifest in a mother's womb until the time of death, here meanwhile he is called a *human being*."[58] But opinions are divided among Buddhist theorists and among physicians as well as to whether life begins at conception, at some time during pregnancy, or at birth.

On the cultural level, there are, for the reasons given earlier, a bewildering variety of meanings attached to the beginning of life or birth, colored by the mores, taboos, customs, and kinship systems of the different parts of the Buddhist world. In Burma, for example, where there is no family name to inherit, less importance is assigned to the birth of a child than in, say, East Asia. However, Burmese Buddhists, like their East Asian counterparts, prefer the birth of a male child but for different reasons. For the Burmese, "only a male child can be initiated in youth into the Buddhist priesthood, and the sponsoring of this ceremony is an important deed of merit on the parents' part."[59] This is just one example of how Buddhist and local cultural features converge in dealing with the phenomenon of the beginning of life.

SEXUALITY

Sexuality, too, has many layers of meaning—religious, cultural, physiological, ethical, and so on—in the Buddhist world. We are told that on his deathbed the Buddha warned his trusted disciple Ānanda against the seductiveness of the female:

> "How should we behave, my lord, in regard to the feminine sex?"
> "Not to see them, O Ānanda."
> "But, Blessed One, if we do see them?"
> "Not to speak to them, O Ānanda."
> "But, my lord, if they speak to us?"
> "Keep wide awake, O Ānanda."[60]

The Buddha warned the monks not only against the female sex but also against masturbation on the grounds that it was not becoming for one who is committed to the goal of stilling passion. Moreover, "it is not for the benefit of unbelievers, nor for increase in the number of believers, but it is . . . to the detriment of unbelievers as well as of believers."[61] "Emission of semen during a dream," however, is not considered an offense.[62] Because monks are to observe perfect chastity, sexual intercourse is, of course, forbidden to them. They are also strictly warned against homosexuality, considered to be a perverted act. Thus we read:

> If there is a man, and thinking it to be a man . . . doubtful . . . thinking it to be an animal . . . thinking it to be a woman . . . thinking it to be an eunuch, if the monk is infatuated and rubs the man's body . . . touches it, there is an offence of wrong-doing.

If there is an animal, and thinking it to be a woman . . . thinking it to be an eunuch . . . thinking it to be a man, if the monk is infatuated and rubs the animal's body . . . touches it, there is an offence of wrong-doing.[63]

Sexuality has different connotations for householders than for monks and nuns. Here again cultural contexts, sexual mores, and social organizations vary greatly in the various parts of the Buddhist world. In much of traditional Asia, polygamy, male and female prostitution, and the institution of the eunuch were tolerated if not officially recognized. The five moral rules that in principle bind all lay Buddhists include abstention from unlawful sexual acts such as intercourse with girls who are still under the protection of father or mother, brother or sister, or relatives; and intercourse with married women, female convicts, and betrothed girls.[64] Otherwise, the Buddhist tradition itself gave no specific injunctions in such sexual matters as masturbation and homosexuality. Evidently, various means of contraception were known and practiced among householders, especially in poverty-stricken areas.

DIGNITY OF LIFE

Inasmuch as Buddhist views of life are permeated by the doctrine of *karma*, the "dignity of life" has very different implications for the Buddhist tradition than for the Western world. This difference probably accounts for its official silence on matters of euthanasia and the prolongation of life. These were considered primarily medical problems to be handled without invoking religious principles. Buddhism has spoken out clearly against injuring, killing, or destroying life in both human beings and animals. But because of the previously mentioned ambiguity about when life begins, there have never been any clear-cut views on abortion. There are canonical references against it, but they seem to condemn monks' involvement with abortion rather than abortion itself.[65] Equally ambiguous is the Buddhist stance on suicide. Some have condemned it, but others have approved it. The ambiguity was evident most conspicuously during the war in Vietnam, when some monks immolated themselves.

DYING

We have already touched upon an important aspect of the Buddhist understanding of death in the discussion on the beginning of life. To be brief, death marks the end of life, which is nothing but a temporary combination of bodily and mental elements. Still, death is the necessary prerequisite for the process of rebirth, which is destined to continue according to the principle of *karma*. Religiously speaking, death is not an evil but an integral part of universal suffering which, according to the first of the Four Noble Truths, characterizes the nature of existence.

> In the absolute sense, beings have only a very short moment to live, life lasting as long as a single moment of consciousness lasts. Just as a cart-wheel, whether rolling or whether at a standstill, at all times only rests on a single point of its periphery: even so the life of a living being lasts only for the duration of a single moment of consciousness. As soon as that moment ceases, the being also ceases.[66]

In a real sense, an essential part of the Buddhist vocation is to reflect on this truth, which will lead one toward the path of ultimate enlightenment and liberation, just as it did the Buddha. Thus, according to Buddhism, a deceased person will be missed but should not be mourned!

Notes

1. Edward J. Thomas, *The History of Buddhist Thought* (London, 1933), p. 14.
2. Benson Y. Landis, *World Religions* (New York, 1957).
3. Isaline B. Horner, trans., *The Book of the Discipline (Vinaya-Pitaka)*, vol. 4, *Mahavagga* 8.26A (London, 1962), p. 432.
4. Ibid., pp. 433–434.
5. A. L. Basham, "The Practice of Medicine in Ancient and Medieval India," in *Asian Medical Systems: A Comparative Study*, ed. Charles M. Leslie (Berkeley, 1976), p. 20.
6. Cited in Nyanatiloka, *Buddhist Dictionary* (Colombo, Sri Lanka, 1956), p. 30.
7. Basham, p. 24.
8. F. Max Müller, trans., *The Dhammapada: A Collection of Verses*, in *Sacred Books of the East*, vol. 10 (Oxford, 1881), p. 54.
9. *The Book of the Discipline (Vinaya-Pitaka)*, *Mahavagga* 1.19; this translation is taken from Earl H. Brewster, *Life of Gotama the Buddha* (London, 1926). See Horner, p. 16; she prefers "ill" to "suffering."
10. Walpola Rahula, *What the Buddha Taught* (New York, 1959), pp. 17–18.
11. Gananath Obeyesekere, "The Ritual Drama of the *Sanni* Demons: Collective Representations of Disease in Ceylon," *Comparative Studies in Society and History* 11, no. 2 (April 1969):175.
12. Nyanatiloka, p. 71.
13. Thomas W. Rhys Davids, trans., *The Questions of King Milinda*, pt.1, Sacred Books of the East, vol. 35 (Oxford, 1890), pp. 191–192.
14. Ibid., pp. 192–193.
15. Obeyesekere, p. 175.
16. Müller, p. 3.
17. Heinrich Zimmer, *Philosophies of India*, ed. Joseph Campbell (New York, 1951), p. 469.
18. Cited in Nyanatiloka, p. 33.
19. Winston L. King, *In the Hope of Nibbana* (La Salle, IL, 1946), p. 31.
20. See ibid., p. 173.

21. Müller, p. 46.
22. Horner, p. 432.
23. Ibid., p. 433.
24. Walpola Rahula, *History of Buddhism in Ceylon* (Colombo, Sri Lanka, 1956), p. 254.
25. Stanley J. Tambiah, *Buddhism and Spirit Cults in Northeast Thailand* (Cambridge, England, 1970), pp. 146–147.
26. Edward Conze, *Buddhist Thought in India* (Ann Arbor, MI, 1962), p. 217.
27. See Kenneth Ch'en, *The Chinese Transformation of Buddhism* (Princeton, 1973), p. 295.
28. Amulyachandra Sen, *Asoka's Edicts* (Calcutta, 1956), p. 66.
29. Ibid., p. 90.
30. Trevor Ling, *The Buddha: Buddhist Civilization in India and Ceylon* (London, 1973), p. 186.
31. See Ilza Veith and Atsumi Minami, "A Buddhist Prayer against Sickness," *History of Religions* 5, no. 2 (Winter 1966):239–249.
32. Rhys Davids, p. 214.
33. Ibid., p. 218.
34. See Tambiah; Obeyesekere; also Nur Yalman, "The Structure of Sinhalese Healing Rituals," in *Religion in South Asia*, ed. Edward B. Harper (Seattle, 1964), pp. 115–150.
35. Joel M. Halpern, "Traditional Medicine and the Role of the Phi in Laos," *The Eastern Anthropologist* 16, no. 3 (1963):195.
36. Sen, p. 78.
37. Horner, pp. 380–393.
38. Basham, p. 20.
39. Zimmer, p. 548.
40. Veith and Minami, p. 243.
41. See Ch'en, pp. 294–303.
42. See Rechung Rinpoche and Jampal Kunzang, *Tibetan Medicine* (Berkeley and Los Angeles, 1973); and Ilza Veith, *Medizin in Tibet* (Berlin, n.d.).
43. Betty Heiman, *Indian and Western Philosophy: A Study in Contrast* (London, 1937), p. 70.
44. T. R. V. Murti, *The Central Philosophy of Buddhism: A Study of the Mādhyamika System* (London, 1955), p. 10.
45. Ibid., p. 17; emphasis mine.
46. Yashapal, "Surgery and Medicine in the Days of Gautama," *Indian Historical Quarterly* 25 (1949):102.
47. King, 136. Although he followed the Pali rendering, *kamma*, I have chosen to use the Sanskrit form, *karma*.
48. Isaline B. Horner, trans., *The Book of the Discipline (Vinaya-Pitaka)*, vol. 1, *Suttavibhanga* (London, 1949), pp. 125–126.
49. Ibid., p. 139.
50. Ibid., p. 143.
51. Ibid., pp. 144–145.
52. H. Saddhatissa, *Buddhist Ethics: Essence of Buddhism* (New York, 1970), p. 71.
53. Rinpoche and Kunzang, pp. 22–23.
54. Thomas W. and Caroline A. F. Rhys Davids, trans., *Dialogue of the Buddha*, pt. 3, in *Sacred Books of the Buddhists*, vol. 4 (London, 1957), pp. 170, 173–184.
55. Sir Charles Eliot, *Hinduism and Buddhism*, vol. 2 (New York, 1954), p. 120.

56. See Thomas W. and Caroline A. F. Rhys Davids, trans., *Dialogue of the Buddha*, pt. 2, in Sacred Books of the Buddhists, vol. 3, *Maha Satipatthana Suttanta* 5, p. 330.

57. Horner, *Suttavibhanga*, p. 126.

58. Margaret Mead, ed., *Cultural Patterns and Technical Change* (New York, 1955), p. 38.

59. Taken from *Mahaparinibhana Sutta*, quoted in A. Foucher, *The Life of the Buddha*, abridged translation by S. B. Boas (Middletown, CT, 1963), p. 109.

60. Horner, *Suttavibhanga*, pp. 193–195.

61. Ibid., p. 106.

62. Ibid., pp. 204–205. The Tantric Buddhist notions and practices regarding sex, which are very different from those of other Buddhist traditions, are not included in this article.

63. See Nyanatiloka, p. 69.

64. Horner, *Suttavibhanga*, pp. 144–145.

65. Nyanatiloka, p. 90.

CHAPTER 2

Chinese Buddhist Traditions of Healing and the Life Cycle

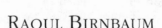

RAOUL BIRNBAUM

Disease is a somber mystery, a powerful transformative process that leads to the gateways of death. Both the physician and the religious specialist have much concern with this boundary between life and death, and those who are especially effective at their callings traverse with respectful familiarity along this distinctive edge. Both seek to provide aid and assistance at treacherous moments in the life cycle, trying to help establish patterns that lead from suffering. It is not surprising that in many societies there is no clear separation between religious and healing traditions, and it is

33

not surprising that often there is no clear separation between the role of religious specialist and that of healer.

Among the international religions—those that reach across cultural and linguistic gulfs—Buddhism has been notable for its intense interest in healing. From the earliest days, Buddhist teachings have been termed a method for gaining freedom from suffering, and within Buddhist traditions much attention has been given to the causes and consequences of disease. In the textual traditions there is a strikingly extensive use of medical terminology in the rhetoric and discourse of spiritual experience. Its first historic teacher, Śākyamuni Buddha, frequently is called the Great Physician, and his teaching is termed a King of Medicines that cures the ills of humankind. Buddhist teachings suggest that all who are not enlightened are considered ill—that is, their full capacities are impinged upon by ingrained habitual faults, their energy flow thus deflected—and the enlightenment process is equated with the healing process.

In addition to metaphorical and symbolic discussion of disease and healing, there are extensive traditions of healing activity in Buddhist history. Since illness is a chief cause of suffering in the world, and the special focus of Buddhist teachings is the methodical elimination of suffering, the causes and treatments of disease have been a topic of special interest among many Buddhist thinkers. While there are some scriptural injunctions prohibiting monks from practicing medicine as a profession, Śākyamuni also charged his disciples with the responsibility of care for each other, including the administration of medical cures when necessary. A materia medica of sorts can be found preserved in a section of the early canon; meditative methods for transcending pain and curing ailments also are detailed, and numerous anecdotes attest to the concern that early monks had for alleviating the distresses of disease. Indeed, Buddhist healers were famous in India and Central Asia in the early centuries around the turn of the Common Era, and such physician-monks were effective transmitters of Buddhist teachings, like the intrepid Christian missionary doctors of recent times.

Physician-monks from Central Asia and India who roamed about the continent were prominent in the process of bringing Buddhism to China in the initial centuries of the Common Era. It appears that the superior healing ability of some of these monks was a significant factor in the spread of Buddhist teachings there. These healers brought to China theories, skills, and medicines different from those of the sophisticated traditions already developed in that land. Their effective healings gained many followers, while texts that they brought from their native lands on healing and extension of the life span were of great fascination to the Chinese, whose native religions placed unusual emphasis on such topics.

In Chinese religious traditions, the ability to heal often has been considered a natural outgrowth of spiritual accomplishment. This ability frequently serves a validating function in the establishment of new cults and religious teachings. In a recurring pattern seen to the present day, charismatic teachers of new religions often are noted for their healing abilities, which serve to validate claims of special insight and access to powerful spirit beings. These demonstrated healing abilities serve in a dramatic way to gain trust for the teachings such persons espouse. Further, in Chinese culture there has been a special interest in longevity and a special respect for those living long lives, with a sense that wise persons are not subject to untimely death but are able to live out a full life span. Teachings brought by healers that devote considerable attention to longevity are assured a wide audience in China; such was the case with Buddhism. These aspects of Buddhism were magnified in China by the intense interest there, and they took on an importance apparently far beyond their role in the Indian homeland of the teachings.

Numerous texts on healing and longevity are preserved in the modern edition of the enormous Chinese Buddhist canon (*Taishō shinshū daizōkyō,* hereafter abbreviated as T). Some of these texts have had a great popularity through numerous centuries, while others faded from sight. The wide-ranging variety of these sources leads to some problems for historical studies, for some of these works were composed in China, others in various parts of Central Asia, and others in India over a period of perhaps ten centuries. At times this diversity of origin is reflected in a diversity of theory, but a set of basic principles can be readily discerned. These basic principles form the core of this present essay.

A brief overview of the most important of these texts provides a sense of their broad range. These works include texts on medical theory, cure by meditative methods, cure through invocation of specific deities, and cure through ritual incantation.

Among the works on medical theory, there is for example the *Scripture on the Buddha's Medicine* (T 793), apparently surviving from the mid-third century in a truncated or condensed version. This text describes the functioning of the body in terms of four elements—fire, earth, wind, water—and the arising of disease, especially in relation to the imbalance of these elements under the influence of their seasonal predominance. This work also lists in brief manner such topics as the nine types of untimely or violent death and the ten causes of disease.

A text entitled *Secret and Essential Methods for the Cure of Meditators' Illnesses* (T 620), translated into Chinese in the fifth century by a noble layman from a text he obtained in the Central Asian state of Khotan, apparently was compiled from several sources. Divided into twelve sections, this work deals with numerous ailments, with special concern for the mental or psychic afflictions occasionally suffered by solitary practitioners of meditative disciplines. These ailments apparently respond to the effective harnessing of the mind for self-cure. Again, as is found in most Buddhist healing texts preserved in Chinese, this work is based on a four-element system (a three-humor system also was important in India).

There are numerous texts brought from Central Asia and India on healing deities. Without doubt, the most important of these is the *Scripture on the Fundamental Vows and Merits of the Master of Healing, the Lapis Lazuli Radiance Tathāgata* (T 450), which reveals the existence of a special healing Buddha who has vowed to help all beings who call upon him for aid. An extended series of related ritual texts also exists, detailing methods for invoking the healing force of this deity and his assistants. (Among the numerous texts on healing deities, see most especially T 449–451, 922–926, 1161, 1331.)

Further, there are texts that provide incantations for relief from various ailments, such as eye disease, childhood afflictions, and dental problems (especially the texts T 1323–1330).

Among the native Chinese Buddhist works on healing, perhaps the most interesting (and certainly the most influential) are the chapters on this topic found in the long and short meditation manuals of the brilliant sixth-century T'ien-t'ai lineage master Chih-i (538–597), the *Mo-ho chih-kuan* (T 1911) and the *Hsiao chih-kuan* (T 1915).

As principal sources for this essay, I have relied most especially on the *Scripture on the Master of Healing* and on Chih-i's meditation manuals. The first, a quintessentially important scripture received from the "western lands," was eventually well circulated throughout China. The second, unusually intelligent syntheses of native Chinese concepts and the received traditions of international Buddhism, transcended lineage boundaries and have been studied by learned clerics and lay practitioners throughout East Asia for fourteen centuries.[1]

Traditionally, Buddhist teachings hold that a complete life cycle is marked by four inevitable sufferings: birth, sickness, old age, and death. For humans with a full span of life, sickness is inevitable. This particular form of suffering constitutes one of the common meeting grounds in the intensely shared reality of suffering that links all humans in an experiential fellowship. In order to perceive more fully the nature of sickness from a Buddhist point of view, it should be considered within its normal context, the life cycle. Here I would like to survey some of these concepts as accepted by Chinese Buddhists. My intention here is not to describe a comprehensive portrait of the concepts and techniques known to have been put into practice by a "typical Chinese Buddhist" of a certain time and place. Instead, I have sought to provide through description and explanation some key elements of the rich array of views and healing practices available to Chinese Buddhists from the sixth or seventh centuries to the present.

Birth

For each individual, birth is not a signal and anomalous event; each individual experiences and endures numerous births, extending back in time to a near-unreachable place and likely continuing in the future to a time beyond reckoning. A single birth constitutes a mere single link of a weighty chain of experiential suffering. One of the goals of Buddhist practice is the achievement of wisdom and insight sufficient to break this chain, sufficient to end the continuous round of birth-death-birth-death-birth.

The chain progressively becomes weaker as the individual cultivates certain enlightened states of mind (through special meditative practices and through general clarification and purification of mental processes), as ways of speech are reformed, and as ways of action are reformed such that they embody the fundamental benevolence that rests at the heart of Buddhist teachings. The patterned currents of these ways of thought, speech, and action—the karmic patterns of the individual—thrust the person into appropriate new situations, including new births.

The conditions for each birth are determined by the amassed *karma* of the individual. *Karma* determines the type of birth—human or nonhuman, the locale for this event, the parents, and their social-economic-educational status. *Karma* determines the physical nature of the child, and so forth.

This karmic judgment can be explained in many ways. As a functioning principle, one might see it operating in an impersonally magnetic fashion. Thus, an angry man may naturally be attracted to a home environment suitably hospitable to his angry nature. Rather more picturesque, the *Scripture on the Master of Healing* describes a scene at the time of death experienced by all humans, at which point the circumstances of the next birth are determined:

> He is seized by the messengers of Yama, who lead his spirit consciousness before that King of the Law. The inborn spirits attached to all sentient beings, who record whether each being's conduct is good or bad, will then hand down these records in their entirety to Yama, King of the Law. Then the King will interrogate this person, and he will sum up this person's deeds. According to the positive and negative factors, he shall judge him.

Auspicious births are described in great detail in a wide range of Buddhist scriptures that became popular in China. First and foremost, human birth is viewed as precious. This mode of incarnation is considered especially fortunate for its particular balance of attendant conditions: suffering enough to awaken the being to the necessity for self-purification, but not so brutish and fear-provoking as that, say, of the animal realms; mental faculties developed enough to embark on that task. Human birth by its very nature is considered auspicious and portentous: it is a fertile ground for planting seeds of enlightenment.

Accordingly, I have not found a Buddhist scripture or a treatise by a Chinese Buddhist monk or nun that condones abortion. To the contrary, the principal texts containing regulations for monks and nuns equate abortion with murder. Those who commit such acts, the texts state emphatically, cannot be considered monks or nuns, nor can they be considered disciples of the Buddha, members of his spiritual family.[2]

While human birth in general is viewed as auspicious, certain qualities are considered particularly fortunate. Often the completeness of the sense faculties and the completeness of the physical nature is remarked upon. It is auspicious to be born physically complete, with all parts functioning in the standard manner. It is auspicious to be born with all six sense faculties complete; according to Buddhist traditions these include taste, touch, smell, hearing, sight, and mental functioning. Any incomplete capacities in these six areas are the result of karmic retribution; thus, any child born with sense impairments or physical handicaps has been born this way not by chance or "fate," but by self-created causation. There is nothing random in the Buddhist universe.

The circumstances of the birth also are determined by karmic retribution. Brutish and ignorant actions lead to rebirth in an outlying region where one rarely gains the opportunity to hear pure teachings of spiritual principles. Unwholesome patterns lead to birth into an unhappy, ignorant, impoverished household. Well-established wholesome patterns lead to birth in a well-situated family where spiritual learning is honored and encouraged, where opportunities for genuine growth are readily made available.

However, no matter how flawed the body, no matter how difficult the circumstances, it is held that all persons have the innate ability to attain enlightenment. Thus, though not always apparent, at a fundamental level there is an equality of potential and of integral nobility.

Disease and Healing

CAUSES

As mentioned above, Buddhists hold that the universe is bound by laws of cause and effect. All sentient beings operate within this web. Buddhist analytical traditions have considered with great care the specific functionings of cause and effect, and much attention has been given to disease, one of the four inevitable sufferings that all sentient beings must endure by virtue of birth in the material world. Those enlightened beings who in acts of great compassion consciously choose birth in this world in order to teach and aid others, having entered into this net of distress also are subject to its conditions and limitations, including disease. However, various authors note that there is a distinct difference between the illnesses contracted by the enlightened, which then are exploited for teaching purposes, and those causing distress to the unenlightened.[3] The cause and cure of diseases of the unenlightened is a principal concern of this present essay.

Most fundamentally, disease is viewed as the direct or indirect result of *karma*, either retribution for specific acts or the ultimate effect of long-established patterns of thoughts, words, and deeds. Since the mind drives the speech and actions that generate *karma*, it is the mind especially that is seen as the root of disease.

In addition to diseases caused by mental states gone awry, according to numerous Buddhist accounts, there may be several other causes. For example, certain diseases are caused by repugnant and evil spirits. Once again, however, persons cannot succumb to such spirit-caused disease if their mental patterns are strong enough to resist the vitality-depleting demon; in order to fall prey to such a demon, one's mental patterns must be confused and weak. I should point out that a variant of the demonic-attack or invasion theory of causation is commonly accepted in modern Western medicine, only here the demons are bacteria and other such creatures who swarm about at strategic spots within the body, causing great distress to those not strong enough to resist their presence.

In Chih-i's long study on meditation, he devotes considerable attention to the causes and cures of diseases. He holds that the unenlightened are subject to a wide range of illnesses that arise from six main categories of causation. In his discussions, we can see a conscious attempt at synthesis of diverse received Buddhist traditions and native Chinese beliefs; this is also a notable characteristic of his teachings on numerous topics in the realms of Buddhist practices and concepts.

Among these six classes of disease, first there is seasonal predominance of the four elements, leading to imbalance within the body and resulting in unpleasant manifestations. Second, there are diseases caused by improper diet, such that one or another of the elements is harmfully increased by the eating of the wrong types of foods. While there is some reference in early Buddhist texts to Śākyamuni Buddha's discussion of proper diet to maintain good health, this also is basic to native Chinese traditions, and even today persons able to afford dietary diversity may plan their meals in accordance with generally accepted principles of the correspondence of foodstuffs to the elements. Third, there are illnesses caused by improper meditative practice (as also discussed in the *Secret and Essential Methods for the Cure of Meditators' Illnesses*). Fourth and fifth are diseases caused by the intrusion of negative spirit forces—demons and the like—into the body or into the mind. Sixth, there are diseases directly related to the *karma* of significant deeds of past lives or the present one. Here Chih-i holds that violation of the fivefold principles of conduct accepted by many Buddhists—prohibition of murder, theft, adultery, telling falsehoods, and ingestion of intoxicants—leads directly to diseases or impairments related to the five sense faculties and to corresponding viscera. For example, murder leads to impairments of sight or diseases of the eye or liver.

CURES

Chih-i suggests methods of cure for these six categories. Diseases caused by element imbalance and improper diet are best cured through ingestion of appropriate medicines and other physical procedures. Diseases caused by improper meditative technique are cured through suitable meditative counterparts. Diseases caused by demonic intrusion are driven out by special meditative techniques and by concentration and recitation of exorcistic phrases, either by the person beset with this trouble or by an able exorcist. Illnesses due to karmic misdeeds should be treated by the cultivation of insight through special meditative techniques, by confession and repentance practices (these also are discussed in great detail in independent texts; for example, the so-called Lotus Samādhi practices for the purification of the sense faculties, which involve a rigorous twenty-one-day exercise[4]), and through wholesome practices of expiation (including charitable works and the like).

These various types of cures can be found in a wide range of Buddhist texts. External cures for ailments include such therapies as hot baths, massage, mudpack, and so forth. Cures using various medicines and healing agents include many types of purgatives and emetics, tonics, some common foodstuffs such as honey and butter, numerous herbal cures prepared in various ways, and certain minerals in powered form. In keeping with Buddhist injunctions against deliberate killing, no medicinal use is made of animal parts. Some Buddhists with medical training, such as the famous eighth-century scholar and traveler I-ching, strongly recommend fasting, together with rest from walking and working, as an effective cure for fevers and colds.

In the context of this essay, internal cures (by internal I refer to the effective harnessing of the mind) hold significant interest. One of the great strengths and glories of Buddhism in the history of religions is its special repertoire of meditative methods, its special emphasis on internal analysis, and the resulting high development of mental control on the part of skilled practitioners. These internal cures may be placed within a larger category of so-called "religion-based" cures, including such following types as: meditation; invocation of healing deities through visualization, prayer, and ritual use of images; confession and repentance; and recitation of potent phrases and scriptures. Such methods are discussed in numerous Buddhist texts of diverse origin, and all these methods are employed by Chinese Buddhists, the more sophisticated practitioners engaging in the more sophisticated practices.

Since it is held that diseases of the unenlightened have a fundamental origin in the crooked twistings and turnings of the mind gone awry, thus both wasting and misdirecting energy as well as perhaps attracting negative forces from the outside, a genuine cure must be effected at the seat of the disease, the mind. Meditative techniques for healing are found in early layers of the Buddhist scriptures, suggesting that they may indeed have been taught directly by Śākyamuni. They are recorded as having been taught by the Buddha only to monks, presumably because at that time only monks had sufficient meditative training to sustain success in this mode of self-healing. This meditation—based on a set of concepts known as the "seven limbs of enlightenment"—proceeds in seven stages, passing in a cleansing and purifying manner through mindfulness, investigation of the rise and fall of all things (thus, awareness of their insubstantiality), striving, joy, tranquility, meditative trance, and equanimity. Numerous cases are cited in early texts of the powerful healing quality of this procedure, as carried out by well-trained meditators.

Various types of procedures for profound calming or settling of the mind are conventionally employed for healing purposes. Chih-i cites several of them as especially useful. Focusing the mind on the site of the ailment can effect a curing. Focusing the mind on the internal energy center just below the navel—a basic practice in Taoist traditions native to China—also generates healing energy throughout the body. A further method involves focusing the mind on the soles of the feet at all times. The view here is that the errant impulses of the mind have caused the four elements to become disturbed; settling the mind in this way allows the four elements to regain their natural harmony without agitated disturbance. Finally, there is the calming meditation in which one achieves profound awareness of the insubstantiality of all things, including disease. Reaching this realization and fully experiencing it, the meditator can then be spontaneously purged of ailments.

Related to this general category above are voidness meditations, in which the practitioner's consciousness is plunged into a calm and blissful sea of light and beyond, that enable the skilled practitioner to transcend pain; in this state some healing of the body may be accomplished.

Observation and visualization meditation may also have a healing effect if properly performed. Mindfulness of the breath—a calming and centering technique involving relaxed awareness of the ins and outs of breathing—is useful for putting inner turbulence to an end as well as for a sense of intake of clear energy and expulsion of stagnant factors. Chih-i discusses types of breath-control exercises at some length, providing a set of six types of healing breath and an alternate set of twelve types, each one correlated to specific problems. This practice involves visualizing the expulsion of the disease as one carries out the specific breathing procedures.

Further visualization methods for healing are detailed at great length in a number of texts. These range from methods of transcending and eliminating pain, to the reorienting of energy flows within the body, to the potent invocation of healing deities through the forming of mental images of them inside or directly outside the body.

The text known as *Secret and Essential Methods for Curing Meditators' Illnesses* provides numerous examples of visualization methods. One group of exercises is keyed to the four elements, with reference to the need to balance out their seasonal fluctuations. For example, spring chills can be cured through entrance into the "fire meditative trance," in which blazing radiance rises within and heats the body. In this visualization, flames in the body create gems that emerge from the body's pores. A golden lotus is created between the flames, upon which a buddha sits, proclaiming the methods to cure disease. Three types of gems then manifest, and these are visualized upon the two shoulders and the crown of the head. Rays of these gems are visualized as emitted from the pores of the body. The result of this process, according to the text, is the relaxation of the body and mind.

To enter into the "wind meditative trance," according to the text, the meditator's body is envisioned as "transformed into a nine-headed dragon. Each one of the dragon's heads has nine hundred ears and countless mouths. The pores, ears, and mouths are like great ravines, and from each comes forth a raging wind." A cure for acute diseases of wind involves a visualization of the body as a diamond throne, with a diamond wheel at each of the four sides. From these wheels grow seven diamond flowers, upon which sit manifested buddhas. These buddhas grasp a water pot in which there is a sixteen-headed dragon. The dragon moves its body and inhales the wind. Throughout the world, the wind becomes tranquil and calm. The seven buddhas then proceed to explain the "seven limbs of enlightenment" and help the meditator gradually enter the eightfold path to liberation.

The meditator who seeks to enter the "water meditative trance" envisions the body as a great bubbling spring, with water flowing out of the 336 bodily joints, covering the earth in all directions. To cure an acute disease of water, the body is visualized as a wish-granting pearl, in the form of an auspicious pot, above which there is a golden blossom. Water from all directions is caused to flow into the pot. Seven flowers arise from the auspicious pot, and their seven stems emit light. Between each stem there are seven springs of water. In each spring, there are seven golden blossoms, and atop each blossom there is a seated buddha, who preaches the "seven limbs of enlightenment."[5]

These several visualizations have been summarized to convey some of the vivid flavor of a particular type of meditative method for alleviating symptoms and curing disease. Buddhist texts are rich storehouses of these methods. The visualizations have specific purposes and—like certain medicines—can have an adverse effect if they are matched to a noncorresponding disease. They are provided here for scholarly purposes only.

In these visualizations, deities are mentioned—manifested buddhas—who play a role in the healing process. There are some very important figures in the vast Buddhist pantheon who are especially pledged to help those who are ill. In addition, almost all of the significant figures in the pantheon have healing abilities and are called upon by devotees in times of need. Here we will discuss the specialists, most particularly the buddha named Master of Healing and his retinue of celestial assistants.

Basic information about this buddha is revealed by Śākyamuni in the *Scripture on the Fundamental Vows and Merits of the Master of Healing, the Lapis Lazuli Radiance Tathāgata*, a text that appears to have been composed in the northwestern borderlands of India around the turn of the Common Era and has been translated into Chinese in several versions. An early cult centered on this buddha was strong in southeastern China in the fifth and sixth centuries. During the seventh and eighth centuries, knowledge of this buddha spread across China, and the cult was integrated into national religious traditions. During this period, Master of Healing was elevated to a principal status in the pantheon, a status that he continues to hold today.

In this scripture Master of Healing is described as lord of a spirit realm located to the east, a land named Pure Lapis Lazuli, with level ground made of that radiantly blue stone, marked by roads of gold and various structures built of precious substances. Like the celestial fields of other buddhas, this realm is a refuge from suffering; it is an ideal site to listen without distraction to the pure principles taught by its lord, Master of Healing, in association with the two leaders of his bodhisattva assembly, Sunlight and Moonglow.

Master of Healing's twelve vows, first made when he set out to gain enlightenment, cover a wide range of benefits to sentient beings. The most widely known is the sixth vow, a pledge to alleviate the sickness and suffering of all beings. The fulfillment of this pledge forms the subject of much of the scripture. In this vow, he states:

> I vow that when I attain enlightenment in a future age, if there are sentient beings whose bodies are inferior, whose sense organs are impaired, who are ugly, stupid, deaf, blind, mute, bent and lame, hunchbacked, leprous, convul-

sive, insane, or who have other types of diseases and sufferings—such beings when they hear my name shall obtain proper appearances and practical intelligence. All their senses shall become perfect, and they shall have neither sickness nor suffering.

The seventh vow is closely related:

If there are any sentient beings who are ill and oppressed, who have nowhere to go and nothing to return to, who have neither doctor nor medicine, neither relatives nor immediate family, who are destitute and whose sufferings are acute—as soon as my name passes through their ears, they will be cured of all their diseases, and they will be peaceful and joyous in body and mind. They will have plentiful families and property, and they personally will experience the supreme enlightenment.

Several other vows are related to his healing functions. The first and second vows describe his appearance and promise to bestow it upon devotees:

First Great Vow: I vow that when I attain the unexcelled complete enlightenment in a future age, a radiant light will blaze forth from my body. It will brilliantly illumine limitless, countless, boundless realms. This body will be excellently adorned with the thirty-two marks of the great man and the eighty secondary marks. I will cause all sentient beings to wholly resemble me.

Second Great Vow: I vow that when I attain enlightenment in a future age, my body will be like lapis lazuli within and without, bright with penetrating and flawless purity. The radiance will be of great merit and will be imposing indeed. My body will be an excellent and tranquil dwelling, adorned with [an aureole like] a glowing net surpassing the sun and moon in its radiance. I will show the dawn to those beings who are completely concealed in darkness, so that they may act in accordance with their desired paths.

While Master of Healing has pledged to aid all beings who are sick and suffering, he must be called upon in order to invoke this potent aid. Methods of effective invocation, according to the scripture, range from the simple expedient of calling out his name to special rites involving prayer and worship before an image of Master of Healing. In the case of life-threatening disease, a complex rite is outlined in the scripture (and described in great detail in special ritual texts) in which forty-nine cart-wheel-shaped lamps are burned before seven images of the Buddha for forty-nine days, with many other ritual acts performed in units of seven or forty-nine. The number seven (with its square, forty-nine) is especially important in the Buddhist healing cults, most likely relating to the number of days in the intermediate state *(antarābhava)* between death and rebirth.

Standard images of Master of Healing—following ritual texts and the basic scripture—depict him as a seated buddha in monk's garb, either having skin the shimmering, rich blue color of lapis lazuli or having a golden complexion with a halo and mandorla of lapis lazuli-colored rays. The buddha holds a bowl or covered medicine jar on his lap with his left hand, while his right hand, resting on his right knee, palm outward, offers the medicinal myrobalan fruit. (Sometimes he stands, holding the medicine jar in his left hand, with right hand upraised in the gesture of banishment of fear.) He is flanked by his bodhisattva assistants, standing in princely garb: Sunlight and Moonglow. Their stately presence may call forth in the minds of Chinese devotees associations with the dynamic harmony of *yang* and *yin* energies that is central to the Chinese worldview.

Below them stand spread out twelve *yakṣa* generals (fierce forest spirits), each of whom commands seven thousand troops, all in aid of the buddha's healing work. Beginning in the ninth century, each of these generals commonly was depicted with a different animal figure on his helmet, each thus representing one of the twelve daily two-hour periods and the twelve years of the Jupiter-based cycle, fundamental units of time in Chinese calendrical and astrological traditions. Depicted in this way, the generals sometimes were shown ranged in a circle around the buddha and bodhisattvas. The pervasive quality of this buddha's healing force may be hinted at by the eighty-four thousand *yakṣa* warriors. Elsewhere in Buddhist texts, this number also refers to the constituent parts of the body ("atoms") and the constituent parts of the buddha's doctrine: the deployment of the *yakṣas* throughout the universe becomes then the extension of the Healing Buddha's body and teachings.

This portrayal of the divine bestowers of perfect health and long life is striking for its sense of cosmic wholeness and harmony—deep blue lapis lazuli radiance at the center like the depths of space, together with the two luminaries, encircled by lords of time—and points to the profound nature of healing, internal and external, provided by this buddha.

The scriptures and ritual texts of the cult recommend creation of images of the buddha and his retinue as effective means of devotional focus and invocation. Such images also can be created mentally, through visualization procedures; in this case there is added emphasis on internal healing, for by this visualization process the buddha and his associates have already been drawn into the mind and held there, their radiating energies infusing the meditator with healing and purifying force.

Spontaneous healings also may occur as a "by-product" of vision quest experiences and other devotional activity. Mount Wu-t'ai in Shansi province has been an important center for Buddhist vision quests in China since the sixth century; aspirants journey to this remote mountain site to gain direct communion and communication with Mañjuśrī, the Buddhist lord of wisdom, who is believed to manifest himself there. In the old chronicles of this site, several spontaneous healings are described (though this mountain does not seem to have been a pilgrimage site for ill persons, as, for example, Lourdes has been for Roman Catholics). A report of one such spontaneous healing is described below; I will admit to having chosen here a bizarre and most unlikely event, thus emphasizing the miraculous quality of such occurrences. The text first discusses the self-immolation in 550 CE of a certain prince of the royal house of the N. Ch'i state which was performed in front of a famous *stūpa*, or reliquary, on Mount Wu-t'ai. (Self-immolation practices are discussed in the next section of this essay.) It continues:

> This prince had a eunuch servant named Liu Ch'ien-chih. This man was sad at having undergone the punishment of castration, and he also was moved by the prince's self-immolation. Accordingly, he petitioned the emperor for permission to enter the mountain precincts to cultivate the Way (that is, to seek enlightenment). The emperor so permitted. Then at this place (where the prince had burned his body) Liu Ch'ien-chih repeatedly recited the *Flower Garland Scripture*, circumambulating the *stūpa* for twenty-one days, praying to see Mañjuśrī. Accordingly, he received a mysterious response: the form of his organs was restored to him. As a result of his expanded awareness and understanding, he then composed a treatise on the *Flower Garland*, six hundred scrolls in length. A synopsis of this treatise, from beginning to end, was brought back (to the capital) and heard by the emperor. Emperor Kao-tsu's reverence and faith were increased as a result of this experience. He had the *Flower Garland* recited every day, and his era was bountiful.[6]

I should note that Mount Wu-t'ai, like many other sacred mountains in China, is famous as a place to gather medicinal herbs. The appearance of medicinal plants at a site is a traditional indicator that divine spirits manifest or dwell at that place. Thus, the presence of healing herbs suggests that a place is sacred and legitimates a visionary experience that may occur there.

Turning to further methods, confession and repentance practices are also employed for healing, as was recommended by Chih-i. Such practices are especially effective for diseases that clearly stem from karmic patterns, including those that may have arisen due to mental anguish or self-blame for faults that have not been resolved. These practices range from very short periods recalling one's faults and pledging not to commit them again, to complex and solemn rites carried out over numerous days or weeks in which comprehensive internal investigation is carried out and solemn pledges against backsliding are made. Deities play an important role in these practices. They are invoked to witness the confessions and repentances, and they are called upon for assistance in maintaining this newly purified state.

In addition to calling upon deities for healing aid, certain diseases may be cured effectively through recitation of potent phrases or scriptures. These practices have roots in the early Indian Buddhist *paritta* traditions of reciting specific scriptures for curing disease, bringing timely rain, and as a defense against noxious snakes. Chinese Buddhist traditions include recitations for such varied problems as eye disease, dental problems, and childhood diseases. In addition, the recitation of certain scriptures—most especially the *Diamond Scripture* and the *Lotus Scripture*—is held to have extraordinarily potent value, including the generation of healings and protection from imminent disaster.

I might add that some of the basic practices of Chinese Buddhism—especially for those leading a monastic life—may assist in maintaining health. The frequent daily devotional exercises involving extended melodious chanting calm the mind and cause the body to relax and resonate in a harmonious way. These services are punctuated by numerous full prostrations (performed in sets of three), done in a graceful manner; this action performed repeatedly on a daily basis throughout the years produces a suppleness of the limbs (and is perhaps also good for the cardiovascular system). These aspects may counter the health-injuring qualities of the notoriously poor food found at less wealthy monastic establishments.

DISEASE AS TRANSFORMATIVE OPPORTUNITY

The scriptures and rituals dedicated to the Master of Healing are pervaded by a sense of transformation, by a sense that healing is a profound process of change. In the texts this buddha continually pledges to assist devotees not only to become healed, but to attain enlightenment in the process. A fundamental feature of the healings bestowed by him is the transformation of karma, a concern for eradicating the patterned causes as well as the visible symptoms of suffering.

In addition, numerous serious karmic faults are described, and in each case this buddha pledges to aid beings in eradicating them so that they can become enlightened. In this context, Master of Healing is especially important for his work in assisting beings to reach a momentous turning point, known as the "aspiration to attain enlightenment," at which the drifting life is cast aside in order to seek spiritual fulfillment. His transformative powers extend to his assistants: ordinarily *yakṣas* are considered fearsome disease-causing spirits, while in the scripture they pledge to assist the buddha in his healing activities. This transforming quality has roots in the earliest textual discussions of healing in Buddhism, where monks advised by Śākyamuni to heal themselves through rigorous meditative effort found that in fact they attained enlightenment in the process.

For Buddhists, sickness may provide a jolt of urgency, a vivid sense of the immediacy of suffering and the necessity of conquering it. It provides a striking reminder of the tenuous grasp one may have on human incarnation, and thus of the importance of forgoing laxity and procrastination in personal spiritual practices. Further, the enormous focused effort required to harness the mind for curing when the body is in a weakened state may be precisely what is required to attain enlightenment. Even further, the physical manifestations of disease may reveal to a patient previously unsuspected karmic currents that have prevented this person from full realization. Revealed, these patterns can be changed or eradicated. Thus, disease—a very great source of suffering—may be viewed as beneficial by Buddhists intent on enlightenment.

Longevity, Extension of the Life Span, and Death

The desire for longevity is particularly strong in Chinese culture. As a result, extensive longevity traditions were developed by Chinese Buddhists and their Central Asian and Indian teachers, and it was perceived that numerous deities included among their functions the granting of long life, or (more properly) genuine protection from a violent or untimely end to the life span. Through fervent prayer or by ritual acts, such deities are invoked for their protective and healing abilities. I have suggested elsewhere, in an extended essay on Chinese Buddhist longevity deities and their symbolism, that analysis of the textual and iconographic traditions of the most important of these deities leads to the view that sophisticated practitioners perceive extension of the life span as a multilayered phenomenon. While the quest for longevity is indeed real, there is profound concern for the *quality* of those additional days and years; the more enlightened one becomes, the more fully and more properly one lives. This understanding constitutes a less materialistic view of longevity.[7]

A full life span is achieved through wholesome living in accordance with spiritual principles. This is not possible for all persons, and even those of extraordinary attainments may be hampered by unexpected karmic retribution stemming from subtle patterns or from acts of the distant past.

Extension of the life span may be achieved by avoidance of the untimely deaths (discussed below) through fervent prayer-pleas to certain deities. Most commonly in Chinese Buddhism, these include Kuan-shih-yin (Hearer of the Cries of the World) and Yao-shih (Master of Healing). Kuan-shih-yin, according to a famous chapter in the *Lotus Scripture*, has pledged to help all beings who call upon him to escape from numerous dangers and difficulties. Yao-shih, as previously discussed, aids in healing; he also rescues devotees from distress.

The Healing Buddha service is a common practice in modern Chinese Buddhism. This is carried out on certain days throughout the year, as well as on the birthdays of elderly devotees. At key points in this service Master of Healing is worshiped, especially by group recitation of the phrase "Na-mo hsiao-tsai yen-shou Yao-shih fo" (Homage to the buddha Master of Healing, who dispels disaster and extends the life span). Sophisticated practitioners carry out a set of visualizations during this service, mentally invoking a conclave of deities who radiate potent healing energies upon the assembled worshipers.

Master of Healing also has the ability to bring the comatose back to consciousness, in response to the prayers and ritual devotion of family and friends. In these cases, according to the *Scripture on the Master of Healing*, the comatose return to this world with a vivid "dream-memory" of impartial judgment based on their *karma*. Upon reawakening, they will change their ways in accordance with this new understanding. Thus, there is a purpose underlying this life extension.

A tradition of seven healing buddhas was introduced to China in the early eighth century and eventually became popular among Tibetans and Mongols. The senior physician in this group is Master of Healing. In Buddhist ritual art this group is often depicted with Śākyamuni Buddha, thus returning to the roots of the Healing Buddha cult in the early tradition of Śākyamuni as spiritual healer. In an eighth-century text entitled *Scripture Spoken by the Buddha on the Extension of the Lifespan by the Seven Stars of the Northern Dipper* (T 1307), Śākyamuni identifies the deities of the seven stars of the Northern Dipper (one of the most important constellations in Chinese astrology, the celestial residence of the "controllers of destiny," who determine the life spans of all persons, according to long-standing native Chinese traditions) with the seven healing buddhas. As leader of the group, Master of Healing is lord of the seventh star, the end of the Dipper's handle. Śākyamuni recommends that in the event of life-threatening disease one should worship the lords of the seven stars, who will cure the patient and thus extend the life span.

Longevity has an eventual terminus, which cannot forever be staved off. Death is viewed as a transition experience leading to a judgment of the *karma* amassed in that particular incarnation prior to entering the next birth. Various types of deaths are discussed in a wide variety of texts, including untimely deaths, suicide, and auspicious deaths.

UNTIMELY DEATH

A number of texts very popular in China discuss different types of untimely death, death that prematurely ends the life span. One of the earliest Buddhist texts translated into Chinese (by An Shih-kao, in the second century) discusses nine types of untimely death. Four arise from problems stemming from improper intake of food: untimely eating, greedy eating, eating of foods to which one is not accustomed, and indigestion. The remaining five include: refraining from natural functions such as urination and defecation, violation of basic ethical principles leading to self-punishment by debilitating remorse, bad company, entering a locale at an inopportune time (and thus being subject to war or other catastrophes), and inability to avoid the inevitable (such as a raging animal).[8]

While the number nine seems to be a constant, the list has many variants. Perhaps most widespread is the list found in the *Scripture on the Master of Healing*. In that text an enlightened hero named Saving Deliverance enumerates circumstances from which devotees of the Healing Buddha will be protected:

> There may be sentient beings who have contracted an illness that, though minor, goes untreated through lack of both medicine and physician. Or, the person may meet a doctor who gives him the wrong medicine. Such persons should not die, yet by these means they are caused to have untimely deaths. Furthermore, a person may have faith in materialistic and demonic heretics, masters of black magic. The false explanations of calamities and blessings that they provide will lead to fearful actions. Since this [misled] person cannot discern correctly with his own heart, he asks divinatory questions in his search for good fortune, and he kills all sorts of living creatures to propitiate spirits. He calls the spirits of the waters and begs for blessings, desiring to lengthen his years. In the end, he is unable to obtain this. Stupid and confused, believing in false and inverted views—it follows that such a person is led to an untimely death and enters into a hell with no definite time of release. These are what is known as the first untimely death.
>
> The second untimely death is by execution according to the ruler's laws. The third is when someone goes out on hunts or pleasure excursions and engages in debauch and drunkenness to excess, with no limits. His vital spirit is snatched away by a [demonic] non-human being, thus causing untimely death. The fourth untimely death is burning by fire. The fifth is by drowning in water.
>
> Some are devoured by wild beasts, thus causing the sixth untimely death. The seventh untimely death is by falling off a mountain precipice. The eighth untimely death is caused by harm from poisonous herbs, hateful entreaties (spells), and magical incantations causing corpses, devils, and other such things to arise. The ninth is caused by starvation and dehydration due to not obtaining food and drink.
>
> This is the Buddha's summary explanation of the nine types of untimely death. Beyond these, in addition there are limitless other untimely deaths that would be altogether difficult to expound upon.

SUICIDE

Suicide is expressly forbidden in Buddhist scriptures, but there are some exceptions that in fact became an honored path in China and other

East Asian countries: self-immolation or self-sacrifice based on religious motivations. Various types of self-inflicted death are recorded in the compilations of biographies of eminent monks, and such acts are accorded special dignity in these works by their recounting in special chapters devoted to notable episodes.

There are at least four distinct categories of suicide practiced by Chinese Buddhists, two of them taking inspiration from scriptural traditions. Of these two sanctioned acts, the first is self-sacrifice to benefit other living beings. Past-life tales of Śākyamuni Buddha are filled with events in which he sacrificed his body to protect others, to feed them, or to ensure that he himself would not harm them. In each case, attachment to the physical body was overpowered by the desire to adhere to the principles of beneficent nonharm that are basic to the Buddhist way of life. In each case, the offering up of one's own body for a specific need was seen as a supreme culmination of the act of charity, a Buddhist virtue. Similarly, there are numerous records of Chinese monks who deliberately gave up their own bodies to protect or feed others, or to avoid harming animals.

Also among the sanctioned acts (although there has been considerable debate regarding its propriety) is self-immolation as a worship offering. Perhaps ironically, this act is specifically linked to healing traditions, for it is modeled on the self-effacing dedicatory offerings of an enlightened hero named King of Healing, who according to scriptures set himself ablaze in two past lives.

In the *Lotus Scripture*, a Buddhist text of special popularity in China, a chapter is devoted to King of Healing and his worship acts of the distant past. From this vantage point, it seems clear that the tale has coherent symbolic meaning. A young man named He Whom All Beings Delight to See attains a meditative trance called "manifestation of all form." Wishing to pay homage to the buddha who is his teacher, he eats incense and fragrant oils for twelve hundred years and then sets himself on fire, standing in flaming radiance for a further twelve hundred years. This conflagration illumines countless worlds throughout the universe, and the buddhas of these worlds appear before him with extravagant praise. They term his self-immolation a supreme gift, more honored than any other, a gift known as "the offering of the Law to the buddhas."

Symbolically, here we see a spiritual individual transcending the world of form by offering up his own body to the buddhas in devotion and service, a supreme act of the sacrifice of self. This helps establish the patterns of word, thought, and deed by which he ultimately becomes the heroic bodhisattva named King of Healing: the turning aside of personal desires and attachments as prerequisite to becoming a great physician.

While literal acts of self-immolation have commanded much respect among Chinese Buddhists through the centuries, some learned masters were staunchly opposed to them. The eighth-century monk I-ching wrote at some length about self-immolation. He held that these practices may be appropriate for laymen, since King of Healing was a lay practitioner in the scriptural episodes of his notable past lives, but in no way are they to be permitted for clergy:

> I hear of late that the youths of China, bravely devoting themselves to the practice of the Law, consider the burning of the body a means of attaining Buddhahood, and abandon their lives one after another. This should not be. Why? It is difficult to obtain the state of human life after a long period of transmigration. Though born in a human form a thousand times, one may yet not have wisdom, nor hear the seven limbs of enlightenment, nor meet the Three Honorable Ones. Now we are lodged in an excellent place, and have embraced an admirable teaching. It is but vain to give up our insignificant body after having studied but a few verses of the scriptures. How can we think much of such a worthless offer, so soon after we have begun to meditate on impermanence? . . .
> We learn from the Buddha's own words the important method of controlling our sensations. What use is it to burn our body in destroying our passions? The Buddha did not allow even castration. . . . The Buddha's word forbids us to transgress a weighty precept and follow our own will. We are disregarding his noble teaching if we take refuge in such a practice as burning our bodies.[9]

Based on the traditions stemming from the acts of King of Healing, some self-mutilation practices also arose in China. Most widespread among these is the burning of several cones of incense upon the shaven pates of ordinands as the final act in achieving full status as a monk or nun. Also, there is the more extreme act of burning off one or more fingers as a penitential act. This act has not been restricted to the fringes of religious practice. For example, the extraordinarily charismatic monk Hsü-yün, a major figure in the twentieth-century renewal and revival of Buddhism whose 120-year life span (1840–1959) served to many as confirmation of his saintliness, burned off a finger at age fifty-eight, with prayers that his dedicatory act would move Amitābha Buddha to assist his deceased mother in the spirit realms.[10]

In addition to acts that some consider sanctioned, there are records of those who died as martyrs, giving up their lives—sometimes in a blazingly effective manner—in order to protect the religion (often against state persecution). Further, there are those who chose suicide from intense dislike for life. In a way, this could be construed as receiving encouragement from the general trend of scriptural traditions, for Buddhist texts continually urge nonattachment to life and include meditative exercises aimed at evoking a sense of revulsion to that which the worldly consider pleasurable. Still, this sort of suicide is not sanctioned by any standard

Buddhist codes. As the learned I-ching wrote in his travel record regarding the taking of one's own life under religious guise:

> In the Ganges River many men drown themselves every day. On the hill of Bodhgaya too there are not infrequently cases of suicide. Some starve themselves and eat nothing. Others climb up trees and throw themselves down. . . . These actions are entirely out of harmony with the Vinaya Canon (monastic rules of conduct). Even those who consider such actions to be wrong are afraid of sinning if they prevent such actions. But if one destroys life in such a way, the great object of one's existence is lost (i.e., the opportunity to attain enlightenment). That is why the Buddha prohibited it. The superior priests and wise teachers never acted in any such harmful way.[11]

AUSPICIOUS DEATH

There is a sense of timely death, of auspicious death, at the completion of a full span of life. Deaths such as these are described as peaceful, the individual retaining full mental capacities to the end. Exceptionally devoted persons may be met at their deathbeds by hosts of deities who will escort them to paradise realms prior to their next incarnation. Such events may be witnessed by others gathered at the bedside, according to traditional accounts. If we accept the stylized reports of the four successive editions of the *Biographies of Eminent Monks*, Chinese Buddhist sages die with foreknowledge of this event. Indeed, this is one means of confirming the spiritual achievement of such persons. Frequently they are depicted as gathering their disciples around them, announcing that their time is fast approaching, enjoining the disciples with final charges, and then shortly afterwards passing away in a peaceful and dignified manner, often while in meditative trance.

Conclusions

The healing traditions of Chinese Buddhism are complex and sophisticated and penetrate to the core of a distinctive religious way of life. The rhetoric of medicine and healing pervades both philosophical discourse and discussion of spiritual experience, while religious rhetoric forms an integral element in discussion of healing. From early times to the present, many eminent monks and nuns have served as healers, using both Buddhist healing methods and native Chinese traditions. Further, an active cult to special healing deities has long been supported in Chinese traditions. An understanding of Chinese Buddhism both as a "functioning entity" and as an abstract set of normative standards is incomplete without clear attention to these healing traditions.

In considering these healing traditions and the drive in Chinese Buddhism toward extension of the life span, it is important to bear in mind
the underlying assumption of causation. All difficulties—such as disease
or disabilities—ultimately stem from self-cause; thus, they are beneficial
as teachers, for they can awaken individuals to faults that must be cor-
rected in order for enlightenment to be attained. Human birth is viewed
as a precious opportunity, for one enters into conditions particularly suitable for this enlightenment quest. Death may be staved off through medical techniques and religious techniques, including prayer and invocation
of potent deities, but the purpose in this extension of the life span should
not merely be more days and years but further opportunity to pursue a
beneficial course leading to more spiritual growth. Since one experiences
incarnation after incarnation, and death is viewed as a transition experience rather than a dark finality, some of the life extensions currently practiced in modern Western hospitals—such as comatose patients suspended
in time for years or forcible procedures carried out in the last moments of
life when the signs of death have appeared and an inexorable progression
is apparent—can only be viewed as perverse and counterproductive.

Postscript: A Contemporary Buddhist Healer

In this essay, I have presented a survey of views and practices associated
with Buddhists in China, most especially in medieval times. Despite some
years of difficulty and turmoil, Buddhism continues to live in China: there
are numerous monks, nuns, and devoted lay practitioners; temples,
monastic establishments, and active pilgrimage sites; vision quests and
visionaries; seminaries and publication programs, featuring classic works,
modern textbooks, and the teachings of twentieth-century masters.

I spent much of the summer of 1986 in Shansi province, visiting historic sites and meeting many monks in rural areas. One man, a monk of
my age (thirty-seven that summer), was strikingly impressive, in many
ways appearing to step out of one of the medieval biography collections
that preserve tales of the eminent monks of the age. I first met him in a
remote mountain temple, an establishment founded in the eighth century,
where he was helping carry some massive timbers as part of a reconstruction project there. His extraordinary measure of vitality and the particular
clarity of gaze that is the hallmark of advanced meditative experience
indicated unusual dimensions to his life.

He invited me to his quarters to chat. We walked past the monks' living quarters to the far north of the monastery complex, reaching the
abbot's private hall. Over the inner doorway there was an elegantly written phrase praising "marvelous hands that renew vitality." Inside, near a
small altar, there were testimonial plaques of the sort that traditional

Chinese physicians receive from grateful patients. We sat by his *k'ang* (an elevated sleeping platform typical of northern China) and chatted, looking over his collection of well-thumbed treatises and scriptures. Finally, after a bit of prodding, he agreed to provide an account of his life. I have deliberately blurred or omitted some personal details, as well as my friend's name, in order to respect his privacy.

He spent his early life in a small city in northern China, leaving senior high school due to the illness and subsequent death of his father. At the time he worked in a factory, but after a few years he found that he could no longer bear the noise, so he stayed at home and grew vegetables. He was fond of social life and enjoyed eating meat and drinking quantities of wine, but suddenly—around the time of New Year's feasts in his twenty-sixth year—he found that he had lost all such desires. He shut himself in a room for twelve days, refusing to eat or speak, clearly in crisis.

An uncle, eighty years old, came to speak with him. He suggested that all these symptoms were characteristics of Buddhist monks. The young man was taken aback, for thoughts about buddhas were far from his mind, and by 1975 the Cultural Revolution had made it difficult to become a monk; it was a hard life, looked down upon by many, especially the young. But he felt a weight lifting from his shoulders, so he sought out this path to alleviate his suffering, going against the tides of the age. Earlier his family had upheld some Buddhist traditions—his great-grandfather and grandfather studied scriptures at home—and he had learned elementary forms of worship in his childhood, but all of that had been abandoned with the changing times in China, so he truly was turning to a new way of life.

He went out in search of temple and master, ending up at the Yün-kang caves, a famous site of rock-hewn sculptures dating to the fifth and sixth centuries, where he met his first teacher. There he received training in Buddhist doctrine and ritual and engaged in meditative practice and in a study of the breath-control techniques *(ch'i-kung)* that are the inner basis for a vast repertoire of esoteric Chinese arts. His master had some traditional medical training but was not willing to pass this on; he tells amusing tales of surreptitious entry into his teacher's quarters to leaf quickly through manuals on herbal healing, and indicates regret that his knowledge of this field remains fragmentary.

After several years of study, he moved to another province, to a temple in a county market town. He was still a novice at this time, for the opportunity to receive full ordination is strictly controlled by the government (as in medieval times). During this period he discovered that he had some healing abilities, and numerous persons came to him for aid. His reputation grew, and local physicians sent him their hopeless cases. Some were healed, others not. Many people from the surrounding countryside came to him for aid, and the temple, in essence, was transformed into a

Buddhist free clinic. Apparently this caused concern among local officials, and he was transferred to a sparsely populated rural area where there were few visitors.

After two years he received full ordination, and two years later he was made abbot of a historically important temple that had fallen into serious disrepair. At this place he supervises the refurbishing and repair work and oversees the training of the twelve resident monks. Perhaps as a result of his supervision, the food at this monastery, though very modest in keeping with the conditions of the region, is notable for its freshness and cleanliness (in this regard, far superior to restaurant meals in nearby market towns). Local people in need are fed at the large noonday meal, together with the monks and construction workers.

He continues to engage in healing practices, apparently with the support of local leaders, judging from the names on the testimonial plaques in his quarters. These healing practices, he explained, are a mixture of prayer, application of ch'i-kung techniques, some herbal prescriptions, and massage. He believes that the healings take place especially through a combination of the force of his concentrated breath-energy and the spiritual force of Buddhist deities. Prior to treating a patient, he recites from memory a long prayer-invocation to Kuan-yin (the "Great Compassion Mantra," a many-syllabled text well known to Chinese Buddhist practitioners), sometimes as many as 108 times. Invocations of Yao-shih fo, the Buddha of Healing, are reserved for life-threatening events. He feels that it is important for him to pray with great concentration, since his medical knowledge is incomplete. During and after these prayer-invocations, he engages in breath-control exercises, generating and focusing internal energy currents. At the appropriate moment, in this heightened state of consciousness with close connections to the compassionate bodhisattva Kuan-yin, he manipulates the body of the patient. When the healings occur, he states, the process is rapid.

Such persons, though rare, provide vibrant examples that point to the experiential reality that underlies the tales and teachings recorded in old books.

Notes

1. The *Scripture on the Master of Healing* and several related works are included in Raoul Birnbaum, *The Healing Buddha* (Boulder, CO, 1979). *The Healing Buddha* provides a cross-cultural view of the cult of Master of Healing, emphasizing its scriptural foundations and iconographic manifestations. Chih-i's comments on sickness and healing, relied on for this essay, are found in T 1911.106a–111c, and T 1915.471b–472b. While mentioning some basic sources, I also should list Paul Demiéville's remarkably thorough cross-cultural essay on Buddhist medical theory and

healing traditions (in French) in *Hōbōgirin,* fasc. 3 (Tokyo and Paris, 1937), pp. 224–265. This has appeared recently in English (trans. Mark Tatz) as *Buddhism and Healing: Demiéville's Article "Byō" from Hōbōgirin* (Lanham, MD, 1985).

2. This is discussed in the *Dharmaguptaka Vinaya (Ssu-fen lü),* the principal regulatory work accepted by Chinese Buddhists, in the section on accepting the ordination precepts; cf. T 1428.815c, 925b–c. Parallel passages can be found in other *Vinaya* traditions preserved in the Chinese canon, as for example T 1433.1054a.

3. For example, the *Scripture Spoken by Vimalakīrti* devotes some attention to this in its fifth chapter. See Robert A. F. Thurman, trans., *The Holy Teaching of Vimalakīrti* (University Park, PA, 1976), pp. 42–49.

4. For a summary with translated excerpts of Chih-i's confession and repentance procedures for purification of the sense faculties, see Raoul Birnbaum, "The Manifestation of a Monastery: Shen-ying's Experiences on Mount Wu-t'ai in T'ang Context," *Journal of the American Oriental Society* 106, No. 1 (1986): 130–134.

5. This material is summarized from T 620.333c–334a.

6. Hui-hsiang, *Ku Ch'ing-liang chüan* (Ancient records of Mount Clear-and-Cool), T 2098.1094c. A somewhat earlier seventh-century text by the famous *Flower Garland Scripture* interpreter Fa-tsang, *Hua-yen ching chuan-chi* (Record of tales of the *Flower Garland Scripture*), also discusses this extraordinary event. Fa-tsang is rather more graphic in his description of the divine restoration and praises the 600-scroll treatise for its orderly exposition of ideas and its penetrating understanding of the mysterious purport of the scripture (T 2073.156c).

7. Raoul Birnbaum, "Seeking Longevity in Chinese Buddhism: Long-Life Deities and Their Symbolism," in *Myth and Symbol in Chinese Traditions,* eds. Norman J. Girardot and John S. Major, special double issue of *Journal of Chinese Religions* 13–14 (Fall 1985–Fall 1986): 143–176.

8. T 150A.880b–c.

9. See J. Takakusu, trans., *A Record of the Buddhist Religion as Practised in India and the Malay Archipelago (A.D. 671–695)* (London, 1895), pp. 196–197.

10. As related in Ts'en Hsüeh-lu, *Hsü-yün ho-shang nien-p'u* (Chronological Biography of Venerable Hsü-yün) (Reprint, Taipei, 1975), pp. 26–28.

11. Takakusu, p. 198. On self-immolation, see Jan Yün-hua, "Buddhist Self-Immolation in Medieval China," *History of Religions* 4 (1964–1965): 243–268; Jacques Gernet, "Les suicides par le feu chez les bouddhistes chinoises de Ve au Xe siècle," *Mélanges publiés par l'Institut des Hautes Études Chinoises* 2 (1960); Jean Filliozat, "La mort volontaire par le feu et la tradition bouddhique indienne," *Journal Asiatique* 251 (1963); and Birnbaum, *The Healing Buddha,* pp. 26–34. Further examples of religious suicides occurring over a period of six centuries at Mount Wu-t'ai in northern China are recounted and discussed in Raoul Birnbaum, *The Sacred Lore of Five Terrace Mountain: A Buddhist Pilgrimage Center in Medieval Times,* forthcoming.

CHAPTER 3

Health Care

in Contemporary

Japanese

Religions

EMIKO OHNUKI-TIERNEY

Meaning and Role of Religions in Health Care

My focus in this essay is on the health care provided at temples and shrines.[1] Excluded from the treatment are the so-called new religions (*shinkō shūkyō*), shamanism, and ancestor worship. Numerous new religions mushroomed in Japan after World War II. They have many adherents, and health-related matters often occupy a central place in their beliefs and practices. They are not included in the discussion, since there are many publications on the subject already available in English.[2] Once

59

a powerful nonformalized religion in Japan, shamanism used to play a significant role in the health care of the people, but much of it has now been transformed into new religions. Consequently, its importance for the general public has been significantly reduced.[3] Although ancestors are said to look after the living, their role in the welfare of the living is a diffused one; contemporary Japanese ask their ancestors only for general welfare but not for cure of specific illnesses.[4] My discussion of the role of temples and shrines in health care first introduces a broader picture of basic concepts of illness and health, then outlines roles played by buddhas and Shinto deities. Finally, I introduce two case studies. The first case exemplifies the use of a shrine, and the second features the use of a temple for medical purposes.

My intention regarding the role of religion in Japanese health care is twofold: (1) a description of Japanese behavior within the context of their worldview and (2) an interpretation of the contemporary phenomenon in historical perspective.

BASIC CONCEPTS OF ILLNESS AND HEALTH IN CULTURAL CONTEXT

Cleanliness, dirt, the body and its parts, illness and wellness, and death are powerfully patterned by culture in any society. Spatial and temporal classifications are especially important for the notion of what is clean and dirty in the daily hygiene of the Japanese.[5] One of the most important cultural rules is the removal of footgear, washing of hands, and, in some cases, gargling, upon returning to "the clean *in*side" (the home) from "the dirty *out*side." The Japanese explain this custom by stating that one gets dirty from germs outside and takes off one's footgear so that dirt from outside does not get tracked into the clean inside. Similarly, one must wash one's hands and gargle to get rid of germs on the hands and in the throat. The Japanese explain these customs in terms of *baikin* ("germs," a term of recent origin, after the introduction of the germ theory from the West). Some even have a visual image of enlarged bacteria, often shown to school children in films. One of the major emphases in child-rearing in Japan is to teach these rules to small children. In fact, mothers often wipe their children's feet before they let the children come in. This is done at an entranceway called *genkan*, where they take off their shoes. It is the vital passageway from dirty outside to clean inside. Therefore, there is always a *genkan* to every house, even in the smallest of apartments. Here the Japanese change into their slippers to walk on the hallway floor, although they must remove their slippers before entering the rooms with *tatami* floors, where they can walk only with socks (including the *tabi*, the traditional Japanese socks), stockings, or barefoot.

A prominent notion behind these hygienic practices is the association of the spatial "outside" with dirt; dirt, expressed as "germs," is the omnipresent "outside." This "dirty outside" does not, however, include all the space outside of the home. It refers to the space beyond the outside wall or hedge surrounding one's house, and, more specifically, it refers to places where people—especially strangers—are located, such as streets, shopping areas, and trains. Nature is not included; it is clean.

The daily hygiene of the contemporary Japanese is related not only to their spatial classification of the universe, but also to their classification of time. Washing one's face and brushing one's teeth are widespread customs not confined to Japan. For the Japanese, however, these commonplace customs are only part of a more complex series of activities that they carry out in the morning, activities that mark the transition from night to day. The most important of these activities is the folding of the mattress *(futon)* and putting it away in the closet. It is often hung outside to dry to get rid of the moisture it has collected from the body of the sleeper and the straw mat *(tatami)* on which it was placed. In most families, the entire house or at least most of it is cleaned every morning. In addition, water is sprinkled outside the entranceway to refresh or purify the area before the other family members (especially the head of the family) go out for the day.

Just as the morning cleaning marks the transition from nighttime to daytime, the transition from daytime to nighttime is also well marked by a bath, which is usually taken every evening and always before going to bed—in sharp contrast to contemporary Americans, who shower just before they go out. The idea behind the Japanese practice is that bathing cleanses the person's body for the night and for the mattress, which must be kept clean at all times.

Just as the cleansing at night marks the transition from day to night, transition from one year to the next is also marked by cleansing activities. The accumulated dirt from the previous year cannot be carried into the New Year. Thus, the Japanese, usually women, thoroughly clean the house on December 31, often until dawn, to welcome the start of the new year in the right way. By the same token, car owners in contemporary Japan, who are usually young people, flock to temples and shrines to have their car "cleansed" during a purification ritual. The car gets "dirty," in the cultural sense of the term, since it always runs outside where dirt is. Thus, it must not only be physically cleaned, but culturally purified as well.

The concept of purity and impurity, which governs the spatial classification of the day-to-day environment of the Japanese, also assigns these values to the human body. The upper half of the body is pure, while the lower half is defiled. Thus, the first rule of laundry is not to mix clothing from the upper and the lower parts; the color of clothes is of little signif-

icance in contrast to this basic rule. Of the lower parts of the body, the
feet are the most defiled.[6] Thus, the removal of footgear at the entranceway derives from the notion of the doubly polluted feet—the lowest and
thus the dirtiest part of the body that touches the ground—the dirtiest
part of the dirty outside. Even without footgear, any so-called proper Japanese should avoid walking on the *tatami* floor on the side of the head of
the *futon* mattress, which is always well marked with a piece of cloth
sewed onto the *futon*.

The Japanese pay particular attention to the *hara* or *ichō*, the area that
includes the stomach and intestines, because it was considered the seat of
the soul. (The well-known *seppuku (harakiri)* is an act to remove one's soul
by cutting into the stomach.) The Japanese are most careful to keep the
stomach warm, and thus many, especially babies, wear a *haramaki* (stomach sash), often made of wool, over the stomach. Laborers who work outside and are thus prone to imbalance of the body through exposure to
outside elements wear a wool sash even on hot summer days. Women
wear the pregnancy sash during the entire period of their pregnancy.
Before the invasion of soft drinks from the United States, the Japanese
used to avoid cold drinks even in the summer and took hot water or tea
in order not to chill the stomach. The Japanese concern about the stomach
is also reflected in their medicine; in terms of types as well as quantity,
stomach medicine far excels any other kind of medicine manufactured
and sold in Japan today. Likewise, of practicing doctors, stomach specialists are the most numerous.[7]

No less strongly patterned than the concept of daily hygiene are the
notions about illness and wellness. The most important principle governing the Japanese concept of health is the dualistic principle of their cosmology, according to which the present life is seen as a constant flux
between health and illness, and between good and evil. In their dualistic
universe, ordinary illnesses are not expelled. Health or wellness is seen
as an ephemeral phenomenon taking place only when the delicate balance of the body with its environment is achieved. One might even say
that the Japanese are fond of illnesses, and consider someone completely
healthy as unintelligent or lacking some desirable quality. Two concepts
illustrate this basic attitude. The first, *taishitsu*, is the constitution one is
born with, and the Japanese meticulously distinguish different types of
taishitsu, depending upon the degree of weakness or strength. The Japanese feel that individuals must adjust to their constitution by diet and
other daily activities, rather than trying to change it completely. Secondly,
there is the concept of *jibyō*, which I once humorously translated as "my
own illness." It is an illness or symptom(s) carried with one (the character
for *ji* means to carry, while the one for *byō* means illness) throughout life;
one "nurses" it, so to speak. The Japanese greeting "How are you?" literally asks the condition of the addressee's health. Talk about one's

health, even minor aches and pains, is not frowned upon. In short, rather than expelling illness from the universe, the Japanese live with it. It must be pointed out, however, that the most dreaded illnesses are often completely expelled, even from daily discourse. These illnesses used to be leprosy, tuberculosis, and madness; now the first two are replaced by cancer.

While the Japanese may accommodate minor illnesses in their daily universe, they nonetheless consider them "liminal" and "dirty." Upon becoming ill, one immediately discontinues the nightly bathing. Recovery from an illness is marked by the resumption of bathing, which often must be signaled by one's doctor. Thus, patients often ask their doctor if and when they may resume bathing. When the doctor gives permission to bathe, it is taken as an announcement of the patient's recovery. Gifts to hospitalized friends or relatives are often items with purifying power, in a symbolic sense, such as soap and cologne.

The Japanese attitude toward death is enormously complex, with a great many differences among individuals. The ideal death to many is *daiōjō*—death at a ripe old age after life has taken its own course, when one's body peacefully leaves this world. Yet, some types of suicide are not only culturally sanctioned but romanticized and beautified. To take one's own life, as long as it is, culturally speaking, for a good reason, can manifest utmost self-control, a taking in hand not merely of life's affairs but of one's own destiny.[8] Death from cancer, on the other hand, is the polar opposite of these types of suicide. That is, cancer eats up one's body beyond human control. One lies helplessly in bed until the disease terminates one's life. So dreaded is cancer that it is chased out of the Japanese dualistic universe in which minor illnesses are comfortably located, as noted earlier. It is still taboo to give the cancer verdict to the patient, although there have been increasing discussions about this topic both among medical professionals and lay people. Typically the fateful news is given to the most important family member or members, who usually keep the news from the patient. This practice derives in part from the Japanese pattern of joint decision making, whereby even the most important decisions are made after a reasonable agreement is reached among the concerned individuals. But it also is due to a large degree to the thinking that such a verdict is so shocking that it undoubtedly will hasten the process of dying.[9] The attitude toward these types of death does not seem to be strongly affected by the Japanese conception of afterlife. Buddhism, both in its institutionalized and folk versions, has stressed heaven and hell. The contemporary Japanese continue to take care of their ancestors, who are enshrined in the family ancestral alcove, by offering them food and water in their daily rite.[10] Yet they do not seem to clearly conceptualize the world after death, and, furthermore, whatever their conceptualization, it does not have strong influence on their attitude toward death, including their own.

PLURALISTIC SYSTEM OF MEDICINE

In contemporary Japan there is more than one system of health care, and most Japanese use several simultaneously or sequentially. The most powerful is the system variously referred to as biomedicine, Western medicine, or international medicine. It was developed in the West and first introduced to Japan by the Dutch during the late eighteenth century. Other important medical systems include: *kampō*, a medical system that originated in China but was introduced to Japan by the sixth century; religious institutions, such as Buddhist temples and Shinto shrines, which continue to play an important role in the health care of contemporary Japanese; a number of powerful new religious sects whose major focus is on health care; shamanistic medical practice, which has declined significantly since World War II; and home care, usually administered by women.

In this brief overview I will discuss only the two institutionalized systems of medicine—biomedicine and *kampō*—and illustrate how these two systems coexist in contemporary Japan despite the contrast of their basic premises. In contemporary Japan, *kampō* comes in all imaginable forms, from the orthodox practice to mass-produced and prepackaged extracts of herbs, to a street-corner computer diagnosis. The orthodox *kampō* practice today is a medicinal system developed in Japan and therefore differing considerably both from the system originally introduced from China and from the medicine practiced in contemporary China. Its treatment consists of moxibustion (herbal cauterization), acupuncture, and herbal and animal medicine. The basic premise of *kampō* is quite different from that of biomedicine in that it does not recognize categories of illness. Each departure from health is diagnosed on the basis of the combined number of symptoms that the patient experiences and those that the *kampō* doctor detects. The sum total, called *shōkōgun*, is carefully evaluated against the gender, age, and constitution of the patient, as well as the climate in which the patient resides, in order to reach a proper prescription for treatment. A *kampō* doctor, using the auditory, tactile, olfactory, and visual faculties to read the patient's conditions, prescribes a specific treatment. In the case of herbs, it is a mixture consisting of a dozen or so. Every patient therefore has a unique illness and requires a unique set of treatments. This premise contrasts sharply with biomedicine, which defines disease in terms of a particular set of symptoms or syndrome; its usual practice is to identify the patient's problem within the biomedical classificatory schema so that a proper treatment for that disease category can be prescribed. Here, any symptoms that do not constitute a part of the symptoms defining the category are often not considered important enough for treatment. Thus, there is often a situation wherein a patient feels the presence of an illness, but is told by a doctor that she or he does not in fact have a "disease" (a term I use to refer to departures from health as defined in biomedicine).

While I have oversimplified the contrast, it is reasonable to conclude that the premise of *kampō* is closer to the way laypeople actually understand and experience their departures from health. It is perhaps for this reason that the Japanese laypeople have supported *kampō* practice even though it has twice been suppressed by the government. First, during the late nineteenth century the Japanese government instituted a rule that one must receive biomedical training in order to practice *kampō*—a rule intended to "modernize" Japanese medicine. Second, the American occupational forces prohibited moxibustion and acupuncture after the end of World War II. In moxibustion, cones made of dried young mugwort leaves (*mogusa* in Japanese) are burned on selected points of the body to provide stimulation from the heat. In contemporary Japan, not only has *kampō* become enormously popular among laypeople, but the government has financially supported research in *kampō* and gradually added *kampō* treatments under health insurance coverage. It exists in a symbiotic relationship with biomedicine in that it specializes in chronic illnesses, especially those accompanied by chronic pain, and new types of illnesses including those caused by environmental pollution and traffic accidents, for which biomedicine has not been successful.

CURRENT POPULARITY OF SHRINES AND TEMPLES: AN OVERVIEW

The current popularity of temples and shrines in Japan is phenomenal, and in fact has been increasing for some time. Many temples and shrines throughout Japan attract literally millions of people each year. In the cities of Kobe, Osaka, and Kyoto, municipal bus companies operate regular tour buses that take people to temples and shrines. The tours are often aimed at older people, many of whom now feel squeezed out of Japanese society, which until recently had formalized ways of caring for them. These bus tours emphasize temples and shrines that specialize in illnesses of older people, such as strokes and hemorrhoids.

The use of temples and shrines is by no means confined to the aged, however. For example, I once attended a New Year's gathering of several related families, all with educated urban backgrounds. A young man of nineteen was late for the New Year's dinner because he was visiting three shrines known to be efficacious in successful passage of the university entrance examination. In fact, Tenmangū in Osaka, which traditionally has been known as a shrine for learning, has been exceedingly popular among students facing entrance examinations, as well as with their families. Similarly, with the strong emphasis on school trips (*shūgaku ryokō*) in Japanese schools, one often sees school tours at temples and shrines, with elementary, middle, and high school students flocking to buy amulets, charms, and other souvenirs for themselves and their families at temple and shrine shops that are usually located within the shrine or temple compound. These are small in size and come in different shapes and materials—wood, paper, and cloth. All have names of the shrine or the temple written on them, together with their purpose, such as for recovery from an illness, health maintenance, protection against traffic accidents, business prosperity, or good luck in general. The youngsters today hang the amulets and charms from their knapsacks or pocketbooks.

This great demand for *omamori* (amulets and talismans) is described by Eugene R. Swanger.[11] He refers to Kōganji in Tokyo, where Toge Nuki Jizō (Splinter-pulling Buddha), noted for its various healing abilities, is enshrined. The temple distributes a small paper image of the *jizō* (a guardian buddha for children) designed to be swallowed or stuck to the skin over the affected area. Swanger describes the demand for the paper amulets as "astronomical"; the temple has even received mail orders from overseas Japanese in Los Angeles, San Francisco, Hawaii, and elsewhere. Not infrequently people purchase a great number of them at a time, although when the supply is short, they are asked to restrict their purchases to only two *omamori* per visit. It should be noted that this temple is located in Tokyo, a city many Japanese consider to be less religious than the Keihanshinkan, the area of western Japan encompassing the cities of Kobe, Osaka, and Kyoto, where the research for this article was conducted. Swanger also reports the existence of factories for manufacturing amulets and talismans; their representatives make the rounds of shrines and temples all over Japan.[12]

One of the most popular uses of shrines and temples in contemporary Japan is for the purification of automobiles on New Year's Day, as stated earlier. With the rapid increase in private car ownership, "my car"—a term borrowed from English and pronounced in Japanese as *mai kā*—is both a popular word and a symbol of a new way of life, as the conscious adoption of the term "my" indicates. The use of the English possessive reflects the recent increased emphasis on the individual, at least on the surface, rather than on the person as defined in Japanese culture—which emphasizes the conception of a person only in the company of others. In addition, the term "my car" symbolizes the new emphasis on nuclear families; the image of young parents with a strong conjugal bond is contrary to the traditional family structure, which has emphasized the extended family and consanguineous ties.

Despite the modern image of these "my car" owners, who are usually young or middle-aged, all flock to shrines and temples on New Year's Day to have their cars purified. According to a report by the *Asahi* newspaper (April 14, 1980), Hiramaji Temple in Kawasaki City purifies cars, as many as forty at a time, every half hour beginning at 9:00 A.M. At a cost of ¥ 2,500 ($11.40 in 1979). The purification service includes a purification rite, a prayer, amulets, and bumper stickers. In 1970, the temple purified 25,000 cars; in 1979, it purified 67,000 cars, bringing in an income of ¥ 167,000,000 ($759,091). The purification rite for cars is not the exclusive domain of temples. Sōzō Taisha, a shrine in Kyushu, recently constructed a hall for the dedication of prayers for cars. It accommodates 200 persons at a time for the purification rite; the shrine also has a parking lot that holds 10,000 cars. Income from the purification of cars alone takes care of 80 percent of the annual maintenance cost for the shrine.

OCCUPATIONAL SPECIALIZATIONS OF JAPANESE SUPERNATURALS

To the Japanese, perhaps the most meaningful feature of the multitude of deities, buddhas, and other supernaturals is their *goriyaku*—the benevolent functions they perform. Table 1 is a translation, with minor changes, of that portion of Mikiharu Itoh's chart dealing with illness and related matters; it provides an excellent summary of these functions in graphic form.[13] I also added to Itoh's list a fourth column, "Taoist Deities," although only one deity is involved. Taoism has remained an important folk belief system in Japan.[14] Although the table by no means exhausts the huge pantheon of Japanese deities, it gives a good example of the functions these supernatural beings perform, which constitute perhaps the most important means of communication between humans and supernaturals.

Itoh's table does not include the frequency with which a particular specialization is assigned to deities and buddhas or the frequency with which any particular deity or buddha is assigned various functions. However, a complementary study that includes these data has been conducted by Ryō Mizobe, who examined the specializations of 103 temples and shrines randomly selected from all over Japan.[15] Mizobe's data consist of specializations officially proclaimed by the temples and shrines themselves. A total of 204 specializations are assigned to the 103 temples and shrines.[16]

In looking at Table 1 and in comparing it with Mizobe's data, we see immediately that deities and buddhas play a significant role in health care. The roles related to childbirth, child welfare, and general matters of illness and health comprise 54 percent (111 out of 204) of the total number of specializations in Mizobe, indicating that these are perennial concerns of the people. Table 1 indicates that deities and buddhas are consulted not only in the care of major illnesses but also for minor aches and pains. Contemporary Japanese seem to place more emphasis on luck and success in life, for these comprise 28 percent of all the specializations.[17] In

Table 1. MEDICAL SPECIALIZATIONS OF JAPANESE DEITIES AND BUDDHAS

Specializations	Shinto Deities	Buddhas	Taoist Deities
	Illness		
Illness in general	Deity of the Kitchen (Kōjin-sama)	"Roped" Jizō (Shibari Jizō)	
	Shibagami Daimyōjin	Substitute Jizō (Migawari Jizō)	
Illness of the face	Wart-Stone Deity (Iboishi-sama)	Lifting Jizō (Mochiage Jizō)	
Illness of the eyes	Deity of the Blind (Mekura-gami)	Konnyaku Enma	Kōshin-sama
	Deity of the Well (Idono-Kami)		
Illness of the ears (running cerumen; ringing in the ears)	Deity of the Boundary (Sae-no-Kami)	Jizō of the Ears (Mimi Jizō)	Kōshin-sama
	Deity of the Ears (Mimino-Kami)		
Illness of the throat	Rooster Daimyōjin (Tori Daimyōjin)	Prayer Jizō (Gankake Jizō)	
Illness of the teeth	Deity of the Toilet (Kawaya-no-Kami)		Kōshin-sama
Illness of the chest and other respiratory organs	Deity of Coughing (Shiwabuki-sama)	"Roped" Jizō (Shibari Jizō)	Kōshin-sama
Illness of the stomach	Tsuri Tenjin	"Roped" Jizō (Shibari Jizō)	
Illness of the hip and the limbs	Deity of the Hip (Koshi no-Kami)		
	Deity of the Lower Limbs (Ashiō-sama)		
	Kōjin of the Limbs (Ashide Kōjin)		
	Deity of the Boundary (Sae-no-Kami)		
Illness of the skin		An Jizō	
Contagious illness	Deity of Smallpox (Hōsoshin)		Kōshin-sama
Illness of women	Awashima-sama		
Illness of children	Deity of Dirt and Poison (Odoku-sama)		Kōshin-sama
	Life Cycle		
Pregnancy and childbirth	Deity of the Broom (Hōki-no-Kami)	Jizō of Easy Childbirth (Koyasu Jizō)	Kōshin-sama
	Deity of Childbirth (Ubugami)		
	Deity of the mortar (Usuno-Kami)		

Table 1. MEDICAL SPECIALIZATIONS OF JAPANESE DEITIES AND BUDDHAS
(cont.)

Specializations	Shinto Deities	Buddhas	Taoist Deities
	Deity of Pregnancy Stone (Yōsekiten)		
	Deity of the Boundary (Sae-no-Kami)		
	Deity of the Toilet (Kawaya-no-Kami)		
	Deity of the Mountain (Yama-no-Kami)		
	Deity of Easy Childbirth (Koyasu-sama)		
Growth	Deity of the Boundary (Sae-no-Kami)	Kannon of Easy Childbirth (Koyasu Kannon)	Kōshin-sama
	Deity of Easy Childbirth (Koyasu-sama)	Jizō of Easy Childbirth (Koyasu Jizō)	
Marriage	Deity of Motherhood (Komochi Gozen)		

Table developed from Mikiharu Itoh, "Shinkō seikatsu" (Religious life), in *Nihojin no Seikatsu* (Life of the Japanese), ed. T. Umesao (Tokyo, 1976).

contrast, functions related to calamities, including traffic accidents, comprise only 17 percent. If we address the issue of what constitutes a religion for the Japanese, these figures demonstrate that the Japanese do not hold rigid distinctions among the "religious affiliations" of their supernaturals—there is often a Shinto deity or a buddha carrying out the same medical function, and the Japanese may choose one or use both.

While the above findings pertain to contemporary scenes, we now turn to historical transformations of these functions. Noboru Miyata provides rich documentation of the histories of popular deities and their medical functions since the beginning of the seventeenth century.[18] The lives and fates of these deities reflect the major concerns of people of the time. Outmoded specializations are often discarded or transformed into new, more meaningful, roles. For example, natural disasters and fire were major concerns in the past, and were reflected in the specializations of deities and buddhas. They are far more controlled at present and therefore do not occupy the central place in people's minds.

The smallpox deity in Table 1 is an example of adaptation of specializations to changing epidemiological patterns. It was of paramount importance in the past, and thus there were elaborate rituals during which villagers ritually sent the smallpox deities out of their settlement. The Deity

of Smallpox is no longer meaningful in contemporary Japan, and its function has been expanded to incorporate contagious diseases in general.
Likewise, the Deity of Coughing (Shiwabuki-sama) was originally a very
popular deity when influenza was a major threat.[19] Since influenza is better controlled in contemporary Japan, the deity is now also consulted for
chronic respiratory illnesses, including asthma. Another example is the
deity of Ishikiri Shrine, not included in the 103 temples and shrines in
Mizobe's study, who used to cure various kinds of boils and growths. As
detailed in a case study presented later in this essay, the major appeal at
present is its efficacy in treating cancer. Cancer as a disease category is a
relatively new phenomenon in Japan, as elsewhere, but no doubt some
of the growths formerly treated at Ishikiri Shrine were carcinogenic. Shōji
Tatsukawa provides a good historical account of cases that were indis-
putably carcinogenic and their treatments, including what was undoubtedly the first radical mastectomy, performed in 1815.[20]

As we have seen, religions play a crucial role not only in the history
of Japanese health care but in contemporary Japan. Temples and shrines
are frequented not only by the aged but by young, urban, educated people
as well. While general trends in people's needs and wishes have been
reflected in the functions performed by deities and buddhas, it is too hasty
to conclude that there have been one-to-one correlations between the
medical roles of these supernaturals and epidemiological patterns. Illnesses that a particular supernatural is said to be capable of healing must
be interpreted broadly. For example, illnesses of the stomach must be
understood to incorporate both stomach ulcers and cancers, as well as any
other illnesses located in the stomach in its broadest sense. As mentioned
above, the stomach receives a special meaning in Japanese culture, and
any interpretation of illnesses of the stomach, therefore, requires a careful
consideration of its symbolic meanings.

Most importantly, some illness labels must be interpreted as being
"metaphorical"—as being expressive of multitudes of physiological-psy-
chological problems, rather than as biomedical disease categories or pathogens. The recent upsurge of concern about aborted fetuses illustrates this
point. Since unborn fetuses commit no sins in this world, they were
thought to be easily reborn. In the past this belief provided the basis, at
least in part, for the ease with which the Japanese practiced abortion and
also for the lack of elaborate funeral treatment.[21] A similar attitude seems
to continue in contemporary Japan. Since the end of World War II, birth
control has been spectacularly effective, owing to a large degree to the
practice of abortion. In 1978, among all married women (including in the
count those who were infertile), a total of 36.1 percent had had at least
one abortion. The total number of abortions between 1950 and 1977
reported to the government by doctors was 24,196,016. The figure was at
its highest in 1955, with 1,170,000 reported cases, and has been decreas-

ing since that time, with 640,000 cases in 1977. Since these figures include only reported cases, estimates of actual cases run two to three times higher. In 1979, the number of abortions was about 100 times greater than the number of traffic deaths.[22]

While abortions continue to be done with high frequency, there has been a sudden upsurge in memorial services. This practice ranges from placing an ancestral plaque with a posthumous Buddhist name for the fetus received from a monk to erecting a tomb. In interpreting this phenomenon, we cannot hastily conclude that it expresses a narrowly conceived concern about the fetus itself. Nor can we interpret that Japanese women perceive the fetus as a pathogen, or as a direct cause of a problem. The fetus is a powerful symbol capable of having several meanings, creating a phenomenon whereby a number of women with various kinds of concerns can relate to it.

The strongest evidence for this interpretation comes from historical data. Abortions have always been performed with a very high frequency, and the memorial service for the water child (aborted fetus) has a long history in Japan. However, it is only recently that it has become the focus of attention. If we expect one-to-one correlations between epidemiology, be it illness or pathogen, and medical specializations performed by supernatural entities, then the frequency of the former should be directly reflected in the latter. In the past, when the number of abortions was much higher because of lack of effective birth control methods, the memorial service was never carried out on such a large scale as it is now. Neither can we rely exclusively on the economic argument that contemporary affluence has suddenly provided people with the means to express their concerns.

Additional evidence for this interpretation comes from the increasing popularity of so-called *kakekomi dera*, or "runaway temples" (*kakekomi*, "to run into"; *dera*, "temple") throughout Japan. These are *amadera* or temples operated by nuns where women seek refuge and help for their problems, often marital. One of these *kakekomi dera* that recently received some attention is Jikishian in Kyoto, which was originally operated by nuns. When a nun by the name of Hirose Zenjun became head of the temple in 1965, she provided a notebook called *Omoidegusa* (Grass of memory) in which visitors were to write down their thoughts. She listened to their problems and gave advice. A young monk, Oda Yoshitake, started more systematic counseling of women when he took over the temple in 1978. Before he was put in charge, he had noticed that the number of women coming for consultation was increasing sharply, and that the problems they wrote down in their notebooks were of a serious nature. It has now become evident that, among the three hundred notebooks already filled since he became director of the temple, the most common concern is the confession and apology to an aborted fetus.[23]

This phenomenon may relate to the changing role of motherhood in contemporary Japan. Traditionally motherhood has received a high cultural value and given women a sense of self-worth and satisfaction. Yet these values are undergoing critical scrutiny and reevaluation. In some cases abortions may reflect marital conflicts, and women may even use the memorial service—at least subconsciously—to draw their husband's attention to their sufferings.[24]

Two cases serve to illustrate the wide range of reasons that prompt people to focus their attention on aborted fetuses. One woman in her early seventies, who has been a widow for some fifteen years, believes that an aborted fetus caused the death of her adult son, although the two incidents occurred several years apart. Some twenty years after the death of her son she acquired a tablet, on which was inscribed a posthumous name for the fetus designated by a Buddhist monk. She has placed the tablet in the ancestral alcove of her house, and she prays to it every morning. The second case is reported by a male novelist whose wife had an abortion shortly after World War II, because they thought two children were enough. Now, after over thirty years, they feel acutely sorry for the fetus as they watch their adult offspring and grandchildren in good health and affluence. The couple obtained a figure of *mizuko no jizō* (a buddha for aborted fetuses) from a temple, and they pray to it every morning.[25]

We must therefore conclude that abortion and the aborted fetus express something beyond the narrowly defined phenomenon of abortion itself. The aborted fetus, like menstrual blood, is a powerful symbol that can embody a variety of meanings and feelings, any one of which may be identified by a particular woman.

Medical Uses of Shrines and Temples—Two Case Studies

CASE ONE: ISHIKIRI SHRINE AND ITS ROLE IN SURGERY

Near the beginning of my fieldwork, I was interviewing a large number of people on the street, on public transportation, at restaurants, and in biomedical hospitals, and I encountered frequent references to the Ishikiri Shrine. One of my sources was an elderly couple, both in their sixties, who were vegetable vendors in front of a railroad station in Kobe. During my frequent stops, I engaged in conversation with them whenever they were free of other customers, and the husband described his monthly trip to Ishikiri Shrine, forty-five kilometers from his home. He had visited the shrine about ten years earlier, when he had a very painful corn on the sole of his foot. His doctor had told him he had no choice but to have it removed surgically. Desperate to avoid surgery, he decided to try Ishikiri

Shrine, on the recommendation of relatives and friends. Although the corn was causing almost too much pain for him to walk, he visited Ishikiri and tried *ohyakudo* several times. The corn miraculously disappeared. *Ohyakudo* literally means "one hundred times" and refers to the custom of making one hundred pilgrimages or visits to a shrine or temple in the hope of recovering from an illness. In front of Ishikiri Shrine are two cylindrical stones, roughly ten meters apart. As one of the practices required for healing, visitors, the sick, or their relatives and friends walk rapidly between these two stones one hundred times, touching them each time. Ever since the miraculous disappearance of his corn, the vegetable vendor has been visiting the shrine once a month.

A career woman in her forties, originally from a rural part of Fukuoka in Kyushu, described her experience at Ishikiri when I joined her at a table in a busy department store lunchroom in Osaka (at most restaurants and other eating places in Japan, one is expected to share a table with anyone who comes along). Six years earlier, when her brother was found to have lung cancer and had to have surgery, she paid her first visit to Ishikiri and gave her brother an amulet from the shrine. The brother's wife later told her that right after the surgery, when he was in great pain, he threw the amulet against the wall of the hospital room, shouting, "A silly superstition!" His operation was a success. Two years after the operation, the man's wife came to Osaka and paid a thank-you visit to the shrine. The woman I spoke to said that her brother's recovery from cancer must have had something to do with the healing power of the deities at the shrine.

A second couple provides another example. This couple, both in their forties, are college graduates who lived in a Western country for several years. At the time of the man's operation for an ulcer, his brother went to Ishikiri to obtain an amulet. After his recovery, the man and his wife went to Ishikiri to thank the deities. I met the couple accidentally on a street just as they were returning from Ishikiri. They were somewhat embarrassed about their visit, and told me that they had gone in part out of gratitude to his brother, who would be happy to hear of their thank-you visit, and in part because they had to pay a thank-you visit to his superior at work, who lived not far from Ishikiri. The attitude of this couple exemplifies one of the typical attitudes of contemporary Japanese toward medical functions of the supernaturals. That is, they "resort" to them when an illness is serious, but they feel somewhat embarrassed about the practice, since "educated" Japanese are not supposed to believe in "superstitions."

As I talked to various people, the magnitude of the shrine's "popularity" slowly but steadily emerged, and its importance was confirmed when I visited a university hospital. During a talk with two surgeons and several nurses, our conversation touched upon the use of amulets, which I had noticed hanging from beds as I visited the patients' rooms. The doctors and nurses confirmed that almost all patients have amulets hanging from their beds, the majority of which come from Ishikiri Shrine. They also commented that many patients forget to take their amulets home; they no longer pay attention to them once their surgery is a success.

Although Ishikiri Shrine was not on the agenda for my fieldwork, its obvious importance compelled me to investigate. The following description of the shrine and its surroundings is a composite of my observations during four visits.

Ishikiri Shrine is situated at the eastern end of the greater Osaka region. This region is at the foot of the Ikoma mountain range, which has retained strong religious meaning to the present day. The Ikoma area is full of shrines and temples, most of which are known to have specific types of healing power. It is also in this mountain range that shamans, whose number decreased drastically in other parts of the Keihanshin cities, are found in the greatest concentration. It should be noted here that the mountains, seen as the residence of deities, constitute the most sacred area of the Japanese universe. There exists an elaborate complex of beliefs about the mountains (sangaku shinkō), although they have lost some of their importance in contemporary Japan.

The formal name for Ishikiri is Ishikiri Tsurugiya Jinja, which means "a stone-cutting sword and arrow shrine." This designation derives from the fact that the shrine keeps as the embodied spirits of the deities (gosh-intai) a sharp sword and an arrow, both "capable of easily cutting even the hardest and largest rock." The two deities enshrined are the grandson and great-grandson of the Sun Goddess (Amaterasu Ōmikami), who is considered the most important deity in Japanese mythology. According to the literature distributed at the shrine, its origin is related to the time when these deities came to the western foot of the Ikoma mountain range to control the area.

The shrine is known to people in the Keihanshin area for its effectiveness in curing illnesses, especially dembo, a term in the Osaka dialect for tumors. The sword and the arrow enshrined as the bodies of the deities are considered analogous to surgical knives removing tumors, since all three cut into the body. In addition, stones traditionally have been assigned multiple symbolic meanings in Japanese culture and have played an especially important role in healing. The Japanese sometimes carry a pebble or write prayers on it and offer it to a shrine. A belief in the effectiveness of stones in curing, especially in the case of warts and excessive discharge from the ears, is found throughout Japan.[26]

One striking feature, obvious even to a casual observer, is the close, long-standing relationship between the shrine and Sakamoto Kampōten, which is the most famous distributor of the aforementioned kampō medicine in the Keihanshin area. Various types of advertisement for this distributor are highly visible not only in the shrine proper but also along the road leading from the railroad station to the shrine. The all-too-conspic-uous presence of this *kampō* distributor indicates that the two medical tra-ditions—*kampō* and religious healing—coexist peacefully and that the two systems recruit in fact similar "clients."

The railroad station is quite a distance from the shrine itself, and an observer notes that the narrow road connecting the two is studded with souvenir stores, vendors, casual eating places, roadside healers, and numerous outfits offering various types of divination. On nice days, one healer spreads a piece of yellow cloth on the roadside near the station. He has a small statue of Kōbō Daishi, a buddha of the Shingon sect, and a scroll on which this buddha's picture is painted. He offers to cure ill-nesses through the healing power of Kōbō Daishi. Every now and then a person stops out of curiosity but usually does not consult him. Finally, however, a woman in her fifties sits down on the piece of cloth and con-sults him about a pain in her knees. Only a short distance away from this healer is another diviner, a man clad in a white kimono. A large piece of white cloth is hanging between two poles, and written on the cloth are the names of a number of illnesses, including neuroses *(noirōze)*, which he claims to be able to treat. When there are no customers, he talks in a loud voice about how he can cure illnesses, hoping to catch the attention of passersby. Eventually a woman in her fifties stops to consult him, and, although the conversation involves interpersonal relationships within her family, she seems unconcerned and talks in a voice clearly audible to those passing by.

Farther down the road, entrepreneurs offering divination services, including Anshindō ("peace of mind store"), advertise "decisive deci-sions" to customers in practically all areas of life, including those related to marriage, entrance examinations, runaways from home, illness, busi-ness, and lawsuits. They do not offer to hold consultations for customers, but offer to hand down ready-made decisions. Nearby, on the opposite side of the street, is another diviner who advertises fees of ¥ 3,000 ($13.60) for divination and ¥ 1,000 ($4.50) for palmistry. Another diviner with a table and a few chairs on the street advertises Takashima divina-tion—perhaps the most widely used "school" of divination in contem-porary Japan. People consult these diviners at times of naming, house-building, marriage, health problems, and so on. Every time I pass the Takashima diviner there are customers, usually women, both young and old.

Numerous other self-proclaimed experts advertise a variety of divi-natory services, including reading personalities through brush strokes *(sumi iro)*, divination using cards *(toranpu uranai)*, character reading by facial features *(ninsō)* or by the shape of the nose, and reading the fortune of a house through its layout *(kasō)*. Reading the character of a house through its shape and directions is still commonly practiced in contemporary urban Japan; many people consult a diviner before they build or remodel a house. On this occasion, the advertisement urges customers to consult before putting a new gas pipeline into the house. By and large, all these divinatory practices are still widespread in urban Japan, and are used not only by older people but also by college students and other young people. Such beliefs and practices are derived from Taoism, originally introduced from China. Although Taoism has never been institutionalized in Japan, it has penetrated deeply into folk belief systems and practices. Kōshin-san, a Taoist god, is assigned numerous healing functions and remains an important deity in Japan today.

Farther along the road to the Ishikiri Shrine, on the left-hand side, there is a large advertisement for the memorial service for *mizuko* (water child, or aborted fetus) at a temple called Yōseien Jizōji. Written on a large advertisement board are these words: "Let us erect *jizō* (the guardian buddha of children), a familiar figure to us all through television, radio, and newspapers. For the memorial service for *mizuko*, choose Yōseien Jizōji." The lower half of the advertisement urges readers to stop at the office located near the sign or at the office at Tennōji in Osaka, and lists the telephone numbers. Behind this sign and the small office is a plot with twenty-one tombs, each with a *jizō* with a red bib, a pinwheel, and flowers. In addition, one medium-sized and one larger *jizō* and tombs are placed farther back, in front of a large mural. As I take pictures of this place, I hear a woman say: "Osaisen ireru toko ga nai ya; sanpuru ya nā" (There is no place to put *saisen* ["money offerings"]; they must be samples [*sanpuru* is derived from the English word "sample"]). This woman, in her sixties, is accompanied by her married daughter, who lives elsewhere but makes a point of going out with her mother once a month to various places such as this one. They inform me of other temples that have recently set up large plots for memorial services for aborted fetuses.

Close to this office is a small shrine specializing in the treatment of ringing ears and excessive discharge of earwax, as the large signs in front of the shrine indicate. In front of the shrine, next to the road, are two piles, one of rectangular pieces of board and the other of small stones. Written on these boards and stones are prayers asking the deity to treat problems, usually problems of the ear, or thanking the deity for effective treatment.

Near this shrine is a large statue of Daibutsu (Great Buddha) erected by the *kampō* dealer mentioned earlier—another example of the peaceful coexistence of Shintoism, Buddhism, and *kampō* in the realm of health care. In the compound are numerous large stone edifices on which the amounts of the dealer's donations to various civic causes are inscribed.

In between these places offering divination, as noted earlier, the road to the shrine is crowded on both sides with stores and vendors—among them the faded shingle of a shaman who moved away some time ago. They sell souvenirs, various kinds of herbs in bundles, and food, particularly local treats such as rice cakes with mugwort leaves in them. (Mugwort is considered medicinally potent, and therefore its leaves are put in rice cakes; its dried leaves are used for moxibustion.) Some people, accompanied by friends and relatives, stop to enjoy themselves in the partly open-air restaurants. Others pause over souvenirs, conspicuous among which are porcelain figures of badgers, frogs, monkeys, and other animals that are familiar figures in Japanese folk beliefs. Called *mayoke danuki* (evil-exorcising badgers), badgers feature prominently in Japanese folk tales and are reproduced as various icons, such as porcelain figurines. Likewise, frogs (*kaeru* in Japanese) are believed to bring good luck to a person. *Hikigaeru*, the Japanese word for toad, includes the term *hiki*, which means "to draw" (draw good luck). Similarly, the word *kaeru* (frog) is a homonym for the word that means "to return." Thus, *kaeru* signifies the concept of returning to a normal condition after a disaster, and the frog symbolically expresses this hope. Also, *gama no abura* (toad oil) has long been a common folk medicine. (Wordplay, with accompanying importance assigned to the power of the word, receives much attention in Japanese culture, a fact as true in the past as at present. Play on homonyms is a part of this cultural emphasis, and it is for this reason that the Japanese painstakingly avoid the number four, since it is a homonym for death—both words are pronounced as "shi.") The three-monkey figure— see no evil, hear no evil, speak no evil—is also prominent among souvenirs. Although meaning assigned to the three-monkey theme has gone through various changes,[27] the underlying notion in the contemporary use of the three-monkey theme is that if one follows these three behavioral taboos, one will live in harmony with other people—a good preventive medicine, at least to some. Many people purchase souvenirs for family and friends. During one of my trips to this site I talk with a woman in her early forties who has purchased a small porcelain badger to place next to her potted plant. She explains that when she last came to the shrine with her teenage children, they forbade her to buy a badger because they did not want her to follow a "superstition." However, she says, since her sister has one and it has brought a string of good luck, she has returned alone this time in order to purchase one in peace.

As one gets closer to the shrine, the presence of the Sakamoto *kampō* dealer becomes even more apparent, for the store sits right in front of the entrance to the shrine and other edifices. The compound, especially toward the front, is also studded with stone pillars. These pillars are covered with engravings of Sakamoto's name, and amounts and descriptions of donations to various causes, which include such civic projects as road construction in Osaka.

As one enters the compound of the shrine, just past a *torii* (the structure signifying a gate to a shrine), one sees a group of people, sometimes as many as thirty or so, walking rapidly between the two aforementioned stone slabs, touching the stones each time they pass. People have a choice of making the rounds either one hundred times or as many times as their age. Elderly people often choose their age, counting one round for every ten years; a person who is sixty-five would go around six times plus five, or eleven times. Some people purchase a bundle of one hundred paper strings, removing them one by one as they complete each round. This practice constitutes a condensed version of actual pilgrimage.

There is an office that registers people who wish to have special prayers (kitō) offered for them by the priest. Those who seek kitō are advised to avoid vinegar and fish with blue-green backs, such as mackerel. The office also sells a number of special items for healing, with instructions on how to use them. For example, after its purchase an amulet must be wrapped in a piece of white paper and rubbed against the ailing part a number of times. Long pieces of white cloth (sarashi) and cotton under-garments to be worn by the patients are also sold. Upon the patient's recovery, items used during the illness must be thrown into a river, burned, or returned to the shrine. Packages of rice are another item sold here. Patients swallow one grain every morning with their first drink of water. In the case of infants, mothers must swallow the rice on their behalf. The symbolic significance placed on rice derives from a belief that every grain possesses a soul, and this belief in turn renders rice a sacred food that is used in almost every ritual and on other culturally important occasions. Even today the Japanese regard rice as a most important source of energy, though they no longer consider it sacred.

To the right of the shrine is an enclosure containing a sacred white pony. Deities are considered to descend from heaven on horseback, and therefore many shrines keep white ponies, since white is a sacred color. There are also a number of structures in the area where prayer boards, paper cranes, and various other items are hung. Written on these boards (ema) are prayers for recovery from particular illnesses and statements of appreciation for recovery, sometimes written by the patients themselves, and sometimes by family members. Many people include their names, especially their first names, and their ages on the boards; a surprising number of them are fairly young. The prayers written on the boards, how-ever, are not confined to matters of illness—some even ask for successful entrance to a particular university. The paper cranes hanging from the boards follow the Japanese tradition in which a woman, in the hope of fulfilling her wish, folds one thousand paper cranes and strings them together into a bundle. Hung among these bundles of paper cranes are various items that have been used in curing, such as underwear in a plas-tic bag or canes used during an illness.

The first time I visited the shrine alone, I rested on a bench in the shrine compound next to a woman of forty-five. Her daughter, twenty, had had surgery two weeks earlier, during which the doctor found a number of small growths in her uterus. The growths were benign, according to the doctor, who did not remove them. Both the woman and her daughter were still apprehensive about the possibility of cancer. The woman stressed that she was concerned because she felt childbearing to be the most important role of women, and any complication of the uterus could affect this vital role. She had therefore visited a male *kamisan* ("deity"; in this case, a shaman) in Kyoto in the morning, and had taken the long bus ride to Ishikiri in order to receive diagnoses from two additional sources besides the medical doctor. The shaman in Kyoto reassured her that her daughter did not have cancer and would have a normal married life with children. The woman explained to me that she had formerly been in the habit of consulting a different shaman, whose spirit was Kōjin-san (the Kitchen God). She switched to her current shaman, who, as she repeatedly emphasized, is very decisive in his proclamations, although she was not sure which spirit possessed him.

Although consultation with shamans is no longer common in contemporary Japan, in other ways this case is illustrative of Japanese culture and requires further "cultural reading." It is all too common for a woman to represent her son or daughter—even when they are adult and married—or even to represent her husband, not only as a patient but also on many other occasions. A woman often visits a doctor on behalf of a family member, describing the symptoms and asking for the doctor's treatment. While such a "substitute patient" may on occasion be a friend of the afflicted, it is usually the mother or wife who stands in; it is rarely a man. Medical doctors are quite cooperative in this matter as long as they have seen the actual sufferer once. There are two cultural factors underlying this practice: the notion of the person in Japanese culture and the tradition of the woman as caretaker of the sick. In Japanese culture persons are defined as humans among humans. The two characters that stand for humans in Japanese are represented by the word *ningen*, with *nin* meaning "humans" and *gen* meaning "among." In other words, persons cannot be conceived of without the company of other human beings. Society, accordingly, consists not of isolated individuals, but of persons as they are related to other persons.[28] A clear-cut boundary between individuals, as is conceived in the individualism of some Western societies, is an alien concept to the Japanese. Thus a mother comfortably substitutes for her family members, who feel no invasion of privacy by this act.

Another woman, aged sixty-two, whom I met on a train, had been a widow since her husband was killed during World War II. Ever since her childhood, when her family lived in downtown Osaka, she and her family had visited Ishikiri Shrine regularly. She remembered one time when she had a growth (*dembo*) and rubbed it with a piece of paper on which the name of Ishikiri Tsurugiya Shrine was written; the growth disappeared in a few days. She visited the shrine always on the first and the fifteenth of the month, and sometimes on a few other days. She usually prayed for the safety and general welfare of the family, but at times she went through *kitō* (special prayers). Sometimes she would pay only about ¥ 1,000 for *kitō*, for which a priest would write her name, age, and her wish on a sheet of paper, which she would then take home. If the matter was more serious, she occasionally paid more and was allowed to go into the *honden* (inner shrine), where a priest offered a prayer to the deities on behalf of all the people gathered there. At one time she used to go around the two stones one hundred times, but now she would go around only eight times (six times for sixty years, plus two).

CASE TWO: NAKAYAMA TEMPLE—ITS ROLE IN OBSTETRICS, GYNECOLOGY, AND PEDIATRICS

As with Ishikiri Shrine, Nakayama Temple was not part of my planned fieldwork. The unquestionable importance of this temple in health care, especially for women and children, became evident during my observations at the hospital obstetric clinic. Many pregnant women in Japan continue to wear the traditional long white sash, called *iwata obi*, over the stomach during pregnancy. Of 106 women who answered my questionnaire, 81 had obtained a sash from Nakayama Temple.

The temple is situated on a large hill not far from a railroad station. According to its own historical account, the temple was originally built by Prince Shōtoku (574–622). Although the origin of its close association with childbirth and child welfare is not well documented, it may date to the end of the sixteenth century, when the wife of Toyotomi Hideyoshi, the military ruler of Japan, became pregnant after offering prayers in the temple. She subsequently gave birth to a son, thus providing the long-awaited heir.[29] The mother of the Meiji emperor, the great-grandfather of the present emperor, also paid homage to this temple before she gave birth to the emperor. Whatever its origin, the temple is known throughout Japan for its role in matters of childbirth and general child welfare.

The following description is based on two visits to the temple, one on an ordinary day and the other on the day of a special ceremony held for the souls of the dead who have no relatives to provide memorial services for them (*muen botoke*).

The major hall (*hondō*) of the temple is situated on top of the hill, and it is flanked by numerous stone statues of *jizō*, the guardian buddha of children, on the hillside. The gate to the temple is situated at the bottom of the hill and is connected to the main hall by a straight path consisting of many stone steps. On both sides of this central pathway are separate temples enshrining various buddhas, each specializing in a certain function. For example, on the left just within the gate is a temple that specializes in success in the university entrance examination. The entrance examination to a good university is a major life passage in contemporary Japan; some children, under the guidance (or pressure) of their parents and teachers, start preparing themselves for this examination extremely early by choosing the right nursery school, and a student's entire school career is devoted to this goal. Another temple enshrines a buddha who specializes in taking care of infants who have temper tantrums, do not sleep, cry at night, and have weak constitutions. Another temple, which bears a sign in the front for traffic safety and the naming of newborn infants, also houses Mizuko Jizō (*jizō* for aborted fetuses). Inside this temple, to the left, are a *jizō* for aborted fetuses and numerous votive plaques hung on two wooden structures. For lack of space, these prayer boards are hung on top of each other in layers, indicating the large number of people who have visited the temple.

At the top of the hill, in front of the main hall, is a large metal incense burner. People buy bundles of incense, light them, and place them in the burner; many then "scoop" up the smoke with their hand and place it on an ailing part, such as the hip, to utilize its "healing power." Visitors, especially women with infants, also purchase white bibs, write prayers and their names and addresses on them, and hang them on one of the stakes surrounding the buddha in front of the main hall. The main hall itself houses two offices. On the right side is a small office where the temple employees sell the aforementioned pregnancy sashes. After purchasing a sash, a woman asks the priest of the temple to write a *sūtra* (verses from Buddhist scripture) on it. On the left is another small office where used sashes must be returned.

As the sketchy description provided here indicates, the central focus of the temple is childbirth and matters related to infancy, including easy and safe delivery, the healthy growth of children, and memorial services for aborted fetuses. According to the people I interviewed, both visitors and temple officials, the temple has long served also as a place for the *shichi-go-san* celebration—a celebration marked by a visit to a shrine, usually on November 15, when a boy is five and a girl is three and seven years old (*shichi-go-san* means seven, five, and three). November 15 is a most auspicious day in the year for, among other reasons intrinsic to the agricultural cycle and the lunar calendar, it combines the auspicious numbers 3, 5, and 7, which mark the growth points of the life cycle. Protection from the guardian deities is sought on these occasions, and they mark the growth of the child in the eyes of fellow members of the community. In the past in some regions a child was not registered in the family registry until reaching either three, five, or seven, depending upon the region, since children younger than these ages were not considered full-fledged humans.[30] In contemporary Japan, *shichi-go-san* remains an important life passage and children dress up to visit the shrines.

Summary and Discussion

The above description indicates that the deities and buddhas in the Japanese pantheon have played a significant role in health care throughout history and are intimately involved in the life cycle passages. Not only does every Japanese start life in a Shinto ceremony at birth and experience Shinto ceremonies of *shichi-go-san*, but contemporary Japanese also seek blessing and protection during more recently created life passages. These include the entrance examination to a university and the entrance to a company, that is, the first employment, which may also be the only employment. At the end of their life, they go through a Buddhist ritual, since most funerals are performed in a Buddhist rite.[31]

In the past, the Japanese sought help from their supernaturals during major epidemics, such as influenza and smallpox, and this practice continues for serious illnesses today, such as cancer. The important role that religious institutions play in contemporary Japanese medicine must be seen as a part of medical pluralism. My own field experience testifies to this. I had not intended to study the role of religion in contemporary Japanese medical systems; however, its importance had to be recognized, since people who were patients at biomedical institutions were simultaneously using religious institutions.

Not only do the Japanese use drastically different medical systems simultaneously, but they also practice different religions simultaneously. In the case of Nakayama Temple, for example, the distinction between Shintoism and Buddhism is of significant concern neither for its devotees nor for the respective religious institutions themselves. The various functions performed by Nakayama Temple are those usually assigned to a Shinto shrine (except for the memorial service for aborted fetuses, which has become important only in recent years). The visitors I interviewed found nothing unusual about the services performed by the Buddhist temple. A few said, however, that although they consider this particular temple to be associated with childbirth, they usually associate the seven-five-three ceremonies with a shrine. They added, however, that since they had come to the temple for the safe delivery of the children, they found it logical to continue to come to this temple for the welfare of the children.

Ishikiri Shrine even more succinctly expresses the comfortable coexistence of supernaturals belonging to different religions. It is a Shinto shrine situated in the mountains, which are considered to be the residence of the deities in folk Shintoism. But we saw that a *kampō* dealer had erected a statue of Great Buddha on the road leading to Ishikiri. In addition, there is an office advertising the tombs for aborted fetuses, characteristically associated with the *jizō* of Buddhism. As a medical institution Ishikiri combines healing by both a deity and a Buddha, as well as the *kampō* treatment, and by numerous types of divination—mostly of Taoistic origins; and its past history includes shamanism.

Simultaneous subscription to more than one religion is a prevalent practice of the Japanese, both in the past and at present. Shintoism and Buddhism have remained distinct in their structural organization and orthodox doctrines; however, even in the realm of "official" doctrines and belief structures, much intermingling and fusion have been apparent. For example, during the eleventh and twelfth centuries various attempts at *shinbutsu shūgō* (joint worship of deities and buddhas) were made by religious specialists. From the perspective of laypeople, the two merge even more. A common explanation for this phenomenon is that these religions have permeated the daily lives of the Japanese. Buddhism is associated primarily with death and the dead; Shintoism is tied to birth, growth, and life in general. Thus all the ceremonies for childbirth are Shinto ceremonies, while most funerals are Buddhist rites, as noted above. Religious practices have become part of the customs of the Japanese without requiring any psychological commitment on the part of the individual to any one religion.[32]

The annual statistics on Japanese religious affiliation consistently list the total membership in various religious organizations as one and a half times the total population of Japan. In other words, over half of the people in Japan belong to more than one religious organization.

While supernaturals of several religions play a part in contemporary health care, there is a wide range of individual beliefs and attitudes underlying visits to religious institutions. Some people do in fact believe deeply in deities and buddhas and in their efficacy in medical and other matters. Other people are halfhearted and pay visits simply because "it does not hurt anything" or because the act pleases someone dear to them who does believe.

Even "true believers," however, believe in the power of a deity to perform certain existential or physical functions, rather than in abstract transcendental power. The use of temples and shrines, both in the past and at present, reveals the very concrete orientation of the people toward their religions. People ask deities and buddhas for health, prosperity, traffic safety, and various other worldly benefits; they do not emphasize their own spiritual well-being or life after death.

In other words, the Japanese visit deities and buddhas to achieve specific goals, for example, the cure of an illness. The underlying attitude therefore is "magical" rather than "religious," if we use the language of past academic discourse. Or Japanese religions are an example of "practical religion," a term used by Edmund Leach in reference to religion that "is concerned with the life here and now."[33] But a pigeonholing of Japanese religions or of the way the Japanese understand them does not lead us to an understanding of the role of religions in the health care of contemporary postindustrial urban Japan.

Basic to the Japanese view and understanding of the universe is the concept of the human being—the self—as defined in the company of other humans *(ningen)*, the Other. The dialectic relation between self and Other at the level of the universe is the collective self of the Japanese as humans vis-à-vis the supernaturals, on the one hand, and the Japanese vis-à-vis other peoples, on the other hand. In this framework, both dialectic relations are hierarchically ordered—the Other, be it deities or foreigners, has the transcendental power to energize the lives of the Japanese. The purpose of ritual is to harness the power of deities, who are considered to reside outside the settlement and visit humans periodically, in order to rejuvenate the lives of the people in a settlement. Likewise, foreigners too bring in positive power for the Japanese, as evidenced by the Chinese, who, from the fifth century onward, introduced writing systems, metallurgy, city plans, Buddhism (originally from India), Confucianism, and a number of other features of civilization. Later, this role was taken over by Westerners, who introduced medicine, guns, and many other technological skills to the Japanese. But unless these outside forces are well controlled, deities and foreigners alike can bring catastrophes—deities by not controlling natural disasters and foreigners by turning into enemies during wars.[34]

I propose that the approaching of deities and buddhas to solicit their power in curing illnesses is an individual enactment of this cosmological scheme. Each individual's act of paying a visit to a deity or a buddha or of consulting a divinatory practice is an act of experiencing personally the universe and its forces. Cosmology becomes a lived experience for the individual, who, at the psychological level, feels that he or she did as well as humanly possible to control universal forces. Seen in this light, a visit to temple, shrine, shaman, or diviner is a *nemawashi* at the level of the universe. The *nemawashi* is a practice whereby an individual in Japanese society who wishes to propose an idea to a group (for example, to coworkers in the company) engages in informal persuasions and negotiations with others so that the decision, when formally made by the group, is a joint, although often compromised, decision. At the time of illness, a human individual visits supernaturals to maximize their cooperation, rather than leaving the course of life up to them; the individual wants the outcome to be a result of joint effort. It is an aggressive act of soliciting the powerful forces of the universe for one's own advantage.

While the cosmological scheme offers a basic explanation, a historical perspective highlights both the specificity of Japanese culture and the scene in contemporary Japan. We might ask: What is the nature of change in the role and meaning of religion in health care when placed in historical perspective? Regarding long-term changes, a more specific question is this: What is the difference between religious healing during the medieval period, for example, and contemporary Japan? Aside from the obvious difference of the absence of biomedicine during the medieval period, our queries must aim in two directions. On the one hand, we must pay attention to such factors as the cultural attitude toward symbols, myths, and religions. On the other, we must examine changes in the ontology that provides the meaning to cultural institutions, such as magico-religious practices. In so doing, we cannot assume "the mechanization of the world picture," "the decline of magic," or "the disenchantment of the world" as the universal development.[35] "Magic" has not declined in Japan; on the contrary, it is prospering. The task then is to examine historical developments and transformations within the context of each society, before imposing these modernization theories, primarily based on Western societies, on other societies. In addition, it is necessary to reassess our assumption of a unilinear model—the idea that secularization or mechanization constitutes a unilinear progression. We are now observing a worldwide phenomenon of "religious revival," in which Japan is taking part. Insufficient notice and little serious study have been given to this phenomenon. Present explanations tend toward the simple and functional. Further studies in this direction will undoubtedly provide us with deeper understanding of the role of religions in health care.

As for recent changes, the popularity of temples and shrines for health care must be seen against the broader background of changes both in the epidemiological pattern and in health care in contemporary Japan, where *kampō* has made a phenomenal comeback. The increased popularity both of *kampō* and religious institutions is in part a symptom of people's dissatisfaction with biomedicine, which not only has failed to sustain its almighty image but has demonstrated its devastatingly negative effects. It is also due in part to the changing self-image of the Japanese vis-à-vis the Other, which has been represented by the West in the recent past. To the Japanese, then, Westerners have represented the Other with dual power, both positive and negative—the source and model of scientific and technological achievements and the destructive power during wars. However, with the success in the world market in high technology, the auto industry, and elsewhere, the Japanese image of the Other has changed, and this change in turn has transformed the Japanese image of self. More than the economic success as such, it is the symbolic nature of their recent achievement that has affected the Japanese concept of the collective self. By superseding the science and technology of the West, the Japanese no longer feel unequivocally inferior to the Other. They no longer have to hold biomedicine in awe, but are comfortable in using their own approach, be it religious healing or *kampō*.

Notes

1. For details of the deities and buddhas and for symbolic analyses of the meanings assigned to these supernaturals, see my *Illness and Culture in Contemporary Japan* (Cambridge, England, 1984).

2. In the study *Religion and Society in Modern Japan: Continuity and Change* (Houston, 1970), Edward Norbeck provides a comprehensive overview; for a detailed case study of one of these new religions, see Winston Davis, *Dōjō: Magic and Exorcism in Modern Japan* (Stanford, CA, 1980).

3. Studies of shamanism are also available in English. See Carmen Blacker, *The Catalpa Bow: A Study of Shamanistic Practices in Japan* (London, 1975); Ichirō Hori, *Folk Religion in Japan* (Chicago, 1968).

4. For an exhaustive treatment of ancestor worship in ancient Japan, see Robert J. Smith, *Ancestor Worship in Contemporary Japan* (Palo Alto, CA, 1974).

5. My fieldwork for this research was carried out in 1979 and 1980 in the so-called Keihanshin area, which encompasses the three major cities of Kobe, Osaka, and Kyoto in western Japan. The people in this area frequently seek their medical treatment outside of their own city yet primarily within this area. My use of the term "the Japanese" throughout this chapter should be taken only to mean those Japanese in this area—although some of my interpretations apply to the Japanese elsewhere as well.

6. The Japanese term *ashi* includes both the leg and the foot.

7. For detailed discussion on the Japanese notion of the stomach, see my *Illness and Culture in Contemporary Japan* (Cambridge, England, 1984), pp. 57–60, 181–184.

8. Ibid., pp. 66–67, 69–70.

9. For actual case histories see ibid., 62–66.

10. Smith, *Ancestor Worship in Contemporary Japan*.

11. Eugene R. Swanger, "A preliminary examination of the *omamori* phenomenon," *Asian Folklore Studies* 40, no. 2 (1981): 242–243.

12. Ibid., p. 240.

13. Mikiharu Itoh, "Shinkō seikatsu" (Religious life), in *Nihonjin no Seikatsu* (Life of the Japanese), ed. T. Umesao (Tokyo, 1976), pp. 226–227; Katō et al., "Kamigami no bungyō" (Division of labor among deities), in *Nihon Bunka to Sekai* (Japanese culture and the world), eds. T. Umesao and M. Tada (Tokyo, 1972), pp. 24–25. Itoh's chart is based on information provided by Kunio Yanagita, *Teihon Yanagita Kunioshū* (Selected papers of Yanagita Kunio), vol. 12 (Tokyo, 1963); see also *Minzokugaku Jiten* (Ethnographic dictionary) (Tokyo, 1951). I have translated the names of Itoh's deities and buddhas only when the translation is meaningful to the English reader; some bear proper names whose translations are meaningless. The recurrent term *sama* is an address form in Japanese used in referring to deities; when particular deities are customarily referred to with this address form, the term becomes, in effect, part of the name, and I have treated it as such.

14. Originally introduced from China, this system has gone through such transformation in Japan that it is misleading to label it Taoism. Its significance tends to be underestimated because it has never been developed into a distinct institutionalized religion. See Katō et al., pp. 69–70; Noritada Kubo, *Kōshin Shinkō no Kenkyū* (Research on belief in Kōshin) (Tokyo, 1961).

15. Ryō Mizobe, "Gendai jiin to gensei riyaku" (Temples and their pragmatic efficacies) in *Nihon Shūkyō no Gensei Riyaku* (Practical benefits of Japanese religions), ed. Nihon Bukkyō Kenkyūkai (Tokyo, 1970), pp. 408–423.

16. What is missing from both sets of data is the frequency of visits by people to particular types of deities and buddhas—in other words, their individual popularity. Ishikiri Shrine, which will be introduced as a case study

below, for example, is exceedingly popular, as we have seen, and thousands of people visit it; but there may be many deities and buddhas who have their shingles up, as it were, and yet are less popular with people.

17. Umesao notes, in Katō et al., p. 76, that one advertisement by a railroad company, urging people to travel by train to different temples and shrines, exhorts seekers, "Be greedy in your wishes and demands," and it lists twenty-seven efficacious functions of these supernaturals, of which only three deal with illness; the majority deal with success in school, work, and life in general. Perhaps this advertisement was aimed at young people, so the emphasis on illness may have been consciously discouraged.

18. Noboru Miyata, *Kinsei no Hayarigami* (Popular gods during the early modern period in Japan) (Tokyo, 1975).

19. Ibid.

20. Shōji Tatsukawa, *Nihonjin no Byōreki* (A medical history of the Japanese) (Tokyo, 1976), pp. 197–202.

21. Yanagita, *Teihon Yanagita Kunioshū,* p. 215, and *Minzokugaku Jiten*, p. 104.

22. Shinichi Fujita, "Usoga ooi jinkō chūzetsusū" (Unreliable figures for abortions), *Asahi*, 21 November 1978; Ayako Sono, *Kami no Yogoreta Te* (Soiled hands of God) (Tokyo, 1980), vol. 1, p. 195 and vol. 2, passim.

23. *Asahi*, 12 April 1980.

24. For a similar analysis of the semantics of a physical illness among women, see Byron J. Good, "The Heart of What's the Matter: The Semantics of Illness in Iran," *Culture, Medicine and Psychiatry* 1, no. 1 (1977): 25–58.

25. Keita Genji, "Mizuko kuyō" (Memorial service for aborted fetuses) *Shōsetsu Shinchō* 36, no. 2 (1982): 46–47.

26. Yanagita, *Minzokugaku Jiten*, p. 22.

27. For an extensive treatment of the historical transformations of the three-monkey theme since its introduction from China, see my study *The Monkey as Mirror: Symbolic Transformations in Japanese History and Ritual* (Princeton, 1987).

28. Robert Smith, *Japanese Society* (Cambridge, England, 1983).

29. Shūyū Kanakoa, *Koji Meisatsu Jiten* (Dictionary of ancient and famous temples) (Tokyo, 1970).

30. For a concise explanation of *shichi-go-san*, see Yanagita, *Minzokugaku Jiten*, pp. 259–260.

31. For information on Shinto funerals, see Smith, *Ancestor Worship in Contemporary Japan*.

32. For a general discussion of this topic, see Itoh, "Shinkō seikatsu," pp. 215–216.

33. Edmund Leach, *Dialectic in Practical Religion* (Cambridge, England, 1968).

34. For details of the concept of self and other in Japanese culture, see my *Monkey as Mirror*.

35. E. J. Dijksterhuis, *The Mechanization of the World Picture: Pythagoras to Newton* (Princeton, 1986); Keith Thomas, *Religion and the Decline of Magic* (New York, 1971); and Max Weber, *From Max Weber: Essays in Sociology*, eds. H. H. Gerth and C. Wright Mills (New York, 1967).

CHAPTER 4

Hinduism and the Tradition of Āyurveda

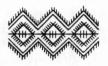

DAVID M. KNIPE

If we were to visit the small town of "Annapuram," located not far from the Bay of Bengal and the eastern seaboard of India, in the Telugu-speaking state of Andhra Pradesh in southern India, we would find a varied array of medical practitioners and healers. On the outskirts of town, in its own enclave composed entirely of the highest caste of Hindus, the brahmans, is a Vedic recitation school consisting of a community of about thirty students and half a dozen teachers, all of them preoccupied with the transmission of an oral tradition that has survived for more than three thousand years. The Vedas, which are the object of their study, comprise a large body of texts containing myths, rituals, speculations, and folklore, and these are believed to be a unitary and eternal revelation, with neither divine nor human origin. Among the many texts that are taught in this school and eventually taken away in the memories of selected, gifted students capable of memorizing thousands of verses is the *Atharvaveda,*

89

often called the fourth Veda—a collection of 730 hymns compiled in
twenty books circa 1000 BCE. Many of these hymns have portions called
mantras extracted from the earliest of the four Vedas, the *Ṛgveda*, which
was composed perhaps two or three centuries earlier.[1] But unlike the
Ṛgveda, and the other two Vedas whose concerns center upon the great
sacrifices that not only regenerate cosmic and human energies and
rhythms but bring the prominent deities into action in the human sphere,
this fourth and somewhat isolated Veda focuses on the family and personal plane, providing invocations, spells, charms, and remedies—all the
arcane and sometimes weird folk traditions that apply to rites of passage
or problem situations (such as the proper way to deal with the powers in
a termite mound that suddenly emerges from your living-room floor).
Until quite recently the *Atharvaveda* was believed to be a relic of a past
age, no longer a living text, but here in this school and in other areas as
well it is not only transmitted but actively practiced. Some individuals
learn the text for what they call its defensive or white magic; others learn
it for its healing mantras. The head of the school is in charge of the cur-
riculum and examining committees, but in addition he is a practicing physician employing selected mantras from the *Atharvaveda* and guaranteeing their efficacy. For example, in cases of difficult child delivery he may
recite particular invocations to lesser Vedic deities and obscure feminine
powers, entirely forgotten by classical Hinduism as it has developed in
the past two thousand years, but some of them traceable by historians
back through their proto-Indo-Iranian counterparts (c. 2000 BCE) to their
possible proto-Indo-European origins in the southwest steppe regions
some six or seven thousand years ago. Or he might apply a particular leaf
described in the *Atharvaveda*, chant the prescribed mantras, and allow the
leaf to ripen and drain an abscess. Most of this Vedic physician's patients
are local people, quite unaware of the fact that their doctor is employing
what may indeed be the world's oldest textually based spiritual healing.
The Vedas are held in such reverent (but imprecise) regard in South Asia
that the mere mention of them as authority causes belief and relief for
some in every class and caste. And subscription to such mantric cures,
whether Vedic or derivative mantras, is widespread among communities
both literate and nonliterate.

   As we proceed along the river into town we pass another community
quite different from the brahman lane with its whitewashed brick houses
and sturdy school. This is a scatter of mud huts belonging to the Scheduled Castes, as they are known to an officialdom that has prohibited age-
old observances of untouchability; Harijans, "the people of God"—
Mahatma Gandhi's phrase—is the label employed for these people by a
few of the educated, but most simply go by the subcaste name within the
larger clusters of two castes, the Malas and the Madigas. In this community, numbering a third of the area's population and constituting its agri-

cultural labor pool, we might find several people specializing in one or another branch of folk healing. For example, one family might be observed stretching great nets between trees on a moonlit night, capturing giant fruit bats, known also as flying foxes, whose parts are ground into cures for asthma. Another family includes a "god-dancer," who moved here from a southern district; he dances himself or a patient into ecstatic trance states and serves as medium or exorcist in communication with an ever-impinging world of demons, ghosts, and unpredictable spirits. Those who come to him for assistance carry a wide range of burdens: sexual impotence, barrenness, repeated miscarriage, increasing blindness or loss of teeth from the curse of an enemy, infections that refuse to heal because of an unfulfilled vow to a god, terror from the nightly actions of an aborted fetus. Most of these clients are illiterate, and there are no texts, oral or written, for the healing techniques applied to them.

Close to the edge of the major settlement areas is a line of small temples and shrines for a number of goddesses, some of them representing epidemic or other life-threatening diseases, all of them important to the area at large during their festival occasions, and a few of them significant to particular communities with their specialist priests. Continuing past these structures and entering the town we move through basic hamlets of the median ranks of the population, the various castes that make up the *śūdra* class—Washerfolk, Weavers, Barbers, Potters, Carpenters, Tailors, Cultivators, Shepherds, and others—some of whom make their living by traditional crafts and specialities, others who in the fashion of modern India have become clerical workers, schoolteachers, social workers, landholders. Here in town there are also sections of smaller, more prestigious communities, minorities such as the Merchants and brahmans, who are among the uppercaste, or "twice-born"-caste, Hindus. Many of the Merchants live in large isolated houses; some of them still are regarded as foreigners although their families came from other regions of India generations ago. The brahmans, on the other hand, who for the most part are engaged in worldly and not spiritual professions, live with few exceptions in quite modest houses and circumstances.

There is a wide range of medical practitioners active in town. With the help of two assistants, one physician in particular maintains a clinic on the main street and offers what India calls allopathy. (Scholars avoid this term as well as the equivalent often given for it, namely, Western medicine. They prefer the term cosmopolitan medicine, since this practice is at once global and syncretic.) Currently this physician is "out-of-station" in Hyderabad, but intends to return. His two assistants, without medical college degrees but with considerable experience and expertise, deal with routine practice, including injections, minor outpatient surgery, the setting of simple fractures, sewing of sutures, and dispensing of medicines through the clinic's pharmacy. (More complicated diseases and surgical cases are referred to the hospitals in one of the neighboring cities, the nearest one being a four-hour journey by bus and train.) On this same street are three pharmacist families that dispense—accompanied by terse, generally knowledgeable but undetailed advice—a wide range of over-the-counter medicines, including antibiotics. In the past five years a dozen other small "medical stores" have mushroomed under English or Telugu signboards in every market and on every major crossroad in town. Many are inexperienced and opportunistic sellers of nationally distributed pharmaceuticals; their advice on dosage and efficacy to the great majority unable to read the English labels can be abbreviated and inexact.

As in the Scheduled Caste communities there are specialists. For example, a member of one of the Cultivator castes is a snakebite curer of wide repute; a Carpenter grinds special wood into a concoction—including pepper, ginger, camphor, plantain juice, and coconut oil—that many regard as the best treatment for bruises, sprains, and swellings; and a popular healer from the Shepherd community uses Sanskrit mantras, both oral and written, as one of several of his curative methods. This last specialist employs a technique used widely among Hindus, Muslims, and some Christians, namely, the insertion of a written word or verse of known power into a silver tube to be worn on a thread around the neck, wrist, or waist of the child, adult, or valuable animal (such as the family cow or buffalo) in need of a cure. He also provides silver rings for alleviating croup in infants and supplies sacred cow-dung ash (*vibhūti*), lime juice, turmeric powder, certain forest herbs, and other items as mantric medication for such varied problems as skin diseases, general fatigue, and effects of the evil eye.

Finally, there is one of the town's best-known astrologers, a brahman, who is considered by his upper-caste clientele to be a well-informed adviser for problems of mental and physical health. In either his town or his home office he draws up horoscopes for clients, then consults a library of Sanskrit and Telugu texts and reveals the correspondences between cosmic elements, deities, celestial bodies, and parts of the human body. If for example excessive sneezing is a problem, then a horoscope may indicate through correspondences of the moment that one of the nine planets, Śani (Saturn), is the cause. The astrologer may then designate rituals that will discharge the evil effects of Śani, whom he depicts as a tall, sturdy, black, cross-eyed godling of considerable power and one whose dangerous shadow may infect an individual for a period of seven years or more.

But all of these authorities, with the exception of the absentee cosmopolitan medical doctor, are part-timers where medicine is concerned. If you ask about *the* physician in town, you will be directed to a particular *vaid*—whose modern Indic designation derives from Sanskrit *vaidya*[2]—that is, one of the practitioners of traditional Indian medicine, Āyurveda. Āyurveda ("*veda* [i.e., knowledge] of life") claims Vedic roots and therefore the same profound heritage as the *Atharvaveda* and *Ṛgveda*. Historically, however, it is a medical tradition that has been part of the fabric of Indian civilization for somewhat more than the last two thousand years, changing with the centuries as the civilization itself underwent gradual transformations but remaining faithful to the Sanskrit texts composed about the beginning of the Common Era. The *vaid* of Annapuram was in fact trained in those ancient texts, as well as in later ones of the medieval and modern periods. His practice in coastal Andhra could easily be shifted, if he were as multilingual as the nation of India, to any other region of the subcontinent, and the physician-patient relationship he now enjoys would remain fairly much the same, with certain adjustments for local customs, ethnic idiosyncrasies, remedies, and dietary restrictions or predilections.

The most prominent of the *vaids* of Annapuram, known locally under the title of *vaidyācārya*, literally "spiritual guide *(ācārya)* of physicians," belongs to one of the highest artisan castes. He is in his early forties. Only recently he performed the last rites for his father, the town's *vaidyācārya* of long standing, whose practice he took over when he graduated from medical college. When the current *vaidyācārya* reflects on how this family practice has changed in a generation he notes the medical pluralism of modern India. Annapuram does not afford the variety of specialists common in many larger towns and all cities, the professionals and semiprofessionals in Hathayoga, certain regional martial arts, Siddha (Āyurveda mediated by Tamil culture in Tamil Nādu and Sri Lanka), Unani (Islamic medicine modified regionally in South Asia), homeopathy and naturopathy (both popular in middle-class urban culture, the former being Samuel Hahnemann's eighteenth-century curative methods, the latter a syncretic medical tradition relying on the body's "natural" healing substances).

But even in such a small town numerous transformations in a single generation are apparent to him. First, the proliferation of medical stores all over town provides occasion for word-of-mouth, relatively inexpensive self-treatment by means of everything from aspirin to antibiotics. Second, the presence of the cosmopolitan medical clinic has fostered a new climate of choice, and its system of referrals to the hospitals of area cities has produced a rapidly growing pool of individuals who have gone and returned with accounts of "modern scientific medicine." Third, only a few years of national television programming have turned health care and preventive medicine into everyday topics of discussion in all sectors of the town.

People generally look for fast relief, says the *vaidyācārya*, and they try the medical stores first. If relief is not forthcoming, then other systems, including the new clinic, might be chosen according to belief and community. Fewer are dependent upon a single tradition today. For example, in his father's practice many of the Scheduled Castes came for Ayurvedic diagnosis and treatment, but now they prefer injections from the clinic for quick results. His father also had many patients come in on foot or by bullock cart from outlying villages, people from all the *śūdra* agricultural and artisan castes. Although there is rapid bus transport throughout the area, his own patients now include fewer *śūdra*s and more of the higher classes, the brahman, *kṣatriya* Landholders, and Merchant communities living here in town. For many of his people cosmopolitan medicine has a good reputation for surgery, and he will recommend a specific eye surgeon, to cite just one example, for treatment of glaucoma or cataracts. Finally, he notes that his practice is far more efficient than his father's in the matter of dispensing medicines. Many items that he prescribes are produced in laboratories and shipped by truck to him in large quantities of plastic or aluminum foil packets, whereas his father's assistants might have spent an hour or more per patient with hand-grinding, mixing, and individually wrapping each newsprint packet, not to mention the constant task of procuring and stocking in tall glass containers more than a hundred different raw materials.

However, the *vaidyācārya* does not wish to overemphasize these changes. The basic practice of medicine today, as in his father's day, is the same as that of the ancient authorities, he insists, and he provides illustrations of some frequently prescribed items that do not come in aluminum foil: turmeric, leaves of the nim tree, *sāmbrāṇi* crystals, as they are known in Telugu, and *pañcagavya*. Turmeric and nim leaves are both prescribed for treatment in one of three ways, by inhalation in steam vapors, ingestion, and external application in paste form. Among other uses, the yellow turmeric and bitter nim are antibacterial, and so indeed are the fumes from burning *sāmbrāṇi* crystals, which when inhaled facilitate the exchange of winds in the body. The five products of the cow—milk, curds, clarified butter, urine, dung—make up a concoction among the most popular in India, *pañcagavya*. Only the urine of the cow has pharmacological use, says the *vaidyācārya*, in the treatment of spleen disorders for example, but belief in the inherent purity and goodness of the cow makes this recipe extremely effective for a wide range of problems. He talks about the use of *sāmbrāṇi* incense to pull a person back from a state of trance or possession by a ghost or spirit, the application of turmeric in marriage rites and of nim in funeral rites, the chemical additives to turmeric that produce the sacred vermilion or deep red colors so important in Hindu worship, and the significance of the nim tree in the ancient myths whose chief repositories are the epics and the Purāṇas. Like the astrologer who described the frequently malevolent planet Śani as sturdy and cross-eyed, this physician moves easily from matters of diagnosis, treatment, diet, and behavior to the myths, deities, rituals, and symbols that structure the Hindu tradition. In fact, running as a thread through his discourse is the same notion as that set forth by the astrologer: the human body is composed of the elements, humors, and qualities that make up the cosmos itself, and specific correspondences, part for part, harmony for harmony, must be realized and regarded if one is to enjoy health and long life.

What we learn from this articulate physician in a small town in southern India is instructive: if we are to appreciate this enduring South Asian system of medicine known as Āyurveda, then we must know more about the traditions of Hinduism.

Hinduism and the South Asian Worldview

Hinduism is the label applied to the dominant religious tradition of South Asia or the Indian subcontinent (the modern nations of India, Sri Lanka, Nepal, Sikkim). With the ambiguous exception of China, whose traditions are undergoing current revivals, Hinduism, of all the world's religions, has by far the largest population in a single cohesive region. It is also the oldest continuous religious tradition, with its roots partially in the obscure antiquity of the Indus Valley civilization (c. 2300–1700 BCE), partially in the Indo-Aryan Vedic civilization (c. 1500 BCE following), and partially in the undated and nonliterate hunting/collecting, nomadic pastoralist, and agrarian folk traditions of the hundred-odd linguistic and subcultural regions of India.

Although there is no question about the location, size, and antiquity of Hinduism, there is considerable debate concerning its definition. Unlike the religions of western Asia (the biblical traditions, Zoroastrianism, and Islam), there is in Hinduism no prerequisite deity, revelation, scripture, ecclesiastical structure, credo, or ritual. Deities, mythologies, sacred texts, god-men, religious communities, vows, rituals, and festivals abound, perhaps more energetically in Hinduism than in any faith, but still there is nothing remotely like a prescription whereby we may locate a Hindu.

What has emerged in the last two thousand years, however, is a general consensus centering on a worldview that embraces certain respected, if not universally shared, notions of Hindu tradition, belief, society, and ritual life. In an attempt to characterize Hindu tradition we may refer to those vast reservoirs of mythologies in the epics, the *Mahābhārata* and the *Rāmāyaṇa*, and in the eighteen great Purāṇas, largely but by no means solely concerned with the gods Viṣṇu and Śiva and the various manifestations of the Goddess. Along with the Tantras, Śāstras, Āgamas, and Yoga treatises, these mythological collections have shaped a common tradition that gradually supplanted the older Vedic heritage.

In seeking the fundamentals of Hindu belief we may isolate in particular the recognition of *karma* (a cosmic, impersonal accounting of individual human "action," by which past and present deeds bear consequences in present and future life conditions) and *saṃsāra* (rebirth, transmigration). For a Hindu they are virtually undisputed facts of existence, although the scope for interpretation is unlimited. As a response to doctrines of *karma* and *saṃsāra* Hindu belief has produced the key notion of *mokṣa* (liberation, release from *karma* and *saṃsāra*). While there are numerous designated paths to this transcendent state (devotion to a deity, meritorious behavior, ascetic technique, soteriological knowledge), there is general consensus that its attainment, even after some remote future existence, is the sine qua non of human life and the solution to the bondage of transmigration.

For a clear understanding of Hindu society we may refer to that vast and complicated hierarchical network of class and caste into which every Hindu is born and outside of which he or she may not be expected to function in the traditional sense. Family, clan, subcaste, caste, and village are the determinative social groups for the great majority of Hindus, although the structure of the hierarchies and the nature of the internal roles may vary from region to region.

In an attempt to explain Hindu ritual life we may speak first of a common set of devotional exercises in temple or shrine worship and to a lesser extent in domestic worship, second of a shared system of life-cycle rites that carry an individual in a single rebirth from conception to death and afterlife, and third of a general festival calendar, all three being universal in outline despite regional variations.

Although modernization and secularization are everywhere in evidence in South Asia today, the rural basis (80 percent) of the subcontinent has allowed Hinduism to exist in the present century in much the same fashion as it has in the previous twenty.

For a brief overview of the history of Hinduism we start by considering the evidence for religious experience in prehistory. In the subcontinent itself there is archaeological testimony for nomadic cattle-herders in the Deccan of South India from about 3000 BCE forward, and for agrarian societies as well, whose appearance is linked to developments in western Asia from the Mediterranean to the Persian Gulf and which underwent a relatively rapid transition from village to urban life along the Indus River and its tributaries by the middle of the third millennium BCE. The Indus civilization, with its major cities of Harappa and Mohenjo-daro, remains just beyond our comprehension, in part because the brief inscriptions that appear in those cities on excavated seals and sealings have not been solved. Great community baths, numerous human figures with animals and plants in apparent ceremonial poses, goddess figurines, a horned-animal deity, humped bull figures, and other items mark the antiquity of many standard elements of historic Hinduism.

Within roughly the same time frame as the collapse of the Indus cities, the middle of the second millennium BCE, successive waves of Indo-Aryan-speaking pastoral nomads arrived in the northwest who over a period of several centuries established themselves across most of northern India. These are the peoples whose oral texts, the Vedas, have already been mentioned. The *Ṛgveda, Atharvaveda,* and two other collections are only the beginning of a thousand-year literary production that lasted almost to the beginning of the Common Era and concluded with domestic ritual manuals as well as speculative texts of great power known as Upan-iṣads. At the very heart of this formative period, circa 1000–600 BCE, early ritual *sūtra*s and lengthy discourses termed Brāhmaṇas spelled out the details of a sacrificial worldview in which every aspect of cosmic and human life was perceived to be mysteriously connected by an intricate code of correspondences and to be governed by the priestly performance of great integrative sacrifices. Knowledge of the rituals and their numinous homologies became for these devotees little short of mastery of the universe.

Three aspects of this formative Vedic period in South Asia are significant for the purposes of this essay. First, and most important, the Vedic perception of the world, of the realm of the deities, and of human society was a tripartite hierarchic one based on a mystical division of the cosmos into earth, midspace, and heaven, of the gods into those resident in each of the three worlds, and of the humans into priests, warriors, and producers (with a subordinate fourth class of subjugated peoples). Our understanding of this Vedic worldview is enhanced by selected comparative studies, for it was the proto-Indo-Iranian pastoral nomads of Central Asia circa 2000 BCE and perhaps earlier who constructed a sacrificial worldview that eventually was to dominate the separate religious traditions of Iran and India. Proto-Indo-European studies of a period at yet a greater remove in time, circa 5000–3000 BCE, permit us an even deeper perspective for this tripartite ideology. Second, in the Vedic process of regenerating the cosmos via great schemes of sacrifices, a discovery was made: the sacrificer's real self, disclosed by ritual action, was perceived to be not only connected with an array of deities (Puruṣa, the original sacrificed person; Prajāpati, the supreme lord of creatures; and Agni, sacrificial fire), but actually to be, like them, impervious to change. Thus human effort, participant in cosmic laws concerning truth and order, apprehended a procedure by which the ravages of ordinary time and space might be overcome. Third, this Vedic sacrificial worldview, fusing convoluted details of ritual performance with speculations about the *results* of ritual action *(karma),* generated over the centuries an entirely new perspective, one that occurred in the Upaniṣads at the close of the period of Vedic textual creativity. This new ideology expressed from a sacrificial context the doctrines of *saṃsāra* and *karma,* closely connected beliefs concerning transmigration and the consequences of human action. While the sacrificial worldview had sought an extension of this good life to a point of cosmic identities, this new teaching of measureless cycles of death-and-births implied that existence itself is problematic. More than this, it also cradled a solution—the hope of salvation or release *(mokṣa)* from the bondage of *karma*. The latter was soon hypostatized as the accumulated binding results not only of ritual action but of all past action surrounding the eternal self.

These new doctrines signaled transformations in the second half of the first millennium BCE that were crucial to the shaping of Hinduism as we know it today. Such teachings challenged or augmented the authority of the Vedas and produced not only schools that quickly blossomed into great competitive religions, Jainism and Buddhism for example, but also experimental modes of thought that led in later centuries to India's six classical systems of philosophy. Among those most influential in their long-range impact on Hinduism were Vedānta, Sāṃkhya, and Yoga. Other post-Vedic categories of oral (later written) traditions included codes of religious law that reflected the new age, as well as the two great epics, the *Mahābhārata* and the *Rāmāyaṇa*. Each genre gave expression in versatile and increasingly popular form to significant ancient themes of deities, heroes, and sacred geographies north and south. In the same half-millennium there was also a rise of sectarian theisms centering upon devotion to two relatively minor Vedic deities, Rudra-Śiva and Viṣṇu, whose varied guises and strong capacities to absorb regional cults and mythologies propelled them eventually into supremacy in the hearts of the Śaivas and Vaiṣṇavas respectively. Further transformations in the society were evident in the solidification of hierarchies; a four- or five-class system proliferated into a network of "kinds of beings" *(jāti*s), resulting in the ranking of individuals into castes (and resulting in a distinct rupture between caste and noncaste status). At the same time that Vedic sacrifice received competition from increasingly complex patterns of worship of deities in homes, shrines, and temples, a program of individual religious life was expanded into stages (the four echelons of student, householder, mendicant, and renunciant), three aims of existence (passion, wealth, and the religious quest or *dharma*), and an increasingly elaborate set of rites of passage that eventually achieved pan-Indian popularity.

By the fourth century CE both Sanskrit epics were well established, thus providing complementary centerpieces of Hindu mythology and folklore that eventually were to gain counterparts in several regional vernaculars. In the same century the Sāṃkhya philosophy was textually grounded, and Patañjali's *Yoga Sūtra*s shortly thereafter became the focus for classical Yoga. These two systems shared many doctrines, including the important notion of three *guṇa*s ("threads," "strands"), the constituents of nature *(prakṛti)* as distinct from pure consciousness *(puruṣa)*. In accordance with other paradigmatic tripartitions, the *guṇas* were hierarchized: *sattva* (brightness, goodness, purity, intelligibility) as the highest constituent, *rajas* (passion, activity) as mediating constituent, and *tamas* (inertia, darkness, impurity) as lowest constituent. As there is in the Chinese yin-yang philosophy a twofold mixture, so in Sāṃkhya and Yoga there is a threefold blend: all of nature is essentially an interwoven composition of three strands, two of them in counterpoint, the third in dynamic mediation and transformation. These strands are associated with the three worlds in hierarchy—sky or heaven above, midspace or atmosphere *(rajas)* as a realm of mediation, and earth or netherworld below.

At this point Indian civilization could be said to have concluded its ancient period and entered a classical era, a "golden age" of Sanskrit literature, art, architecture, and philosophy, due in large measure to the creative prosperity of the Gupta dynasty, circa 300–500 CE. This was a period in which additional collections of mythology, folklore, and temple-centered rites and symbols were assembled as Purāṇas, a specific genre in Sanskrit that remained vigorous through the medieval period. The circulation of these Purāṇas throughout the subcontinent permitted regional voices to harmonize in a pan-Indian faith. As one example, thousands of local cobra *(nāga)* cults and lores were eventually shaken down to a few basic myths and to a recognized date in the lunar calendars, Nāgapañcamī, the day when everybody worships and honors serpents. A second example is the pan-Indian recognition of great pilgrimage goals, or *tīrthas*—temples, cities, mountains, and rivers of fabled power that had to be seen and experienced by devout Hindus. Late in the classical age appeared the *Devī Māhātmya*, a text elevating the Goddess in her numerous manifestations. Also in the sixth century another genre emerged: the Tantras, reflecting not only the increasing popularity and institutionalization of South Asia's age-old Goddess traditions, but also an increasing preoccupation with the body as the locus of liberation and transcendence. Ancient statements of divine androgyny, for example, were stirred into a blend of esoteric philosophy and symbolism, antinomian ritual, and radical yoga that typified tantric Hinduism.

The medieval period, circa 700–1750 CE, witnessed the continued aggregation and circulation of Purāṇas until a collection of them existed that rivaled the epics and attained a mystical number of eighteen texts. By this time their sectarian tendencies were pronounced. For example, the *Bhāgavata Purāṇa*, among the most popular of all, favored a cycle of myths concerning the Kṛṣṇa *avatāra* (incarnation) of supreme Viṣṇu, just as the Śiva Purāṇa brought into view the several *avatāra*s (among whom was the terrifying Bhairava) of that outsider deity of asceticism, death, and destruction, namely, the great lord Śiva. In this period also came numerous poet-saints to sing the praises of gods and goddesses in regional languages, augmenting the Sanskrit Purāṇas, Tantras, and Śāstras with their emphases on devotion *(bhakti)* as the path to liberation, a path already illuminated in the *Bhagavadgītā,* the classic treatise incorporated in the *Mahābhāabarata* epic, and in the vivid poetry of classical Tamil in southern India. Philosophical syntheses, particularly those generated by Hinduism's two prominent religious thinkers, Śaṅkara in the eighth century and Rāmānuja in the twelfth, were responsible for much of the intellectual framework for medieval and modern Hindu thought. Finally, it was also in the medieval period, beginning in the eighth century and accelerating in the sixteenth and seventeenth centuries during the Mughal dynasty, that Islam worked its creative impact upon South Asian history and culture.

Modern South Asia, circa 1750 to the present, is coterminous with the advent of European colonial powers, the British Rāj (until independence in 1947), and the formation of several new nation-states, including Sri Lanka, Pakistan, Bangladesh, and others. A number of reform movements, particularly evident in the nineteenth century, were concomitants of the new cosmopolitan atmosphere of the modern era and of a new self-consciousness confined for the most part to urban India. The arrival of the age of television in the 1970s and 1980s may signal radical changes, but still evident in the late twentieth century are the remarkable durability of the Hindu tradition and of devotional theism in particular, as well as a striking capacity for self-renewal and reintegration. Modernism and secularism seem at times to be not so much threats as challenges to creativity, and such appears to be the case in urban areas today as well as in villages and towns.

In sum, this capsule overview of significant periods in the history of Hinduism calls attention to a constructive and transitional age following the completion of Vedic oral traditions with the Upaniṣads. In this era the basic doctrines of *karma, saṃsāra,* and *mokṣa* were maturing, the great epics were in creative oral process, and sectarian literatures, institutions, arts, and iconographies were ripening. Although historians uniformly locate "classical India" in the period 300–700 CE, we note here that Hinduism received its definitive texts and characteristics in this late ancient and preclassical period, in the last few centuries before, and the first few centuries after, the Common Era began.

Medicine and the South Asian Worldview

South Asian prehistory has provided us with scant evidence for medical traditions in either the civilization of the Indus Valley or the post-Harappan settlement areas of the subcontinent. We must turn again to the Vedic tradition for the oldest expressions, particularly in the period of oral textual creativity from about 1400 to 300 BCE, with its tighter focus on the shaping of a sacrificial worldview about 1000 to 600. Once again there is the benefit of comparative studies, the attempts to reconstruct the proto-Indo-Iranian and much deeper proto-Indo-European evidence. These include, for example, the micro-macrocosmic elements of wind, fire, and water; the trifunctionally hierarchic social classes and their three methods of healing—oral (pronouncing mantras), surgical (employing knives), and pharmacological (applying herbs and spells); and the close correlation of the third estate, the producers, involved in animal husbandry, agriculture, and crafts, with the healing arts. There too one finds the mythologies of the divine physicians, as well as myths and cults centering upon a sacred celestial plant of remedies, poetic visions, even immortality. In a different set of myths, more shadowed and uneven, one finds as well individual and aggregate feminine powers of disease, death, and destiny.

In the *Ṛgveda* there are numerous hymns to and about the divine twin physicians known as the Aśvins (or Nāsatyas), who are embedded in the mythologies of horses, the sun and the dawn, immortality, the healing of the gods, restoration of the head of the sacrificial victim, and the deliverance of humans from the pit of old age, disease, and death. Reflected herein is the mortal counterpart of this divine role, the human physician (*bhiṣaj*) with his healing charms, remedies, and techniques. The entire ninth book of the *Ṛgveda* is devoted to *soma*, the divine plant of poetic inspiration and regeneration and the primary victim, along with domestic animals, of the great cosmogonic sacrifices. Thus human transformations, according to the Vedic myth-ritual system, are inextricably bound to the deliberate (ritual) transformations of both plant and animal substances, and Brahmanic correspondences could not fail to highlight the mystical exchanges involving breath, heat, waters, food, speech, and being in all the three worlds. But it is in the *Atharvaveda*, as we have noted above, that the earliest literary evidence for traditional medicine occurs. Its 730 hymns in twenty books include descriptions of diseases and prescriptions of magical-ritual remedies and charms. The *Kauśika Sūtra*, a text preserved by a later Atharvan school, is a lengthy handbook that unravels much of the mystery and ritual context of this fourth Veda.

Although it seems clear that already in the late centuries before the Common Era a proto-Āyurveda slowly began to compete with and then replace Vedic traditional medicine, including this thousand-year-old Atharvan medical lore, the latter did not disappear completely, and it is known in remnant form in Annapuram, as we have had occasion to see. And there are in the vicinity of Annapuram today brahman *soma*-sacrificers who still perform the animal sacrifices according to the earliest Vedic ritual texts: they themselves—not their nonbrahman assistants—carve the goats or other victims for offering-pieces "like doctors," as they say, for their ancient art of dissection is subsumed into the higher purpose of reintegration, wholeness, perfection. The perfect sacrifice does not degenerate. There is no doubt that such meticulous sacrificial practices in antiquity, with careful attention to enumeration of parts and their human as well as cosmic correspondences, produced a developing sacred lore of anatomy. In addition, certain ancient Vedic ascetic techniques appearing in rituals such as the *dīkṣā*—an intense preparation for and transformation into the consecrated statuses of sacrificer and sacrificer's wife—allowed for considerable yogalike physiological experimentation in the long history of Vedic spirituality.

The Indian heritage, with an eye that is characteristically more observant of mythic than historic continuities, regarded Āyurveda as an extension of the Atharvan or other schools. But for the greater part of its long history Āyurveda has properly recognized a set of three basic texts as authoritative. The earliest of them was post-Vedic by a century or more, and none of the three holds any historic position in the multiple textual and scholastic lineages of the Vedic tradition. Each, however, stands clearly in a recognized textual tradition that is perhaps no later than the final two centuries BCE. All three were transmitted in Sanskrit, the classical language of the Dharmaśāstras, epics, philosophical schools, and Purāṇas. It is important to note here that the last two or three centuries BCE in which the roots of proto-Āyurveda were taking hold are the same centuries credited with the consolidation of classical Hinduism. By this time the Vedic sacrificial worldview had given space to evolved doctrines of *saṃsāra* and *karma*; epic traditions were well underway toward pan-Indian textual prominence; sectarian traditions of the great deities Viṣṇu and Śiva were productive mythically, iconographically, and architecturally, with new temple traditions to support them; and foundations were in place for a later synthesis of multiregional Purāṇas that eventually were to comprise a pan-Indian faith. It was in this same milieu, wherein worldview, myth, and cult were redirected and reshaped, that Āyurveda blossomed. Texts known as the Vedāṅgas, "limbs of the Veda," containing ritual and textual sciences such as astronomy, metrics, phonetics, and etymology, had long since added to this climate of inquiry and experimentation. Another lengthy textual tradition culminated in the *Yoga Sūtra*s of Patañjali, including archaic techniques of asceticism and meditation concerned with recognition of the body as cosmos, bodily postures (*āsanas*), interior correlations of triadic and pentadic winds, control of the breath (*prāṇāyama*), and so forth.

Out of this multifaceted environment came the earliest of the three most authoritative texts of Āyurveda, that of the writer Caraka, a work known as the *Caraka Saṃhitā* or "collection."[3] (Among surviving texts the *Bhela Saṃhitā* may possibly be older, but it is known only in one incomplete manuscript.) Caraka, by tradition the editor of an older text known as the *Agniveśa Tantra*, covers subjects recognizable to any student of comparative medicine who begins with Mediterranean nomenclature: pharmacology, dietetics, therapeutics, physiology, anatomy, embryology, pathology, epidemiology, diagnosis, and prognosis. But laced into these discourses are other subjects—for example, accounts of longevity (Āyurveda being the knowledge, *veda*, of a life, *āyus*, that is hopefully prolonged); relationships between the five sense organs (eyes, ears, nostrils, tongue, skin) and the five elements (*bhūtas*) of the cosmos; basic human desires; types and qualifications of physicians; lists of tastes; types of patients; correspondences between the gods and the ages of the worlds on one hand and the emotions of a human and his phases in a single life cycle on the other; the soul and its liberation (*mokṣa*) from bondage to transmigration; and the many signs and portents of a patient's death.

As an example of the Ayurvedic tradition to be found in the *Caraka Saṃhitā*, chapters 2–4 of the fourth section (which is on the Śarīrasthāna or division of medicine concerning the body, *śarīra*) discuss the formation of a human embryo and the evolution of the fetus. This new being is described as a replica of the cosmos (4.4.13; cf. 4.5.1–26) and thus an embodiment of all aspects of the universe, material both in gross form (the five elements of space, wind, fire, water, and earth) and in subtle form (consciousness, described in this section of the text as a sixth element). The self or soul (*ātman*) of this being, engaged in the process of transmigration from material body to material body and determined by the results of its past actions (*karma*), takes up residence in an embryo (*garbha*) in the mother. This embryo or incipient fetus is a composite of organic contributions from the mother (blood, skin, flesh, fat, heart, and other internal organs) and from the father (semen, bones, teeth, nails, hair, veins and arteries, ligaments), a composite now placed under the direction of a consciousness associated with the *ātman*, but never the same as the *ātman*. The discussion then continues with a month-by-month evolution of the fetus during the constant transformation of food into essential bodily fluid (*rasa*).

The second of the three traditional texts of classical Āyurveda is the *Suśruta Saṃhitā*,[4] a work displaying the same range of subjects as *Caraka* but going beyond the latter in its expansive discussions of surgery (*śalya*, "arrow," so named because of the frequency of military patients' need for skilled attention). Surgical techniques gave Āyurveda great fame in the early medieval world, and the name of the surgeon Suśruta became known from the Mediterranean to Southeast Asia. After establishing surgery as the most ancient and pivotal branch of medicine and reminding the hearer or reader of the myth of the Aśvins wherein these divine surgeons restored the severed head of the Sacrifice (a mysterious and life-maintaining cosmic entity) Suśruta proceeds to detail the types of surgical instruments, such as forceps, tongs, and tubes, and to give instruction on incision, cauterization, extraction, piercing, tying, and so forth, advising that these procedures be carried out on such practice objects as full water bags, animal bladders, gourds, and other nonhuman materials. It might be mentioned here that dissection of a human corpse was accomplished, according to *Suśruta Saṃhitā* 3.5.49–56, by securing it for seven days in a river, then brushing away the decomposed flesh in order to observe the details of each organ. A remarkable passage (4.29), ritualistic in structure and symbolism, deals with rejuvenation of a patient (who must necessarily be from one of the privileged three twice-born classes) by means of the sacred pressed *soma* juice, whereafter the patient might enjoy his new body on the full-moon day of the fourth month of treatment.

The "eight limbs" *(aṣṭāṅga)* or divisions of medical science—*aṣṭāṅga* is a popular synonym for medicine still employed today—were perpetuated in the third and latest of the three great traditional texts, the *Aṣṭāṅgahṛdaya Saṃhitā* of Vāgbhaṭa II, dated within the seventh or eighth century CE.[5] Yet another compendium of these limbs was the *Aṣṭāṅga Saṃgraha* of Vāgbhaṭa I, compiled perhaps a century or more earlier but not as illustrious a text in the tradition of medical literature.

Subsequently in the medieval period other Sanskrit medical compilations appeared. Chief among them was the *Mādhava Nidāna*, a systematic enumeration of diseases and the principal Ayurvedic text on diagnosis *(nidāna)*.[6] Written by Mādhava about 800 CE, it remains the most significant work outside of the three classics. By this time the texts of both Caraka and Suśruta had been translated into Persian and Arabic. Other important medieval works included the *Siddhiyoga* of Vṛinda, a text on therapeutics; the *Cikitsāsāra Saṃgraha*, another work on therapeutics written about 1060 CE by the prolific Bengali author Cakrapāṇidatta (who also composed the *Āyurveda Dīpikā*, an influential commentary on the *Caraka Saṃhitā*, as well as the *Bhānumatī*, a commentary on *Suśruta*); the *Śabda Pradīpa* of Sureśvara, circa 1075 CE, a dictionary of medical botany in the genre of glossaries; and two twelfth-century works, one the *Śārṅgadhara Saṃhitā*, a treatise in which diagnosis by pulse rate was first described in South Asia, the other the *Nibandha Saṃgraha* of Ḍalhaṇa, another important commentary on the *Suśruta Saṃhitā*.

In the medieval period of South Asian history there appeared two substantial medical traditions to rival Āyurveda. One of these, Ūnānī medicine, an eclectic tradition based upon Arabic and Persian texts, called "Ionian" because of its dependence on Greek medicine, was established in western Asia by a combination of Nestorian Christian and Muslim translators and physicians. Textual and oral traditional knowledge of Āyurveda was already a part of the milieu in Baghdad in the early Abbasid caliphate prior to the entry of Ūnānī medicine into South Asia via various Arabic, Turkish, Afghan, and Persian Muslim migrations. Ūnānī medicine and the *hakīm*s who practiced it became widespread, particularly during the expansion of the Mughal empire in the sixteenth and seventeenth centuries. *Tibb* became a term for a South Asian synthesis of Hindu and Muslim folk or popular medical traditions. The other rival to Āyurveda, Siddha, was derived largely from Āyurveda itself in Sri Lanka and Tamil Nadu but it proceeded from a unique philosophical perspective and depended upon Tamil as well as Sanskrit textual transmission.

Modern South Asia, from about 1750 to the present, has witnessed the proliferation of a cosmopolitan medicine established by European and then American missionaries and physicians from the late sixteenth to the twentieth centuries. For the past hundred years some Indian physicians have received part or all of their training in the West. Certain anomalous Western systems such as homeopathy were also imported and then variously modified by Āyurveda, Ūnānī, and Siddha. As in the case of its predecessor from western Asia, Ūnānī, homeopathy fares well in South Asia today, whereas both are virtually extinct in their respective lands of origin. In the fertile soil of medical pluralism in traditional India Āyurveda thus faced powerful new competitors once again in the modern period, in addition to the constant pressure through the centuries from a vigorous battery of nontextual and largely noninstitutional folk medical traditions. Hinduism as a pan-Indian faith was itself under attack from both religious and secular ideologies from the West. And yet Āyurveda, like Hinduism, actually experienced a revival in the nineteenth century that continued into the late twentieth century, with particular expansion in the decade following Indian independence, that is, in the 1950s. This revival assured South Asia of a dual medical system with hospitals, clinics, medical colleges, and registration of physicians for both indigenous medicine, including Āyurveda, and for modern cosmopolitan medicine.

In sum, a chronological ordering of the medical traditions that appeared in South Asia would have to include the Vedic, Ayurvedic, Ūnānī, Siddha, "allopathic" or cosmopolitan, and homeopathic systems, all with substantial classical and popular literatures and institutional structures. A sixth tradition, which may be classed under the umbrella of folk medicine, is more or less visible as an amorphous and eclectic substratum throughout this chronology, a substratum largely discovered in regional oral traditions that occasionally intersect with the literate ones. Of these six it is Āyurveda (and its regional variant, Siddha) whose history and development are inextricably linked with Hinduism. Again it is instructive to note that classical Hindu medicine produced its basic traditions and texts in the very period, the late centuries BCE and early centuries CE, in which Hinduism found its own definitive statements. The particular human physiology that undergirds classical and modern Āyurveda cannot be understood apart from the Hindu worldview. It is that physiology, a product of combined religious and empirical inquiry, to which we now turn.

Āyurveda in Theory and Practice

If Āyurveda is sought as an independent, secular science of medicine, the picture that emerges is surrealistic and incongruous, a tradition front and center stage with the South Asian or Hindu worldview as remote backdrop. If on the other hand the focus is first upon the worldview, then Āyurveda is more correctly perceived as participant and interdependent, a tradition responsible to its cultural matrix because of its several charters—mythic, ritual, and social. Let us examine these charters, beginning with the mythic function and employing Suśruta's chapter on *soma* as an illustration. Āyurveda, as an extension of the sacred cosmic utterance *brahman*, can be appreciated as an oral textual lineage descended from the *Atharvaveda*, whose wisdom is originally derived from the creator god Brahmā. Again, the god Dhanvantari, divine physician, is connected to the primordial event of the churning of the cosmic ocean, one of the most prominent of all motifs in the epics and Purāṇas (*Mahābhārata*, *Matsya Purāṇa*, *Viṣṇu Purāṇa*, etc.). Dhanvantari emerges as divine provider of a bowl containing the *amṛta* or *soma*, the liquid essence of immortal life. As pupil of both great deities, Viṣṇu and Śiva, Dhanvantari thus embodies the wisdom of healing and is regarded as the crucial link to the practical world of the human physician. The eight branches of medicine are thus according to Suśruta a divine provision for humankind.

A second charter of Āyurveda is its context of ritual, which at times seems more properly called magico-ritual. The symbolic use of *soma* for rejuvenation has already been described. Suśruta, like a well-trained pharmacologist, lists no fewer than twenty-four types of *soma* and goes on to a generic description of season, color, smell, and other characteristics. His eye for detail is not that of the Vedic ritualist—rather that of the physician, always on therapy and its course; but his charter is formulaic action in faith, faith in the context of myth. If his patient does not win immortality, as guaranteed by the ritualist, at least he will have ten thousand years. And the *soma* so carefully described, according to Suśruta, is entirely invisible to one without faith.

The third charter for Āyurveda is social. The *vaidya*s of Caraka's and Suśruta's age were drawn from the three basic social classes, the *brāhmaṇa*s (priests), *kṣatriya*s (warriors), and *vaiśya*s (producers), and the same three classes, as we have seen, were alone eligible for therapy by *soma* juice. Of these three charters set in the classical context of an archaic *soma* myth and ritual it is perhaps the last that is least apparent in the modern period, as we have observed in the practice of the *vaidyācārya* of Annapuram.

More significant is the manner in which Āyurveda has redirected the archaic and hierarchic tripartite worldview, with all of its mythic, ritual, and social constructs, to serve the purposes of a new post-Vedic medical tradition and its newly articulated physiology.[7] The central concern of Āyurveda is management, that is, maintaining or restoring order in the body system. The body of disease (*vyādhi*) is one in disorder and imbalance; the challenge to the physician is one of recalling harmony. Moving with, and then beyond the triadic, pentadic, and septadic symbol systems of the Vedic worldview, the epic and Puranic cosmographies, and the Sāṃkhya, Yoga, and Vaiśeṣika philosophies, Āyurveda retained the notion of micro-macrocosmic correspondences but employed them for other ends. The *vaidyas'* consuming preoccupation with the components of the body, the materia medica, and the typologies of symptoms directed them to take the body for real, and to abandon older notions in which the body and its processes were metaphors. Like the Greek physicians no longer stirred by the Eleusinian mysteries, Caraka and Suśruta withheld credit from the transcendent, transformative powers of sacrifice.

Basic to their scheme is the theory of the three humors (*tridoṣa*). The body consists of wind (*vāta*), bile (*pitta*), and phlegm (*kapha* or *śleṣman*), all in equilibrium in the body of health, just as the cosmic body of three worlds (*loka*s) and the human social body of three classes (*varṇa*s) are hierarchically triadic in world-maintaining harmony. The five elements (*bhūta*s)—earth, water, fire, air, and space—make up each of the three *doṣa*s or humors. Each *doṣa* is related to one of the three universal qualities (*guṇa*s), again a hierarchical set (*sattva, rajas, tamas*), and, furthermore, each *doṣa* is itself pentadic. For example, the human correspondent to cosmic wind, *vāta*, is not respiration dependent upon the lung-organ, but rather an entire system of five breaths with specialized functions and locations. Such duties and positions are critical, for loss of performance or separation results in system breakdown or confusion—and because humoral balance is difficult to maintain, an extended meaning of *doṣa* is in fact "fault." An additional pentad in this Hindu physiology is the set of five sense organs (*indriyas*) and five perceptions associated with them. Finally, in the same period in which the Yoga and Vaiśeṣika philosophies and Puranic mythologies expanded the Vedic cosmos and human body-as-cosmos from three or five levels to seven-leveled entities, employing septadic expressions for general categories or for micro-macrocosmic correlations, Ayurvedic tradition, not content with retaining the three pentadic *doṣa*s as humors and the five *bhūta*s as elements in the body, recognized seven substantial constituents (*dhātu*s): nutrient fluid obtained from digested food (*rasa*), blood (*rakta*), flesh (*māṃsa*), fat (*medas*), bone (*asthi*), marrow (*majjan*), and semen (*śukra*). All seven develop in sequence, via internal transformations, from *rasa*, which, incidentally, is an ancient epithet of *soma*. *Rasa* is the sap or essential fluid of the mortal body, *soma* the divinely obtained essence of immortality. The circularity of cosmic essence is further reinforced by the fact that *śukra* is also equivalent to *soma* in ancient reference.

Thus an archaic physiology concerned with the flow of breath, semen, and blood and with the interaction of cosmic and human substances was modified for centuries by a South Asian propensity to experiment with the body (through Vedic sacrifice, animal dissection, the *dīkṣā* consecration rite, yogic postures, breath-control, diet, and purifications); and a propensity as well to transcend the body and its limitations. This physiology finally established itself in the classical Ayurvedic treatises that still are the students' handbooks. Side by side in Annapuram today are the priest—who refers to *amṛta* ("nondeath") on the transcendent plane of *mokṣa*, final liberation from *saṃsāra*, the endless round of births and deaths—and the physician—who refers to long life *(āyus)* on the immanent plane of *dharma*, ordered existence that is firmly set *within* the confines of *saṃsāra*.

Notes

1. See Kenneth G. Zysk, *Religious Healing in the Veda*, Transactions of the American Philosophical Society, new ser., vol. 75 (1985), pt. 7. This volume includes translations and annotations of medical hymns from the *Ṛgveda* and *Atharvaveda* and renderings from the corresponding ritual texts. Other sources that explore the worldviews and medical traditions discussed in this chapter are: "New Research on Traditional Medicine in South Asia: A Symposium," *Social Science and Medicine* 17 (1983):933–84; *South Asian Systems of Healing*, eds. E. Valentine Daniel and Judy F. Pugh, Contributions to Asian Studies 18 (Leiden, 1984); Daniel C. Tabor, "Ripe and Unripe: Concepts of Health and Sickness in Ayurvedic Medicine," *Social Science and Medicine* 15B (1981):439–455; Jean Varenne, *Yoga and the Hindu Tradition*, trans. Derek Coltman (Chicago, 1976); Margaret Trawick Egnor, "Death and Nurturance in Indian Systems of Healing," *Social Science and Medicine* 17 (1983):933–984; Charles Leslie, "The Professionalizing Ideology of Medical Revivalism," in *Entrepreneurship and Modernization of Occupational Cultures in South Asia*, ed. Milton Singer (Durham, NC, 1973), pp. 216–242; Surendra Nath Dasgupta, "Speculations in the Medical Schools," vol. 2, chap. 13 of *A History of Indian Philosophy* (Cambridge, England, 1932); Julius Jolly, *Indian Medicine*, trans. C. G. Kashikar (Poona-New Delhi, 1951); three works by Priya Vrat Sharma, namely, *Indian Medicine in the Classical Age* (Banaras, 1972), *Introduction to Dravyaguna (Indian pharmacology)* (Banaras, 1976), and *Dravyaguna-vijñāna*, 6 vols. (Banaras, 1977–1983); David M. Knipe, *In the Image of Fire: Vedic Experiences of Heat* (Delhi, 1975); Bruce Lincoln, *Myth, Cosmos, and Society: Indo-European Themes of Creation and Destruction* (Cambridge, MA, 1986); Jahn Puhvel, "Mythological Reflections of Indo-European Medicine," in *Indo-European and Indo-Europeans*, eds. G. Cardona et al. (Philadelphia, 1970), pp. 369–

382; Ellison Banks Findly, "Breath and Breathing," *Encyclopedia of Religion* (New York, 1986); Karl H. Potter, "Guṇas," *Encyclopedia of Religion*; Mitchell G. Weiss, "Caraka Saṃhitā on the Doctrine of Karma," in *Karma and Rebirth*, ed. Wendy D. O'Flaherty (Berkeley, 1980), pp. 90–115; and three studies by Francis Zimmerman, "Ṛtu-sātmya: The Seasonal Cycle and the Principle of Appropriateness," *Social Science and Medicine* 14B (1980):99–106, *The Jungle and the Aroma of Meats: An Ecological Theme in Hindu Medicine* (Berkeley, 1987), and "Le discours des remèdes au pays des épices: Recherches ethnologiques et epistémologiques sur la tradition classique de la médecine hindoue chez les brahmanes *ashtavaidya* du Kerala," 2 vols. (unpublished manuscript, Paris, 1986).

2. All technical terms mentioned in this essay are in Sanskrit, the major literary language of Hinduism and of the classical medical traditions, unless another language is specified (as in this case, *vaid*, which is employed in all the modern vernaculars).

3. *Agniveśa's Caraka Saṃhitā*, ed. and trans. Ram Karan Sharma and Bhagwan Das, 2 vols. (Banaras, 1976–1977).

4. *The Suśruta Saṃhitā*, ed. and trans. Kunjalal Bhishagratna, 3 vols. (1907–1916; reprint, Banaras, 1981).

5. *Vāgbhata's Aṣṭāngahṛdayasaṃhitā*, ed. and trans. Claus Vogel (Wiesbaden, 1965). This volume contains the first five chapters of its Tibetan version.

6. *The Mādhavanidāna and its chief commentary*, ed. and trans. Gerrit J. Meulenbeld (Leiden, 1974), chaps. 1–10.

7. See further my *In the Image of Fire: Vedic Experiences of Heat*, pp. 1ff., 90 ff.

CHAPTER 5

Health and Medicine in the Living Traditions of Hinduism

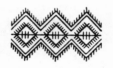

SUDHIR KAKAR

Ramnath is a fifty-one-year-old man who owns a grocery shop in the old-est part of the city of Delhi. When he came to see me he was suffering from a number of complaints, though he desired my help for only one of them—an unspecified "fearfulness," which became especially acute in the company of his father. This anxiety, less than three years old, was a relatively new development. His migraine headaches, on the other hand, went back to his adolescence. Ramnath attributed them to an excess of "wind" in the stomach, which periodically rose up and pressed against the veins in his head. This diagnosis had been arrived at in consultation

111

with doctors of traditional Indian medicine, Āyurveda, and the condition was treated with Ayurvedic drugs and dietary restrictions, as well as liberal doses of aspirin.

Ramnath had always had a nervous stomach, though it was never quite as bad as in the early months of his marriage some thirty years earlier. Then he had suffered from severe stomach cramps and an alarming weight loss. He was first taken to the hospital by his father, where he was x-rayed and tested. Finding nothing wrong with him, the doctors had prescribed a variety of vitamins and tonics that had not been of much help. Older family members and friends had then recommended a nearby *ojhā*—"sorcerer" is too fierce a translation for this mild-mannered professional of ritual exorcism—who diagnosed his condition as the result of magic practiced by an enemy. The enemy was further identified as Ramnath's newly acquired father-in-law. The rituals to counteract the enemy magic were expensive, as was the yellowish liquid emetic prescribed by the *ojhā* which periodically emptied Ramnath's stomach in gasping heaves. In any event, he was fully cured within two months of the *ojhā*'s treatment, and this particular problem had not recurred.

For the gradually worsening arthritic condition of his right arm, Ramnath had turned to homeopathy after the obligatory but futile consultations with the "allopath," as the Western-style doctor is called in India in contradistinction to practitioners of other medical systems. Homeopathy, too, had failed, and Ramnath had then consulted the priest-healer of a local temple who was well known for his expertise in curing pains of the joints. The priest prescribed a round of *pūjā*s or prayers together with dietary restrictions, such as the avoidance of yogurt and especially butter. The remedies had not worked.

Ramnath's "fearfulness" had been treated with drugs by various doctors—allopaths as well as homeopaths, the *vaid*s of Hindu medicine as well as the *hakim*s of Islamic tradition. He had consulted psychiatrists, ingested psychotropic drugs, and submitted to electroconvulsive therapy. He had gone through the rituals of two *ojhā*s and was thinking of consulting a highly recommended third one.

The only relief came through the weekly Satsang, the gathering of the local chapter of the Brahmakumari (literally, "Virgins of Brahma") sect which he had recently joined. The communal meditations and singing gave him a feeling of peace, and his nights were no longer as restless. Ramnath was naturally puzzled by the persistence of his anxiety state and by his other ailments. He had tried to be a good man, he said, both according to the *dharma*, the "right conduct" of his caste and the limits imposed by his own character and predispositions. He had worshiped the gods and attended the services in the temple with regularity, even contributing a generous sum toward the consecration of the Krishna idol in the temple of his native village in Rajasthan. He did not have any bad habits, he asserted. Tea and cigarettes, yes, but since a couple of years ago he had abjured even these minor though pleasurable addictions. Yet the anxiety persisted, unremitting and unrelenting.

In this essay, contrary to my actual handling of Ramnath's case, I am concerned neither with a psychological understanding of his symptoms nor with the tracing of their genesis in his life history. My purpose is to understand Ramnath's ailments and his efforts toward the restoration of his well-being against the background of his cultural tradition. In other words, the aim is to essay a cultural analysis rather than a psychoanalysis of Ramnath's condition, which will help us in becoming explicitly aware of the nature of health and illness in the Indian setting.

At first glance, Ramnath's cognitive space in matters of illness and well-being seems incredibly cluttered. Gods and spirits, community and family, food and drink, personal habits and character, all seem to be somehow intimately involved in the maintenance of health. Yet these and other factors such as biological infection, social pollution, and cosmic displeasure, all of which Hindus would also acknowledge as causes of ill health, only point to the recognition of a person's simultaneous existence in different orders of being. To use Western categories, from the first birth cry to the last breath, an individual exists equally in his or her *soma, psyche,* and *polis;* in other words, a person is simultaneously a body, a self, and a social being. Ramnath's experience of his illness may appear alien to non-Hindus only because of the fact that the body, the self, and the polis do not possess fixed, immutable meanings across cultures. The concept of the body and the understanding of its processes are not quite the same in India as they are in the West. The self—the Hindu "subtle body"—is not primarily a psychological category in India, though it does include something of the Western psyche. Similarly, for most Hindus, the polis consists not only of living members of the family and community, but of ancestral spirits, other spirit helpers, and the familiar gods and goddesses who populate the Indian cosmos.

Subjectively, then, a Hindu is inclined to believe that his or her illness can reflect a disturbance in any one of the orders of being, while the symptoms may also be manifested in the other orders. If a treatment, say in the bodily order, fails, one is quite prepared to reassign the cause of the illness to a different order and undergo its particular curing regimen— the *pūjās* or the exorcisms, for instance—without losing regard for other methods of treatment.

A pluralistic openness and a willingness to accept all orders of existence as possible sources of ill health, however, does not mean that each can indiscriminately substitute for the other in case of a particular disease or class of diseases. For example, until recently most Hindus assumed that the occurrence of measles, smallpox, chicken pox, and cholera was due to the visitations of certain disease-specific goddesses. The propitiation of these goddesses—who were known by different names in different parts of the country—was the main method of treatment.

The involvement of all orders of being in health and illness also means that a Hindu is generally inclined to seek more than one cause for illness in especially intractable cases. A Hindu tends to view these causes as complementary rather than exclusive and arranges them in a hierarchical order by identifying an immediate cause as well as others that are more peripheral and remote. The causes are arranged in concentric circles, with the outer circle including all the inner ones. To continue with our example: Ramnath, in concordance with Ayurvedic theory, which provides the governing paradigm for the explanation of physiological processes in Hindu India, may identify his arthritic pain as a humoral disequilibrium, say an excess of *vāyu* or wind, which needs to be balanced through diet, drugs, and external applications. The disequilibrium may be further felt to be compounded by personal conduct—bad thoughts, habits—which, in turn, demand changes at the level of the self. The fact that the disease persists or is manifested with such stubborn intensity may be linked with his astrologically bad times, requiring palliative measures, such as the *pūjā*. The astrological "fault" will probably be further traced back to the bad *karma* of a previous birth about which, finally, nothing can be done— except, perhaps, the cultivation of a stoic endurance with the help of the weekly meetings of the Brahmakumari sect.

Like most Hindus, Ramnath's image of his body and bodily processes in which he would locate the first circle of any physical illness is still governed by the precepts of traditional Indian medicine, Āyurveda. Āyurveda, of course, is more than a system of physical medicine. Its notions of the constituents of the person; one's limits and extension in time; the nature of one's connection with the natural environment and with the psyche (and soul); the nature of the body's relationship with the psyche, the polis, and the cosmos in determining health and illness—Āyurveda comprises all of these, though in the individual they may not always be at a conscious level. Yet these ideas constitute the cultural prism through which men and women throughout South Asia have traditionally viewed the person and his or her state of well-being. As Gananath Obeyesekere has remarked: "Without some awareness of the theory of Ayurvedic medicine it is not possible for us to understand much of what goes on in the minds of men in the South Asian world."[1]

Body, Nature, and Health

Following the Indian philosophical tradition, Āyurveda holds that everything in the universe, animate or inanimate, is made up of five forms of matter—earth, fire, wind, water, and *ākāśa* (roughly translated as ether).

Under certain favorable conditions, matter becomes organized in the form of living creatures. These living creatures constantly absorb the five elements contained in environmental matter (nutrition), which is transformed by the fires in the body into a fine portion and refuse. Successive transformations of the fine portion of food produce the seven physiological elements—"organic sap," blood, flesh, fat, bone, marrow, and semen—as well as the substances constituting the sense organs, body joints, ligaments, and so forth. Nutrition, then, is of critical import. "Food sustains the lives of living beings. Complexion, clarity, good voice, longevity, genius, happiness, satisfaction, nourishment, strength, and intellect are all conditioned by food."[2]

The body, like nature with its ceaseless transformations of matter, is in a perpetual state of flux. The ancient physicians believed health to be a state of dynamic equilibrium of the bodily elements. The Ayurvedic theory especially emphasizes the equilibrium of the three humors—wind, bile, and phlegm. Illness occurs when any one of the three humors becomes excessively "agitated" and increases disproportionately in relation to the others. The imbalance of humors occurs (and this is the general theory of the causation of disease in Āyurveda) due to the excessive use, deficient use, or misuse of (1) the objects of the senses; (2) actions of body, mind, and speech; and (3) time, that is, the different seasons.

The restoration of the balance of bodily elements and thus of health rests on the consumption of environmental matter in the right form, proportion, and combination, and at the right time. After ascertaining the nature of any imbalance in the body, the doctor identifies a substance (or a combination of substances) in nature—drug or diet—which, when transformed within the body, will correct the humoral disequilibrium. This is why "there is nothing in nature without relevance for medicine" and why Āyurveda has collected an enormous amount of data on the therapeutic efficacy of all kinds of natural substances. In Āyurveda, seasons, plants, natural substances, and constituents of the body are all integrated in a complex yet aesthetically elegant theory of physical health as an equilibrium of somatic and environmental elements.

Food and Health

In the popular understanding of Āyurveda today, the use and misuse of environmental matter in the form of food has come to be regarded as the primary cause of health and illness. The Ayurvedic theory of food is an elaborate one. Various methods of food classification—by taste, by heating or cooling properties, by mode of cooking, and so on, all have an intricate relationship to the humors and their equilibrium. Of course, most people in Hindu India do not know all the details of this theory. They do

know, however, that a balanced diet is one that consists of all the six
tastes—sweet, sour, salty, bitter, pungent, and astringent. They also know
that certain foods produce heat in the body, other foods produce cold,
while yet others give rise to "wind." According to the prevalent belief,
eating the wrong kind of food is the most common cause of disease. Acid-
ity, diarrhea, dysentery, blood in the stool, and jaundice, for instance, will
be attributed to an excess of "heat" in the body. Fever, headaches,
asthma, bronchitis, and typhoid, on the other hand, are examples of
"cold" diseases; while pains in the joints, paralysis, and polio are several
of the "wind" diseases.

The heating effect of "hot" foods or the cooling effect of "cold" ones
has nothing to do with the temperature or degree of spiciness, but is a
description of the effect produced in the body. Hot and cold foods are to
be chosen judiciously, especially in certain physiological states. For example, in pregnancy or during lactation, states which are associated with
heat, hot foods like meat and eggs are to be avoided; while cold foods
such as milk or its products must be eschewed for any type of fever.

Besides the properties of taste and "temperature," most Indians know
that the distinction between cooked and uncooked food is also important
for the maintenance of health. Though there are many exceptions, generally cooked food—implying an adequate ripening in the field and cooking in oil (rather than in water)—is preferable to the uncooked.

Given the widespread acceptance of the Ayurvedic model, one would
expect that Hindu patients would primarily seek treatment from *vaids*, the
practitioners of Ayurvedic theory. Yet all the recent studies on "health-
seeking behavior" in both rural and urban India show that in case of illness, a great majority of the patients, of all castes, prefer first to consult
doctors of Western medicine rather than their indigenous colleagues.[3] The
explanation for this apparent cognitive dissonance is, I suspect, simple,
and gives further testimony to the reputed Hindu capacity for the assim-
ilation of alien systems and modes of thought. Western medical drugs are
generally considered "strong" in the sense that the "hot" drugs are hotter
and the "cold" drugs colder than their Ayurvedic counterparts. The preference for Western-style medicine is thus not due to an Indian's acceptance of the Western medical model's greater explanatory powers. Rather,
this preference is due to the superiority of the Western system's drugs, a
superiority, however, that is understood in Ayurvedic terms. This is also
the reason why many families limit the ingestion of Western drugs to
men, considering them too "strong" and "hot" for women and children.
(Others, more skeptically inclined, will argue that since Western medicines are generally more expensive, it is natural that in a patriarchal society arranged for the convenience of adult men, women and children are
excluded from all expensive modes of treatment.) The "strength" and
"heat" of these medicines—like the reputed attributes of India's ex–colo-

nial overlords—is also the reason why many traditional *vaid*s, though explaining and treating a disease in terms of the Ayurvedic model, have little compunction in prescribing or dispensing drugs derived from penicillin, sulpha, or cortisone.

Sexuality and Health

Besides food, evil spirits, infection, and pollution, sexuality can also be the cause of ill health. In the narrow sense of ill health, that is, disease with objective, physical symptoms, "overheating" due to too much sexual intercourse can, in the view of many Hindus, lead to venereal disease. However, there are others who would trace venereal disease to an infection, the carrier of which is invariably a woman. Indeed, in Tamil the popular name for VD is "woman's disease." In addition, forbidden sexual intercourse with a menstruating woman and adultery are held to cause a few other diseases, including a couple of mental ones.

The relation between sexuality and health, however, is infinitely more complex than a simple matter of the sexual origin of diseases. Sexuality—whether in the erotic flourishes of Indian art and the Dionysian rituals of its popular religion or in the dramatic combat of Yogis with ascetic longings who seek to conquer and transform it into a spiritual power—has been a perennial preoccupation of Hindu culture. In this resides the reason, puzzling to many non-Indians, why in spite of the surface resemblances between Jungian concepts and Indian thought, it is Freud rather than Jung who fascinates the Indian mind. Many modern Indian mystics feel compelled, in fact, to discuss Freud's assumptions and conclusions about the vagaries and transfigurations of libido while they pass over Jung's work with benign indifference.

Indian "mysticism" is typically intended to be an intensely practical affair, concerned with an alchemy of the libido that would convert it from a giver of death to a bestower of immortality. It is the sexual fire that stokes the alchemical transformation, wherein the cooking pot is the body and the cooking oil is a distillation from sexual fluids. The strength of this traditional aspiration to sublimate sexuality into spirituality, semen into the elixir Soma, varies in different regions with different castes. Though only small sections of Indian society may act on this aspiration, it is a well-known theory subscribed to by most Hindus, including nonliterate villagers. In its most popular form, the Indian theory of sexual sublimation goes something like this.

Physical strength and mental power have their source in *virya*, a word that stands for both sexual energy and semen. Either *virya* can move downward in sexual intercourse, where it is emitted in its gross physical form as semen, or it can move upward through the spinal cord and into the brain in its subtle form known as *ojas*. Hindus regard the downward movement of sexual energy and its emission as semen as enervating, a debilitating waste of vitality and essential energy. Of all the emotions, it is said, lust throws the physical system into the greatest chaos, with every violent passion destroying millions of red blood cells. Indian metaphysical physiology maintains that food is converted into semen in a thirty-day period by successive transformations (and refinements) through blood, flesh, fat, bone, and marrow till semen is distilled—forty drops of blood producing one drop of semen. Each ejaculation involves a loss of half an ounce of semen, which is equivalent to the vitality produced by the consumption of sixty pounds of food. On another, similar calculation with pedagogic intent, each act of copulation is equivalent to an energy expenditure of twenty-two hours of concentrated mental activity or seventy-two hours of hard physical labor.

If, on the other hand, semen is retained, converted into *ojas*, and moved upward by the observance of celibacy, it becomes a source of spiritual life rather than a cause of physical decay. Longevity, creativity, and physical and mental vitality are enhanced by the conservation of semen; memory, will power, inspiration—scientific and artistic—all derive from the observation of celibacy. In fact, if unbroken celibacy in thought, word, and deed can be observed for twelve years, the aspirant will obtain *mokṣa* or "salvation" spontaneously.

The "raising of the seed upward," then, is a strikingly familiar image in the Indian psycho-philosophical schools of self-realization commonly clubbed together under the misleading label of "mysticism." Wendy O'Flaherty remarks: "So pervasive is the concept of semen being raised up to the head that popular versions of the philosophy believe that semen originates there."[4]

The concept is even present in the *Kāma Sūtra*, the textbook of eroticism and presumably a subverter of ascetic ideals, where the successful lover is not someone who is overly passionate but one who has controlled and stilled the senses through *brahmacarya* and meditation. Indian mythology, too, is replete with stories in which the gods, threatened by a human being who is progressing toward immortality by accruing immense capacities through celibacy and meditation, send a heavenly nymph to seduce the ascetic (even the trickling down of a single drop of sexual fluid counting as a fatal lapse) and thereby reduce him to the common human, carnal denominator.

Of course, given the horrific imagery of sexuality as cataclysmic depletion, no people can procreate with any sense of joyful abandon unless they develop a good deal of skepticism, if not an open defiance, in relation to the sexual prescriptions and ideals of the "cultural superego." The relief at seeing the ascetic's pretensions humbled by the opulent charms of a heavenly seductress is not only that of the gods but is shared equally by the mortals who listen to the myth or see it enacted in popular dance and folk drama. The ideals of celibacy are then simultaneously subscribed to and scoffed at. There are a number of sages in the Indian tradition (Gandhi is only the latest one to join this august assemblage) who are admired for their successful celibacy and the power it brought them; there are, however, also innumerable folktales detailing the misadventures of randy ascetics. In the more dignified myths, even the Creator is unable to sustain his chastity and is laid low by carnality.

The ultimate if ironic refinement of celibacy is found in the tantric version, where the aspirant is trained and enjoined to perform the sexual act itself and the "spilling of the seed" without desire, thus divorcing the sexual impulse from human physiology and any conscious or unconscious mental representation of it. The impulse, it is believed, stirs up the semen in this ritual (and unbelievably passionless) sexual act and evokes energy forces that can be rechanneled upward.

There are germs of truth in the signal importance Indian cultural tradition attaches to sexuality. The notion, arising from this emphasis, that sexual urges amount to a creative fire—not only for procreation, but equally, in self-creation—is indeed compelling. Further, a tradition that does not reduce sexual love to copulation but seeks to elevate it into a celebration, even a ritual, that touches the partners with a sense of the sacred and in which orgasm is experienced as "a symbolic blessing of man by his ancestors and by the nature of things," is certainly sympathetic. Our concern has to do with the concomitant strong anxiety in India (seen elsewhere mostly among adolescents) associated with the "squandering of the sperm" and "biological self-sacrifice." Indeed, there is a particular cultural disease called *svapanadoṣa* (literally, "dream fault"), a young man's complaint of body aches and headaches, increasing enervation, and feelings of unreality about the body scheme because of the loss of semen in nocturnal emissions.

Mental Illness in the Hindu Traditions

Broadly speaking, mental illness in the living Hindu traditions is ascribed to two sets of causes: humoral disturbance and spirit possession. Whereas the first is the healing concern of the traditional medical practitioner, the second is generally an object of "shamanic" healing, a term that includes the practice of exorcists of various persuasions as well as the healing rituals that take place at specific religious shrines and temples.

In traditional Hindu medical theory the locus of mental illness is *manas*. Often translated as "mind," *manas* has in fact a more concrete and limited meaning than the corresponding Western concept.[5] Psychologically a mediator between the "inside" and "outside," metaphysically *manas* is also the barrier between the two, the sheet covering the "true" nature of reality.

The functions of *manas*, corresponding to the psychoanalytic notion of ego, are: (1) activation, direction, and coordination of the sensory and motor organs; (2) self-regulation; (3) reasoning; and (4) deliberation, judgment, and discrimination. Mental illness, in the traditional medical idiom, refers primarily to the impairment of these functions.

Given the Ayurvedic thesis of a psyche-soma identity, *manas* is naturally influenced by the humoral imbalance that also disturbs the gross body. There are, for instance, different types of insanity linked with the disturbances of wind, bile, and phlegm. Besides being affected by disturbances in the bodily humors, *manas* is permeated by three "qualities" (*guṇas*) of purity/light, activity/passion, and darkness/inertia. These qualities wage a constant struggle for supremacy and therefore keep *manas* in an ever-changing state of restlessness. Of the three qualities, the latter two are called the humors of the *manas*. They are, so to speak, mental humors whose excitation and disturbance lead to mental illness, or, more exactly—remembering the principle of psyche-soma identity—to illnesses whose origins are chiefly mental. Of course, the vitiation of the mental humors will also be reflected and expressed in the bodily sphere. In the etiology of epilepsy, for instance, it is pointed out that the vitiation of the heart and sense organs by the mental humors leads to an obstruction of the bodily humors, which can no longer travel in their accustomed channels, thus giving rise to the morbidity typical of epilepsy. Āyurveda, we must again remember, is truly dialogical: body and mind make up a whole *simultaneously*, not sequentially, each being of *equal value* (with no claim to superiority). In the ultimate analysis, there are no such things as "physical" illness and "mental" illness; there is only illness.

What are the reasons for the disturbing increases in the mental humors? Hindu psychology has singled out desire and repulsion as the twin causes. As a category desire is defined as the wish to obtain an object which has pleased the body or the mind, and includes the emotions of lust, elation, and covetousness. Of course, to be desirous of certain objects is natural. It is only when desire oversteps the bounds of "propriety" (*maryādā*) inherent in the object and becomes its slave that the humors become excited. The second category, repulsion, is defined as the avoidance of an object that has caused pain to body or mind, and is associated with the emotions of anger, fear, and envy.

For the Hindus, the roots of desire and repulsion have little to do with the individual's life experience. One root extends down to the prenatal stage, around the third and fourth months of pregnancy. In this period the unfulfilled longings of the mother and her unrelieved fears are said to be transmitted to the newly activated psyche of the fetus, where they are stored and thus create the source of its eventual suffering. The other root of desire and repulsion goes back even farther in time to a previous existence. It is postulated that the unfulfilled longings and unresolved traumas at the end of a previous life enter the fetus as a "memory-trace" which, in time, will rise to the surface, demanding completion and closure, and thus increase both the mental humors.

Possession, by spirits and various heavenly and demonic beings, is perceived as the second cause of mental illness. Its treatment, through various magical means and exorcism rituals, belongs to an old tradition, going back to the *Atharvaveda*, that still flourishes in all parts of India, rural and urban.

The common thread running through the many manifestations of possession and the variety of its treatments is the disturbance and restoration of the patient's bond with his or her polis, especially with the family and the village or caste community. The exorcism therapies, then, invariably take the form of a polyphonic social drama that attempts a ritual restoration of the dialogue, not only within the patient, but more importantly, with the family, the community, and its gods. In contrast to the more individualistic premises of most Western psychotherapies, the underlying values of the traditional Indian healing of the shamanic sort seem to be that faith and surrender to a power beyond the individual are better than individual effort and struggle. They affirm that the source of human strengths lies in a harmonious integration with one's group, in the individual's affirmation of the community's values and its given order, in the individual's obedience to the community's gods, and in his or her cherishing of its traditions.

What about the shamans themselves? Can any generalizations be made about these curers, who are ubiquitous in Indian villages, towns, and cities and who are typically the first ones to be consulted by those showing symptoms of mental illness? Many of these shamans follow a hereditary profession, having learned their craft from their fathers. Others have had a long period of apprenticeship with a guru, living according to the prescribed conduct and rules that govern the shamanic training of the guru's particular school. In addition to performing shamanic roles, most work in other professions such as farming and shopkeeping. Religious symbols and rituals are an invariable part of their practice, employed both in the diagnostic phase and in the process of cure. Most shamans, according to this writer's experience, are honest professionals, deeply religious and generally more devout in their life-style than most of their neighbors.

Typically, among the many people waiting to see the shaman on a particular day, it is not easy to distinguish the patients from those who have come for some other purpose. Among those waiting, there may be one or more former patients who have dropped in to greet the shaman, who generally tries to maintain a close contact with his ex-patients. In addition, there are always a few spectators present: some have come to witness the excitement of a healing drama, while others presumably attend to fulfill their own deeper needs to be near the sacred. To obtain an amulet from the shaman as a protection against unknown future threats may be one person's purpose, while yet another may consult him about a recent theft or loss. Shamans not only take care of mental illness in the community, but are usually also general practitioners of reassurance and specialists in faith.

Passages: The Cycle of Life and Death

The first stage of the Indian life cycle coincides with the period of pregnancy, especially after the third month (or the fifth, depending on the region), when the "subtle body," comprising the mind, the soul, and the karmic memory-traces from a previous life, becomes conscious. In this stage of *dauhṛdaya* (literally, a "bicardiac" state), where one heart belongs to the fetus and the other to the mother, the unborn child and mother are said to function psychologically as a unit, mutually influencing each other. The feelings and affects of the fetus—a legacy from its previous birth—are transmitted to the mother through the channels of nutrition. For the future well-being of the child it is imperative that the cravings of the pregnant woman be fully gratified (since they are those of the unborn child) and that the unit of pregnant mother and fetus be completely indulged.

With birth begins the second stage of the life cycle, infancy or the *shishu* period, which extends for the first three to four years of the child's life. In a central myth of the Hindu tradition, with the cutting of the umbilical cord, the original divinity within each person is cut off from its fountainhead by human beings' active or passive interactions with a polluting world, as *karma* begins to be generated and stored.

In the Hindu view the newborn infant, as we saw above, is not a *tabula rasa* but comes equipped, as it were, with a uniquely personal psyche. In other words, the *karma* of a previous life, in the form of innate dispositions, and the embryonic experience, especially during the *dauhṛdaya* stage, have already laid down the basic contours of personality *in utero*.

Moreover, the child's temperament and nature are believed to be influenced by the configuration of planets and lunar mansions (*nakṣatra*) at the moment of birth. Hindus do not view infant nature as universal or infinitely malleable. Thus, there is little social pressure to foster the belief that, if only the caretakers were good enough and constantly on their toes, the child's potentialities would be boundlessly fulfilled. With the emphasis on human beings' inner limits, there is not the sense of urgency and struggle against the outside world, with prospects of sudden metamorphoses and great achievements just around the corner.

If the rites are any guide, the period of infancy is deemed complete by the third or fourth year, to be followed by *bala*, an early childhood stage. Whereas until this age the rites have been the same for both male and female infants, the life cycles of boys and girls now begin to diverge. For a boy the gender differentiation is marked by the rite of tonsure; while for girls, in many parts of the country, the social recognition of the beginnings of her gender identity is through the rite of piercing the earlobes.

It is, however, only in the stage of late childhood, which begins around the age of five to seven years, that cultural expectations and experiences of boys and girls begin to diverge markedly. For the boy the world of childhood widens from the intimate cocoon of maternal protection to the unfamiliar masculine network woven by the demands and tensions of the men of the family. The most striking feature of his experience is the contrast between an earlier, more or less unchecked benevolent indulgence and the new inflexible standards.

The Hindu daughter, on the other hand, is not severed from the other women in the household although she is given new, grown-up household tasks and responsibilities, especially in the care of younger children in the family. Her childhood, as compared to her brother's, is shortened in the sense that she takes on domestic responsibilities at an age when her brother is still playing in the streets or, at most, running small errands.

The end of childhood stages is heralded by the initiation ceremony for boys *(upanāyana)* and marriage rites for girls *(vivaha)*. For the boy initiation marks what the Hindus call his "second birth," his birth into the community as a social being.

The life tasks of the four stages that now follow, as outlined in the tradition, have a much greater social and, in Western terms, ethical content. The stages are thus ideal in the Platonic sense, with prescriptive contents that reflect the tradition's view of the "good," fulfilled life.

Brahmacarya, the stage after the initiation ceremony, is a stage of apprenticeship, where the task lies in learning the craft skills of the community (family, caste) in which the individual is born. The development of competence and of devotion to the teacher are the primary gains of this stage of life.

The next stage is that of the *gārhasthya* or householder, where the primary task has been defined as the establishing of a family and the production of the means of maintaining the social order. In short, "maintenance of the world" is the householder's chief duty and "care" his primary virtue. The importance placed on the adult householder's caring function is reflected in such passages from the Hindu scriptures and law books as the following: "And in accordance with the precepts of the *Veda* and of the *Smṛti,* the householder is declared superior to all of them; for he supports the other three. As all rivers, both great and small find a resting-place in the ocean, even so men of all orders."[6]

In the next stage, *vānaprastha* or withdrawal, the individual is supposed to detach himself gradually from the affairs of the immediate family and extend care to the community at large; a man's interest now turns from the sphere of the family to the sphere of public affairs. If the primary task of the householder can be said to lie in the practice of *dharma*—a multivalent concept that denotes "right living" in this particular context—then the task of the *vānaprastha* stage lies in the teaching of *dharma*.

The last stage in the ideal Hindu life cycle is that of *saṁnyāsa* or renunciation, in which all worldly ties are renounced in a concern for self-realization and the preparation for death. The detachment from the world and the renunciation, according to the *Bhagavadgītā*, does not pertain to all action, but only to selfish actions and the fruit of all actions. It is the surrender of the notions of *I* and *mine*, which is considered the hallmark of the last passage of human life. The "good death" is then prepared for throughout life, the quality of life determining the quality of death. Conversely, the bad death is life cut short or inadequately lived according to the traditional image of the cycle.

The View of Death

In a society whose thinking is so much dominated by its mythological images and ritual, a myth of death perhaps best conveys the way Hindus have sought to contain its terror.

> Out of the happiness of his heart, Prajāpati began to create. Each of his creations was unique and wonderful. The one on earth had everlasting life. Then, one day, a sound of pain reached his ears and a smell of something rotting assailed his nostrils. He saw that a large part of his creations on earth had become old, weak, almost lifeless, and the stink arose from the creation's aged body.
>
> Prajāpati lost himself in meditation. His forehead creased in worry, his smiling visage gave way to an unhappy one as if clouds were drifting across the fresh blue sky. At that particular moment, a shadow emerged from inside him and slowly took on a body. A woman, with hands folded in supplication, was standing in front of him. "Who am I, father? Why have I been created? What is my work?"
>
> Prajāpati replied: "You are my daughter—Death. You have been created to do the work of destruction." The woman said: "I am a woman and yet you have brought me into existence for such heartless work! My woman's heart and woman's *dharma* will not be able to stand such cruelty."
>
> Prajāpati smiled and said: "You must do this work. There is no other way." Death protested but the Lord was unbending. She engaged in *tapas* (ascetic practice) and carried out its hard austerities for many years till Prajāpati was forced to appear before her.
>
> "Ask for a boon," he said. "Please release me from the difficult *karma* you have given me as my lot," Death said.

"That is not possible," said the Lord and returned to his abode.

Death undertook further *tapas* with even harder austerities till Brahma once again appeared. On seeing him, Death began sobbing uncontrollably, her tears an unstoppable stream. From these tears, terrifying images rose up one after another.

"These are diseases. They are your creations and they will be your helpers," said Prajāpati.

"But, being a woman, how will I ever be able to take away a husband from the side of his wife? How will I snatch an infant from its mother's breast? What about the sin of this heartless work?"

Prajāpati gestured her to stop. "You are beyond sin and virtue. You will not be touched by sin. People will call you only through their own *karma*. Human beings will be victims of wrong conduct and bad conduct, and you will only give them release from pain, peace from storm, a new birth from an old one."

"But," said Death, "when wives, sons and daughters, mothers and fathers are in full throes of grief, how will I witness such heartrending scenes?"

God said, "I shall take away your sight. From now on you will be blind."

"And their weeping and wailing?" asked Death, "the heart-wrenching cries of men and women?"

"You will also be deaf. No voice will reach your ears."

Thus Death is blind and deaf; diseases lead her by the hand toward those people who have summoned her through their *karma*.

Death is the end of a body *(dehanta)*, a passage into the next life, and an interval between lives, not the termination of life itself. Till the final release of *mokṣa* or *mukti* from the cycles of life and death, humans are destined for repeated rebirths, and texts enjoin one to view death with equanimity if not in celebration. Life and death, the tradition reassures the mourners, are not different ontological entities in polar opposition to each other, but facets of a single, seemingly endless cycle. Krishna's words to a mourning Arjuna, often repeated to those who are left behind, have been culturally charged with a consoling power for centuries: "For death is a certainty for him who has been born and birth is a certainty for him who has died. Therefore, for what is unavoidable, thou shouldest not grieve."[7]

Moreover, the mourning rituals, which may extend over a year, seek to underline a continuing bond between the dead and the living. Death is not a final separation to be suffered passively. In fact, for a very long time to come, the family will remain actively responsible for the dead soul's future welfare. Family bonds and obligations, in effect, transcend death. Before the rebirth can take place, the dead person's spirit has to be helped by the family members to reach and progress through the three worlds of ancestral spirits till the time of rebirth draws near. Every day immediately after the death the vulnerable spirit is offered a *pinda*—a ball of rice or flour—which reconstitutes a specific limb until the ethereal body is completed by the tenth day. It is now able to rejoin the other ancestral spirits. The ritual bond between the living and the dead is emphasized again and again in household rituals and sacrifices when *pinda*s are offered to at least three generations of ancestral spirits in order to aid their progress toward rebirth, and, ultimately, toward salvation—the release that is every individual's final aim, his or her birth- and death-right.

In conclusion, I shall only reiterate that in the living traditions of India, health and healing are intimately related to the central postulates of Hindu religiocultural thought. As one would expect, this connection is most clearly evident in the postulated relationships between food, sexuality, and health, as well as in the images of the life cycle, that is, in the connection between health and right living in the different stages of life. Indeed, as we saw, the impact of the Hindu tradition extends further to the very processes of the body, which then becomes as much a cultural as a biological construction. In emphasizing the intimate connection of the body with its natural environment on the one hand and its social and cosmic environments on the other, the Hindu cultural tradition does not see the bodily order as the sole repository of health and disease, but it gives equal weight to other orders of individual existence. It is thus understandable that healing efforts in India follow the culture's "center of gravity" and manifest the culture's major themes in their practices and goals, and it is an axiomatic truth that the character and value of a therapy, easily misjudged if subjected to some abstract, universal criterion, become understandable only if one grasps the central thrust of the culture from which that therapy ultimately derives.

Notes

1. Gananath Obeyesekere, "The Theory and Practice of Psychological Medicine in the Ayurvedic Tradition," *Culture, Medicine and Psychiatry* 1 (1977): 155.
2. R. K. Sharma and Bhagwan Dash, trans., *Caraka Samhita* (Banaras, 1976), pp. 349–350.
3. See, for instance, M. E. Khan and C. V. S. Prasad, *Health Seeking Behaviour and Adoption of Family Planning in Himachal Pradesh* (Baroda, 1984); H. Ramachandran, *Environment, Health and Health Care System: A Study of Rural Households in Tumkur District* (Bangalore, 1984); D. Banerji, "Formulating an Alternative Rural Health Care System for India," in *An Alternative System of Health Care Service in India*, ed. J. P. Naik (New Delhi, 1977).
4. Wendy O'Flaherty, *Women, Androgynes and Other Mythical Beasts* (Chicago, 1980), p. 45.
5. For a detailed analysis, see Sudhir Kakar, *Shamans, Mystics and Doctors* (New York, 1982), pp. 243–247.
6. G. Bühler, trans., *The Laws of Manu* (Oxford, 1886), pp. 214–215.
7. *Bhagavadgītā* 2.27.

CHAPTER 6

Despair and Recovery in Sinhala Medicine and Religion: An Anthropologist's Meditations

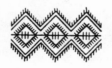

GANANATH OBEYESEKERE

In this chapter I shall examine the manner in which the existential condition of hopelessness and despair is articulated in two forms of cultural expression in Sinhala-Buddhist society in Sri Lanka. In one form despair is given ethical meaning and significance through the practice of a popular form of meditation, which in turn leads the sufferer to a realization of the nature of life and of salvation, or *nirvāṇa*. The other form of life is spirit possession, in which despair is defined as an attack by a malevolent spirit. Spirit possession is both a reaction to despair and an expression of it.

The former is rooted in the Buddhist doctrinal tradition, whereas the latter is part of the spirit cults that exist on the popular level in all Buddhist nations. I chose meditation and spirit possession because they present radically opposed reactions to despair in antecedent history, soteriological goal, ethics, and style of performance. While exploring these differences, I shall pose this fundamental question: What are the implications of defining despair as existence in the one case and illness in the other?

In both cases my focus is on ordinary individuals engaged in extraordinary practices, rather than on religious specialists, be they monks or shamans. The cries of despair we utter and the sense of hopelessness we feel are a part of our species condition. And where there is despair, there is also hope—at least sometimes. Though despair and hope are universal, they are expressed and embedded in forms of life that are historically and culturally constituted. But this does not force us to adopt a naive cultural relativism, for both history and culture may exhibit similarities from one society to another and may even be amenable to tentative generalization. The cry of hope and despair, however, in whatever cultural form it is expressed, cannot fail to move us, whether we are Buddhists or Christians or living in the Dream Time in the Australian bush. So I think it right that I preface my discussion with the poignant cry of despair in Gerard Manley Hopkins's "Carrion Comfort":

> Not, I'll not, carrion comfort, Despair, not feast on thee;
> Not untwist—slack they may be—these last strands of man
> In me or, most weary, cry *I can no more.* I can;
> Can something, hope, wish day come, not choose not to be.

"I can no more" is the universal cry of despair; "I can" is the cry of hope. I shall explore how cries of despair and of hope are expressed in the two radically contrasting forms of life known as "meditation on revulsion" and "spirit possession."

For a full clarification of these two forms of life it may be useful to sketch for the reader the background of Sinhala medicine and religion. Prior to the introduction of Western medicine, the Sinhalas had a system of physical medicine borrowed from the ancient Sanskrit medical corpus known as Āyurveda. Ayurvedic medicine was fundamentally a humoral theory, closely allied to Hippocratic medicine. The medical theory, and often its practice, tended to eschew supernatural agencies in the causation of disease or its cure. It was thoroughly grounded in conceptions of bodily function and physiology—however wrong they may seem from the modern Western perspective. But Āyurveda does not exhaust the sphere of medicine in the history of Sri Lanka, since there were also a great number of diseases that were caused by bad planetary conjunctions or by the actions of spirits.

Neither spirit possession nor meditation can be properly understood without a preliminary grasp of the religious tradition in which they are encompassed. The Sinhalas of Sri Lanka are mostly Theravāda Buddhists. They, like other Theravāda peoples of South and Southeast Asia, have incorporated a variety of non-Buddhist, often pre-Buddhist, religious beliefs into their practical religion. These beliefs pertain to the gods, major and minor, and to evil spirits like demons, ghosts, and the greedy spirits of dead ancestors known as *preta*s. Astrology is another major component of their practical religion, but it is not relevant for the present discussion. The "spirit cults" have been assimilated into a Buddhist framework over a long historical period by a variety of techniques.

According to Sinhala Buddhism, the Buddha is a kind of superdeity at the head of the pantheon, and the Hindu-derived major gods are there by his permission or warrant. The lesser gods and demons have obtained their warrant from the major gods or directly from the Buddha himself. Ultimately, therefore, all authority devolves on the Buddha and is delegated by him to those below. The Buddha, however, gave his authority when he was alive; nowadays the major gods act on his behalf as guardians of both the church and the state. The idea of warrants and that of the territorial jurisdiction exercised by the gods are all derived from the idiom of Kandyan "feudalism." For example, there are four major guardian gods and in the Sinhala low country they are generally Viṣṇu, Saman, Skanda, and Pattinī (a goddess). Each deity has his or her sphere of territorial jurisdiction and authority. But beyond each specifically demarcated domain, a major deity has a more general role as overlord of Sri Lanka and of the world. The pantheon, then, as a totality is integrated into a hierarchical structure defined by the political idiom of the Kandyan state.

The pantheon is also a moral order. Buddhist ethics and doctrinal values define the roles and attributes of gods and demons. Gods and demons are there by virtue of their good and bad *karma*. The karmic load that these deities bear is increased by the good or ill they do, as well as by the merit transfer of devotees. Thus, there is long-term mobility in the pantheon fueled by *karma*. People will often say that Viṣṇu and Saman are in the first stage of *nirvāṇa* and therefore not always as effective in helping the devotee. They are aloof and, like all Buddhist renouncers, tend to be uninterested in the world. When this happens the more world-involved deities from the lower ends begin to ascend into the upper reaches of the pantheon.

The morality of *karma* rationalizes the attributes of the deities in the pantheon. The gods are wholly just and will punish those who transgress the values of the society. Demons by contrast are irrationally malevolent and can cause harm without just cause or principle. If the gods represent the positive Buddhist values, the demons represent the negative, embodying such things as greed *(lobha)*, attachment *(tanha)*, anger *(kōpa)*, and cruelty *(krodha)*. Consequently, the activation of the pantheon in a healing ritual produces simultaneously a cosmic drama and a morality play.

In addition to ethics, soteriology also affects the pantheon. The Buddha, in Theravāda thought, is no longer alive and consequently incapable of changing the world. His religion or *dharma* is essentially concerned with otherworldly matters. Thus, in Sinhala culture the Buddhist aspect of public belief and worship has to do with the otherworld or with soteriology, while the gods and demons have to do with this-worldly interests. When Buddhist laypersons go to a temple they do not generally ask for favors from the Buddha; nor do they when they meditate. But when they propitiate the gods they do so for purely pragmatic, worldly reasons. Hence, an interesting feature of the practical religion of Sinhala Buddhists is that people propitiate Hindu Gods like Viṣṇu and Skanda, but unlike the gods of Hinduism these gods have no say over human salvation. They are there to get things done in an imperfect world no longer blessed with the Buddha's living presence.

One must not overdraw the this-worldly/otherworldly distinction in respect to Buddhism by equating it with a distinction between material and ideal interests, for otherworldliness has its material side as well. It is common enough for Buddhists to pray at a temple or perform meritorious acts in order to ensure material happiness in a future existence, even if such happiness is rarely requested in one's present existence—the present is the provenance of the gods, not of the Buddha; yet, in a general way, the distinction is valid. The allocation of religious roles is also based on this distinction. The Buddhist monk's work has almost exclusively to do with nonworldly matters, and hence he is the most respected member of society. By contrast, the work of the god is by a priest known as a *kapurāla*, and that of the demons by a *kaṭṭaḍirāla*. The distinction between these two roles is often blurred, and both varieties of curer or healer are sometimes given the common term *ädura* ("teacher"). In conformity with this division of labor, monks are not supposed to deal with demonic curing or with rituals for gods, and in fact this ideal rule is rarely breached in actual practice even today.

A Fragment of a Buddhist Meditation on Despair

In 1970 I asked three students at the University of Sri Lanka (Peradeniya) to administer a questionnaire to thirteen persons of advanced years who came to meditate in a Buddhist temple regularly on holy days. The questionnaire was designed to investigate the typical activities of these virtuosos during these days. All these respondents were over the age of fifty except one aged forty-four; the mean age was sixty-seven. These were old people who had practically retired from active life. Let me give some representative statements from their interviews.

Case 1 (age 61, male)

> I try to control my body. I think: my hair, teeth, nails, nerves, bones, and so forth are impermanent. Why? They are not mine. They are of no use. There is no point in all of this. Though one enjoys life and dresses well while living in the world it is of no use for the other world. . . . My body is revulsive like a corpse, like feces. [Then the generalization:] The bodies of others are also foul. So's the female body. I care not for women. I feel nauseous towards them.

Case 2 (age 80, male)

> By meditation on revulsiveness I mean the thirty-two defilements of the body. . . . It is not my body alone that is foul: so are the bodies of others. Though you apply talcum powder and scent on the body it is like feces; it is like a clay pot full of feces.

Case 3 (age 66, female)

> [After describing the techniques of meditation this woman said:] One must separately control all parts of the body, from the hair to the teeth. I list the thirty-two parts of the body separately and say this part is impermanent, it has no soul. . . . This body is like a lump of feces. I think then of urine and feces. When you remove the skin from that lovely body it is like a *domba* seed [veined and shriveled]. The whole body is a heap of dirt. It is like a bag of millet which, when you untie it, leaves you nothing. . . . When I think of my mother or my children, they too are like this. I think: their bodies are dirt also.

Case 4 (age 85, male)

> I reflect on the thirty-two parts of the body from my hair to my bones. . . . I think that my teeth and wrinkled skin are impermanent. So is my life. My body is revulsive. I think: when my bowels are stretched out, my, how long they are! I feel I want nothing of the human body. Why think of one's wife

and children? They too have bodies like mine. All persons are like this: no finality.

Case 5 (age 86, male)

I meditate on the body. The body is a heap of dirt. It contains thirty-two heaps of dirt. It is something covered by skin. . . . This is what I'll be when I die. I think: it is transitory. The body is a hell. A heap of dirt.

[Interviewer:] Why do you think that the body is dirt? [Response:] It breathes, it eliminates. It is filth, filth. You rub soap to get rid of its dirt. . . . This dirt does not belong to me. It is transitory. It dies. The body is a heap of feces. Impermanent. A few years after I got married I did not care about women. After my two children were born, I felt that sexual intercourse was useless.

Case 6 (age unknown, female)

When I meditate I feel no fondness for my body. With the feeling of useless-ness of life [kalakirīma] I lose my liking for my body . . . I feel the impurity of the body and hence no desire for it. I become aware of dukkha, suffering. I think: the bodies of others are like mine also. When I think of my body it is thus: I think it is a heap of dirt. It is surely like a heap of feces. I think the same of the inside of my body. It is as if a pot containing feces has been pol-ished on the outside.

Only two of the respondents stated that their activities on holy days were precipitated by specific antecedent events. Case 6 stated that she was regularly beaten and abused by her husband, who subsequently abandoned her and her children. He used to have flagrant liaisons with other women. Then her father died: "The sorrow [sōkaya] of my father's death was such that I took the white cloth that he wore during sil [the practice of Buddhist precepts] and his rosary and his books and I started observing the precepts myself." She did not wish to remarry: "If this man was bad, so must they all be. The married life is troublesome. Several proposed marriage to me but I refused. There is no freedom here." The other respondent was a seventy-two-year-old man who claimed to have practiced the precepts from childhood. However, he began to observe the precepts regularly four times a month when the head monk of his village died sixteen years earlier. He loved this monk, he said, and suffered great shock (kampanaya) at his death. In both cases the pain of mind and sorrow were articulated in Buddhist terms and expressed in the activity of sil and meditation. The signs of sorrow (unlike the symptoms of "depression") are not free-floating; they are expressed in Buddhist terms. In all of the other cases there were no specific antecedents; rather sil was a response to old age. It is likely (though no direct evidence is available from the interviews) that old age produced in some of these respondents a sense of hopelessness and loss ("depressive affects"), but these feelings were generalized and given Buddhist meaning. The problems of personal sorrow, due to the conditions of old age with its attendant ills, became a problem of existence in its ontological sense.

These respondents were neither laypersons nor monks nor novices, but an intermediate category known as *upāsaka*s, generally, older people who have partially renounced the world and are preparing themselves for death. These people have seen friends and peers die, and they are aware of the key motif that runs through the Buddhist sermons about dying and in their funeral rituals: "Impermanent are all conditioned things." These *upāsaka*s wear white clothes, in contrast to the yellow robe of the monk, and observe the eight or ten precepts (the ethic of the novice) known as *sīla* ("precepts") on holy days known as *pōya* (the four phases of the moon in the lunar month). In popular Sinhala usage their activities on *pōya* days are simply called *sil*. During *sil* these old persons practiced various types of meditations, but two were especially popular—meditation on universal kindness-compassion (*maitrī bhāvanā*) and meditation on mindfulness (*satipaṭṭhāna bhāvanā*), which is based on a text known as *satipaṭṭhāna sutta*. The latter meditation is a very complex exercise, and only part of it is generally practiced by those observing *sil*. This section is known as *pilikul bhāvanā* ("meditation on revulsion"), probably the most common form of meditation practiced in Sri Lanka. It is the significance of "meditation on revulsion" that I shall examine here.

Meditation on revulsiveness has a long and ancient tradition in Buddhism and is known in the texts and commentaries as *asubha bhāvanā*, *asubha* meaning "foulness" or "impurity."[1] In the monastic tradition meditation on "foulness" pertained to the actual contemplation of the corpse in ten separate stages of decay, each stage associated with special techniques of meditation and goals of realization of the nature of life. The general intent of *asubha bhāvanā* is to produce in the meditator a sense of disgust for sense pleasure, which will then lead him or her to realize the sense of the transitoriness of the body. In the lay tradition this is not the case; one does not meditate on an actual decaying corpse, but one conjures in one's own mind the putrescence of the body, which in turn will eventually lead to a knowledge of the transitoriness of the body and the world. The layperson has an especially difficult task, having no physical object at hand in order to conjure up the body's putrescence. The layperson has to evoke this putrescence through various metaphors of revulsion, the most conspicuous being that of feces. Feces is the one object par excellence that everyone in the society is familiar with as a revulsive object. It then becomes a metaphor for the revulsiveness of the body in the meditation on revulsion.

The Buddhist situation can be better appreciated if one compares it to what happens in the West. In Sri Lanka persons faced with despair at the loss of a loved one or confronted with the specter of death looming ahead may cry with the poet: "I can no more." But they are not stuck at this level. They can express their despair in a cultural idiom, and in a set of practices derived from Buddhism. In the modern West despair has been medicalized; it has been converted into an illness labeled "depression." The label "depression" is in turn articulated by a larger vocabulary of despair borrowed from the technical language of psychiatry; the label also locks the sufferer (now defined as "patient") into a set of practices derived from clinical psychiatry. The power of this language, together with the Western praxis of despair, is such that it can swallow the ordinary language used to describe similar affects—despondency, melancholy, feeling low, and so forth—by treating them as "symptoms." The previous idiom, derived largely from Christian notions such as sin, loss of self-worth, alienation from God, and loss of grace, has in contemporary times practically lost its application and relevance for depicting despair. The person suffering from "depression" is stuck like an old record at "I can no more."

This has not happened in Sri Lanka in any serious sense, though it eventually might with increasing urbanization and the concomitant medicalization of existence. For the most part, the Sinhala vocabulary of despair is linked inextricably to the Buddhist tradition. It is almost impossible for a Sinhala person to use words expressing sorrow without relating them to the Buddhist tradition. Even if all the words used do not come from that tradition directly, the larger context of usage will eventually embody it in the doctrinal tradition. Let me give some examples of Sinhala words employed to express sorrow with a rough approximation in English.

I have already mentioned *sōkaya*, sadness, sorrow and *kampanaya* or *kampāva*, the shock of loss; another word is *saṅvēgaya*, pain of mind. The Buddhist term *dukkha* also has a variety of meanings ranging from ordinary sorrow to suffering in its doctrinal sense. One of the most common terms in the lexicon of sorrow is *kalakirīma*, a sense of hopelessness, or despair of life. Etymologically *kalakirīma* is derived from the words *kāla* and *kriyā*, "the termination of time," that is, death. When the word is used in its formal etymological sense as *kālakriyā*, it refers euphemistically to "death." However, in its popular form as *kalakirīma*, it refers to a sense of hopelessness, but not a free-floating one; it is a reaction against life itself. Specific emotional words for sorrow and loss—such as *sōkaya, kampāva, saṅvēgaya*—are easily assimilated into more general terms that express an attitude to life in general, such as *dukkha* and *kalakirīma*. This is reflective of the Buddhist orientation of the culture. The situation is such that any kind of sorrow or despair can and must be expressed in ordinary language that is itself for the most part derived from Buddhism or can be articulated in Buddhist terms.

Moreover, one is socialized into myths, parables, and legends that deal with the phenomenon of personal loss and sorrow as part of the nature of existence in general. One of the most famous is the parable of the mustard seed, familiar to most Buddhists. This text deals with the story of Kisā Gotamī, whose first and only child died in infancy. Distraught with pain and grief she went from place to place seeking some medicine to resurrect her child. She eventually came to the Buddha and asked the sage whether he could revive the dead child. The Buddha said that he could if only she would bring a mustard seed from a house in which death had not occurred. Elated, Kisā Gotamī went from one house to another seeking for the impossible mustard seed, and soon she came to the realization that her own personal grief was simply a part of a larger universal problem of suffering. In this recognition of the nature of life lay her salvation. The parable of the mustard seed could as easily serve as a parable on the nature of depression.[2]

The lay virtuosos or *upāsaka*s discussed earlier have read texts such as that of Kisā Gotamī, and they have resorted to *sil*, a temporary movement away from domestic living, and to meditation. The text of *pilikul bhāvanā* deliberately denigrates the body in order to deny the self itself as real. The metaphor used in the denigration of the body and the self is feces. In the Western illness known as depression the self is also denigrated; lowering of self-esteem and self-worth is conspicuous in this state. But in Buddhist virtuosos this is deliberately undertaken. I do not know whether a person who suffers a sense of worthlessness can overcome it by techniques like "meditation on revulsiveness." Perhaps some do and others do not. In some situations it is likely that a person who has not been afflicted by negative sorrowful affects may be encouraged to cultivate or resurrect them deliberately through meditation—that is, meditation itself may create the "depressive affects" as a way station in the larger quest for understanding the world. One thing is clear enough: that which may be labeled as depression in the West is given a radically different form of cultural canalization and expression among the Sinhala Buddhists. Furthermore, the idiom of feces is especially effective in conveying the emotional quality of the horror of putrescence. The meditation is designed to make meditators feel that their bodies are objects that belong to them yet are outside of them, so that they can view them (and their parts) in detachment; these bodies also exist in others and in the world. It is likely that the ideal virtuoso, once full detachment is effected, can transcend both feces and body, so that these become neutral objects existing outside oneself. True detachment must free a person from both disgust and attachment. However, I believe that for most persons the situation of meditation sends taproots into the life of infancy and childhood: to the infant fecal matter is part of the self yet is also something differentiated from the self. In other words, the detachment of the self from the self—in order to deny its ontological reality—is facilitated by the metaphor of feces.

The metaphor of feces as putrescence is also implicated in the values of Sri Lankan society and the socialization of its children. In Sri Lankan society, as elsewhere, what is important is not the technology of child care—its time and place—but the maternal attitude, which in turn expresses the values of the culture. Freud noted this in *Civilization and Its Discontents*, observing that the socialization of the anal system is linked with the values of Western civilization: order, cleanliness, routine, and ultimately, through a long detour, aestheticism.[3] In Sri Lanka the formal techniques of toilet training are similar to those in many parts of the non-Western world. There is extreme permissiveness: time and place are not defined; children gradually move from the home to the backyard and, when old enough to look after themselves, to the outhouse or bush. But this idyllic picture is soon dispelled when we focus on the maternal attitude toward feces. The mother's reaction is one of horror if the child attempts to play with it. "Chi!" is the typical Sinhala expression of revulsion, meaning, prototypically, feces. In socialization the child is soon made to feel that all dirt is feces: thus when a child plays with mud, the exclamation "Chi!" is used to express the same disgust. Indeed, in child-training the mother may even rebuke a child by addressing it as *chi*—an early use of the metaphor of feces in order to lower the child's self-esteem. The idiom of feces and foul smells is extended to other contexts also, for example, the idea of shame. Thus, a person who has lost face is someone who "stinks"; dirt, mud, and bad smells all appear in the idiom of shame. All of these feelings are activated or reactivated in "the meditation on revulsion" in order to convey the horror of putrescence, which is a preliminary step in one's transcendence of the body and leads to a recognition of the impermanence or transitory nature of life itself.

A Fragment of a Possession Episode

In Sri Lanka, spirit possession is well known, but is never viewed as part of Buddhist teaching. In traditional villages people may become possessed by evil spirits, and when they do, they are generally exorcised in colorful rituals by the demon exorcist or *kaṭṭaḍirāla*. However, over the last few decades there has been a dramatic rise in spirit possession in urban areas. While in the village rituals the demon is exorcised and banished from the body of the patient, it is not so in the city. In city rituals the priest exorcises the demon, but this exorcism is often only a preliminary to substituting a divine possessing spirit for the demonic one. Very often the patient who has been afflicted by an evil spirit later becomes a priest or priestess who acts as a medium for a benevolent deity or a god. The priest officiating at these city exorcisms is a *kapurāla* or *sāmi* ("lord"). Buddhist monks or *bhikkhus* never officiate at (or even witness) these rituals.

In September 1968 I studied a shrine located in Nāvala, an urban suburb a few miles outside the city limits of Colombo. The shrine itself is a tiny, unimpressive building with a large sandy compound that serves as a dancing area for large-scale rituals of exorcism. The priest lives with his mother, two wives, and several children in a tiny thatched wattle-and-daub house across from the shrine on the other side of the compound. These unimpressive features stand in sharp contrast to the large houses of middle-class professional people in the neighborhood. However, none of the rich neighbors ever visits the shrine. It is unobtrusively located in a quiet cul-de-sac, though the periodic beat of drums announces its presence.

The shrine, like almost every shrine in urban Sri Lanka, renders two standard services to its clientele:

1. Every morning at 11:05 A.M. the priest or an assistant gets into a trance and acts as a vehicle for one of the deities in the pantheon, male or female. This again is a departure from tradition. Whereas in the village of Sri Lanka a priest may get possessed by the spirit of *one* of the lower gods (known collectively as the Twelve Gods), here in the city the priest can act as a vehicle for *any* of the major (higher) gods housed in the shrine. Clients visit the shrine and tell the priest their problems. He often utters *śāstra*s, "divine utterances" or "prophecies" from the deity. These prophecies in general diagnose the client's troubles, prescribe medicine if the client is sick, and give advice of a general kind.

2. In addition to these regular sessions, the priest has occasional rituals of countersorcery to cure clients who are the victims of sorcery, as well as rituals to exorcise persons possessed of evil spirits and demons. Such rituals start at around 6:00 P.M. and continue until 9:00 or 10:00 A.M. the next day. They are known as *kāpilla*, "cutting," since in most instances their aim is to "cut" the evil bondage of the sorcerer's magic.

I tape-recorded every ritual session held in the shrine during the period from 17 September to 18 October 1968. During this month seventeen regular sessions were held at the *śāstra* hour, 11:05 A.M., and two major *kāpilla* rituals were held. A fragment of one of these rituals, the exorcising of an evil spirit from the body of a female patient, is described below.

The subject of this exorcism was Sumanāvatī, a forty-five-year-old woman married to a postman working at Piliyandala, ten miles from the city limits of Colombo. She had had several spirit attacks since puberty, but the serious ones started in 1966 when her dead grandmother—whom she loved very much—possessed her in the form of an evil spirit. Several demonic exorcisms were held to banish the spirit but to no avail. Eventually she was taken to Nāvala, and during a preliminary prophecy the priest, with considerable insight, told her that she had the magnetism (*ākarṣana balaya*) of the goddess Pattinī. She was not only possessed of the spirit of her dead grandmother but she also had the propensity to a Pattinī *ārūḍē*, that is, the capacity to be possessed by a good deity. Indeed, for several past births she had been meditating on this wish and she would now realize it in her present life. An exorcism was performed for her on 24 September 1968. In the early part of the ceremony the priest became the medium for Īśvara (Śiva). About 8:15 P.M. a dialogue ensued between god and evil spirit, acting through the bodies of priest and patient. Excerpts from this dialogue follow:

God Īśvara: With joy I say that the reception of the garland of magnetism [*ākarṣana mālāva*] of the Seven Pattinī is near, and, as a result, when you leave this human body you can achieve a great deal of merit. . . . From the vast store of merit you two will have your share. . . . Hence you must swear that you will leave this human body at 4:20 in the morning as you promised us earlier.

Spirit: God, I will leave [this body] for a period of three years.

God: Verily! Not for just three years. Hah! This human body has to be consecrated to Pattinī and so, especially, that the Seven Pattinī Goddesses' magnetism will raise this body into high [status] . . . will you [therefore] leave this body? Hah! *(He orders roughly)* Speak at once.

Spirit: Is that true? Will you raise me [my status]?

God: Yes!

Spirit: Lord God, are you saying the truth?

God: Yes. . . .

Spirit: If that is true I'll leave [this body] for good. . . .

God: Yes! Verily I am the immortal Īśvara, yes! Meditate on my truthfulness, yes! Are you going to respect this rise [in status]?

Spirit: (In humble tones) I respect it.

(An assistant brings a picture of the Buddha and Īśvara asks the spirit to swear before the Buddha that it will leave the body of the patient.)

God: Again place your hands together on your head and swear that this human body is now consecrated to the goddess Pattinī. Touch [the picture] three times and say that this body is consecrated to the goddess Pattinī. Swear three times!

Spirit: This human body is consecrated to the goddess Pattinī.

God: Saying in that manner won't do. You must touch this "Buddha-picture-shadow" . . . touch this picture and swear . . .

Spirit: I am loath to leave, O lord God.

God: If so, I'll have to punish you . . . swear and say that this body will take on a noble character.

Spirit: May this human body take on a noble character.

God: . . . You must swear and say that never again will I enter this human body.

Spirit: (Touching the picture of the Buddha) Never again will I enter this human body!

God: Yes, especially say, "As long as this human body exists I will not cause it suffering." Yes!

Spirit: (Swears) As long as life lasts in the body I will not afflict suffering on this human body.

God: Verily may this noble human body be consecrated to the goddess Pattinī.

Spirit: (Swearing) May this noble human body be consecrated to the goddess Pattinī.

After this the god Īśvara gave a series of ritual instructions, interdictions, and medicines for the patient. Three days after the exorcism (27 September 1968) Sumanāvatī sent her brother for further instructions during the 11:05 sessions; she came personally for instructions on 3 and 10 October 1968. An important incident occurred on the latter date. The priest was possessed by Gaṇeśa, and while he was uttering *śāstras* Sumanāvatī got possessed again, but the deity told Sumanāvatī that she was ready for the Pattinī *ārūḍē* (since the grandmother's spirit was no longer in her). "The time for keeping the company of the dead is over, now finally . . . time for keeping the company of the goddess." In his *śāstra* he instructed her in precise detail to sew a gown, belt, blouse, and so forth, to wear as the vestment of the deity. He told her that within thirty days she would have a "great victory," namely, *mukha varam* or "mouth warrant," the power to utter prophecies. The reference is to the formal installation: within thirty days the woman was to be given permission to speak on behalf of the deity.

On the day of Sumanāvatī's exorcism a classificatory (not blood-related) brother's daughter was present. This girl, Kusumāvatī (aged twenty years), had a similar history of possession. During her aunt's exorcism she too got into a trance and started yelling and dancing. According to the priest she had a similar power. Thus she too had an exorcism. During Kusumāvatī's exorcism her aunt got possessed again and danced in the ritual arena with the priest who looked upon it as an expression of Pattinī's magnetism. Kusumāvatī was also given instructions, similar to those given her aunt, and she was formally installed as a priestess about three months later.

Both were highly intelligent women. Initially each worked as a priestess for one or two days of the week in the Nāvala shrine; subsequently they received instructions to establish shrines in their own houses. Kusumāvatī's parents at first objected to this, but the deities, speaking through the girl, forced them to agree. When I interviewed them on 1 June 1970, both women were fully involved in their new roles. My impressions of the two women were then as follows:

When Sumanāvatī was a patient she could not bear to hear the sound of drums or the chanting of Buddhist texts (*pirit*). Now she can, and she has never been troubled again. She now utters prophecies and performs exorcism; she speaks with pride of her achievements. Since obtaining *mukha varam* she has uttered over one hundred prophecies and has performed seven exorcistic rituals. She described them well, and told me that two of her patients—thirty-year-old and eighteen-year-old females— will acquire power from the god Skanda of Kataragama. Her husband stated that he was pleased with her transformation, not to mention the added income.

When I first met Kusumāvatī as a patient she was extremely thin, shy, withdrawn, and very depressed and lethargic in appearance. The contrast now was truly impressive: she was energetic and talkative, and she spoke to me with considerable self-assurance. Also she was no longer anorexic; she looked physically attractive and had a healthy complexion. Her new role had given her a new self-image and had also enhanced her status and given her fame. Two weeks earlier, she said, many people came to see her possessed by the spirit of the goddess Sarasvatī. She no longer fell ill and could calmly hear drumming and Buddhist *pirit* chanting.

Although Kusumāvatī started with a Pattinī possession, now she can take the spirit of any deity. During such sessions people from neighboring villages come for consultations; she prescribes medicines, utters prophecies, and gives the blessings of the deities. She told me that she has performed at least four exorcism rituals during the last few months, assisted by her aunt Sumanāvatī. All these rituals were performed at home in her parents' house; the Nāvala priest was present, but only as a witness. She, however, offered him the client fees from these rituals as a token of her gratitude.

Kusumāvatī's mother said that she has had four proposals for marriage and that the parents will soon select a suitable partner for her. Kusumāvatī also wants to get married and settle down. She said that when she gets married she will give up her priestly role and settle down to a "normal" existence.

The Specificity of Illness and the Generality of Existence

I want to bring out some contrasting features of the two different types of cultural reactions to despair presented above. None of the meditators perceived their life crises and their despair as "illness." They had defined despair in ontic terms, as a problem of human impermanence and suffering as Buddhists see it. The conditions of old age were also not given a specificity so familiar to Western usage in such terms as "mid-life crisis," "old-age crisis," "menopause," "male menopause," and so forth. Quite the contrary; they saw it not as a crisis, but as an emerging condition of

existence that produced problems of meaning pertaining to human fini-
tude and death. Even when the movement to adopt meditation was a
response to a specific event such as bereavement and loss, the event was
immediately perceived in more general terms as epitomizing the human
condition. Such generalization can occur because Sinhalas are Buddhists
and they have myth models, such as the parable of the mustard seed
quoted earlier, which permit spontaneous and immediate generalization.

Contrast the situation in Western depression. We know from clinical
studies that even modern depressives tend to *generalize* their despair;[4] but
they cannot *universalize* it and give it ethical and soteriological significance as, for example, their forebear Hopkins could in the latter part of
the nineteenth century. At that time it was still possible to escape the
medicalization of despair (and the increasing medicalization of existence),
but it is near impossible now. While contemporary depressives attempt to
generalize their despair (that is, give it ontic significance), they can no
longer express it in Christian existential terms, for these no longer have
any significance, having been eroded by psychiatric terminology and,
behind the terminology, by the power of modern medicine. For most purposes depressives must become patients and be forced to accept the psychiatric view of their condition as illness, not existence. But illness (or disease), I submit, must for the most part be specific, since specificity is
necessary for diagnosis and treatment. Associated with specificity, and
intrinsic to it, is causation; the antecedent causes must be identified and
they too must possess the quality of specificity. Patients cannot maintain
their urge to generalize their despair for very long; they must be brought
to the specificity of the psychiatric definition of their illness. The increasing medical definition of despair must also mean an increasing specifica-
tion of the antecedent causes, the symptoms, and even the prognosis of
the disease. Thus most research work aims at isolating a specific neuro-
logical, genetic, or biochemical cause to explain the genesis of depression.
The irrelevance of existence cannot be underscored more clearly.

There is then a fundamental difference between existence and illness.
One must not confuse the metaphor of illness with illness itself. When
Pope said, "this long disease, my life," he was for the most part talking
about his body, beset by illness in its literal sense; when the Buddha
defined life as illness, it was in a metaphoric sense entirely. Christ and
the Buddha may occasionally help heal a specific disease, but they are not
curers, as shamans are; they heal life's ills in the metaphoric or symbolic
sense. The great historical religions deal with problems of existence, not
illness; and I shall soon show that when they deal with illness, they must
of necessity convert it to problems of existence. We have to take the cultural definition of a condition as illness or existence—or as both—seriously. The analyst may see "illness as metaphor," but another culture for
the most part may see it as reality. In my view a metaphor that is gener-

ally recognized as such can be "unpacked" by members of a society; people *know* the significance of a metaphor. Thus it does not make sense to say that "spirit possession" is a metaphor, whereas we may be conscious of metaphor when we say that "life is a disease" or that "Buddha is a healer." If spirit possession (and illness in general) is not a metaphor, it can be a symbol or symbolic system or a field of symbolic meaning. A symbol like a metaphor possesses polysemy, but not all the meanings are readily grasped by ordinary people. Its meaning must be unpacked by exegesis, which is for the most part a professional activity engaged in by a scholar or perhaps a religious specialist like Muchona, the hornet among the Ndembu.[5]

The symbolic meanings of illness are readily apparent in the case of "spirit possession." In Sumanāvatī's case I noted that she was possessed by the spirit of her dead grandmother who loved her. But Sumanāvatī cannot understand why someone who loves you must inflict suffering, leading you to a state of despair. The analyst must supply the interpretation by unpacking the unconscious meanings of spirit attack. In *Medusa's Hair* I described the significance of spirit attack in great detail. In these cases, as in Sumanāvatī's, the individual experiencing a spirit attack—most often a woman—withers away, becomes skin and bone, and sees terrifying visions. Her body shakes as she becomes possessed, she runs away from home and acts very much like the demon within her. I have interpreted this type of experience as a product of primary guilt and expiation.[6] In all of these cases the patients had a common antecedent history: the betrayal of a loved one. Typically this betrayal was not a childhood one, but one occurring in later life, especially a failure to attend a loved relation's funeral. But this in turn was based on earlier betrayals, some of which perhaps may have had ontogenetic roots. In the typical case the possessing demon is the dead relative, who punishes the patient for betrayal; the patient in turn suffers pain of mind and body, and gradually overcomes this dark experience, through a kind of penance and expiation. After the expiation of guilt, the attacking, hostile ancestor takes on a benevolent and loving form and becomes a guardian spirit of the patient. The patient herself ultimately triumphs over privation, guilt, and "evil" and becomes a priestess. Her possession was initially demonic; it is now converted to a divine propensity and is so legitimated by the gods themselves. She has also effected a role transformation, giving up her earlier mundane roles and role relationships to become a priestess, helping others in misfortune. She renounces ordinary domesticity and her ordinary sexuality for a devotional-erotic relationship with a divinity. She lives in grim physical surroundings in the slums of the city, but this everyday physical and social reality is of little consequence, for the true reality is her spiritual experiences with the gods in such ecstatic states as visions and trances.

When a particular culture defines a problem as illness, it is deliberately, though temporarily, isolating the illness from its larger existential context. However, most non-Western cultures (unlike Western biomedicine) eventually put the illness and the patient back into their existential context. The process of isolating the illness and then putting it back into its larger context varies with the type of illness and the culture; one can therefore only give some examples. In cases of possession anywhere in the world, the possessing spirit (or spirits) is identified and exorcised from the body of the patient. But the individual has not exorcised the spirit from the world it inhabits: spirits continue to exist, the patient remains vulnerable. The intruding spirit is part of a cosmos or worldview shared by the patient and others in the society, including the curers. Spirit attack can be terribly traumatic, alienating the patient from the group. But it does not necessarily alienate the group from the patient, for they are all bound by a common idiom and worldview. When Sumanāvatī fell ill and said "I am possessed by a demon," her family tended to agree with her; they also knew how to act in the situation. If she went to a Western psychiatrist her condition would have been diagnosed as "hysteria" or "paranoia" or whatever. Such labels are incomprehensible to ordinary people and result in patient and group alienation at every level.

Sometimes the exorcism of the spirit from the body of the patient and her eventual reintegration into the group constitute the finale of the cure. But I have noted that recently in Sri Lanka, there is an increasing tendency for a patient to convert the evil spirit to a benevolent deity and for the patient to be converted to a priestess. In this situation one can infer certain principles underlying the whole process of exorcism and its cure.

1. The individual's propensity to possession by a demon is utilized in the postexorcism proceedings. The negative spirit is expelled and a positive deity is substituted.

2. The patient is given a new role and a higher status. For a woman the status is striking; she has a new freedom. This is a "role resolution" of a psychological conflict: in her new role she can put her conflicts to creative use. Her earlier sickness had impaired her role performance; the new status provides an opportunity for role performance more congruent with her inner needs.

3. The individual has, in her own estimation, developed spiritually. She lives in a spiritual world to which few have access and continues to interact with the deities of the shrine. This gives meaning and direction to her life.

4. Not all patients take over the priestly role; some simply join the cult group and get into occasional trances during celebrations at the shrine or on trips to pilgrimage centers. Some who become priests may eventually give up the role, as Kusumāvatī planned to do after marriage. In such a

case, the exorcism and investiture help the patient overcome a difficult
personal crisis and put her back on her feet to function normally.

One striking feature about spirit possession is that it can exist without
"trance." The patient may be diagnosed as being possessed by a spirit,
but the spirit does not cause the patient to act out her possession in seemingly bizarre behavior. When the spirit is dormant, there is no active possession trance and the prognosis for a cure is poor. I think that those who
are extremely inhibited and who are socialized in terms of middle-class
values cannot act out their inner suffering and despair in the outer drama
of spirit possession. Often when spirit attack occurs the patient does not
eat, and this results in anorexia. We noted that Sumanāvatī was thin when
she first came to the shrine; but after she was initiated as a priestess she
not only gained weight but also regained personal attractiveness and self-
confidence. Middle-class women, socialized in notions of decorum and
propriety, cannot act out in this fashion. I have seen plenty of middle-
class anorexics in Sri Lanka, but they rarely appear at exorcisms. They
generally consult Ayurvedic physicians, who almost inevitably diagnose
the disease as a loss of *dhātus*, or the vital essences of the body.

Medicine, Ethics, and Soteriology

I would now like to reexamine the two types of reactions to despair, spec-
ulating on the manner in which medicine and existence have been given
ethical significance in a great historical religion like Buddhism. I have
argued elsewhere that one of the features of the great historical religions
is what one might call "radical ethicization"—a process whereby an ordinary secular morality is invested with soteriological significance.[7] There is
nothing unique about the Buddhist precepts or Christian commandments,
since similar injunctions are found in many preliterate religions. What is
unique about Buddhism or Christianity is that the public morality or ethics is inextricably implicated in soteriology, so that a violation of a moral
norm is *ipso facto* a violation of a religious norm, and this in turn is an
obstacle to salvation. Alongside this radical ethicization characteristic of
the world religions is a related process whereby folk beliefs and practices
are invested with symbolic and ethical significance. We noted that in the
Buddhist case this ethical thrust of the great tradition resulted historically
in drawing the pre-Buddhist folk–healing traditions into an ethical and
symbolic framework legitimated by Buddhist values.

The meditation on revulsion, we noted, was a response to a life crisis
that did not entail healing except in a metaphorical sense. The activities

of the meditators take them into the heart of Buddhist ethical and soteriological values. Meditation is a technique that was devised by the great
tradition itself and is integral to it. Not so with spirit possession, which
exists in many societies independent of soteriology and, to a great extent,
of ethics. It is not only characterized by possession trance but is overwhelmingly dominated by women. The specialists of the cult may be
male or female (or transvestite) exorcists or shamans. What then happens
when a cult that existed (and exists) in many preliterate societies independently of any soteriology confronts a great tradition—in our case Buddhism? How does the Buddhist confrontation differ from the Christian?
To answer this question one must examine both the nature of the soteriology and the nature of the confrontation with spirit possession in the
two religions.

The Buddhist soteriological stance in respect to possession (and other
practices) is that these have little negative or positive value in respect to
salvation. Salvation lies in following a specifically Buddhist path, and this
effectively means world renunciation. Ideally it is monks who pursue this
goal, but lay virtuosos like our meditators have also made a preliminary
move. Ordinary laypersons, because they are involved in the world, cannot achieve *nirvāṇa* except in some distant rebirth. They can at best lead
ethically meaningful lives and achieve the secondary soteriological com-
pensations of heaven and a happy rebirth. Lay life, then, is an impedi-
ment to salvation. How does all of this affect healing? Insofar as healing
is a lay activity, the monk is not involved in it. Hence monks never officiate at rites of passage, except at funerals, where the soteriological welfare of the deceased has to be assured. Exorcisms, village harvest rites,
and so forth are officiated by shamans, exorcists, and similar priests. Yet,
as Sri Lankan Sinhalas are Buddhists these healing rituals must conform
to Buddhist values. Thus in Sri Lankan history there is a constant ethical
and symbolic transformation of possession trance in a Buddhist direction—not by monks, but by the Buddhist lay public and the local priests,
who of course are also Buddhists. Let me give two examples of such
transformation.

1. In many cultures possession trance is associated with animal sacrifices. This simply cannot occur in any village ritual in Sri Lanka without
producing serious reactions. Hence, a little bit of blood is used instead
of an animal, and sometimes a substitutive admixture that resembles
blood; or a burnt feather of a chicken may be used as a symbolic substitute.

2. The demons who possess the patients are invested with Buddhist
ethical values such as craving, hate, greed, envy, and so forth and are
integrated into the Buddhist pantheon. The local specialist can then carry

on his or her traditional role of exorcist without challenging the monk, who is the guardian of Buddhist doctrine. The monk is a healer in a metaphoric sense alone—of life's ills rather than illness. In his confrontation with spirit possession the monk's posture is determined by the Buddhist soteriology; he leaves it alone as long as its practices do not violate Buddhist ethics. The Christian soteriological posture is different, since the salvation of the laity is intrinsic to its soteriological quest. Here also the lay practices are ethicized, but more than that, they must be given soteriological direction and purpose. Consequently, the intruding spirit becomes the devil, the embodiment of evil in it radical soteriological sense. This must result in an alienation of the patient from the religion—a situation quite impossible in Buddhism. In fact, the soteriological redefinition of spirit attack in the history of Christianity means that the sufferer ceases to be a patient; rather he or she is a sinner whose salvation has been jeopardized. Once again it is interesting to note that what might be defined as illness in one culture is converted to an existential condition in another once it is incorporated into the great tradition. The Christian priest, even when he expels the intruding spirit from the body of the patient, retains his role as a curer of an existential condition rather than a curer of an illness, that is, a physician pure and simple.

Beneath the contrasts in the style of confrontation is an ethical and psychological posture common to both great traditions (and perhaps to all). In both, the agents mediating the confrontation are literate; and, if monks and nuns, they are also celibate. Even when no celibacy is required as in Protestantism, there is at least a rigid ethicization of sexuality. The rationality of these literati is in a fundamental sense opposed to the seeming irrationality of spirit possession. Doctrinal Buddhism and Christianity alike emphasize the rational control of drives and place a premium on decorum, self-possession, and rational discourse. In spirit possession the very opposite seems to prevail: the patient loses control and autonomy by being the vehicle of an intruding spirit, which, in Buddhism, violates the doctrinal principle of the self-reliant individual pursuing his or her salvation quest lonely as the single horn of the rhinoceros.

Buddhist and Christian rationality is not simply a matter of discourse but of morality as well. Not only does spirit possession violate doctrinal rationality but proximity to it has psychological implications for the clergy. Celibate monks cannot be confronted with the orgiastic—and sometimes orgasmic—convolutions of the body of female possessees. The possession condition not only undermines the clerical view of rationality and control but also threatens to undo the control of their own drives and loosens their own precarious repressions, especially that of sexuality. The Buddhist monk is in a better position, however, than his Christian counterpart. The soteriological duty of the Buddhist forces him to avoid confrontation whereas the Christian priest's experience of confrontation, we know, can be quite brutal.

What then is the Buddhist monk's rational alternative to possession trance? The answer to this question brings us back to the beginning of this essay: meditation. Meditation, insofar as it entails the calming of desire and the autonomy of the individual, is the very opposite of spirit possession. If spirit possession involves healing, meditation involves existence, if spirit possession pertains to worldly desire, meditation pertains to its transcendence. The calm and serene expression of the meditator (monk or *upāsaka*) contrasts with the violence of the person possessed by spirits. One involves silence, the other involves noise.

I think anyone living in Sri Lanka cannot but be impressed by this relational contrast, and I believe it is this relation that gives each tradition its full range of meaning. I also think that the contemporary relationship of the two traditions in Sri Lanka could give us a clue to their historic evolution in human culture. Spirit possession came first in the evolution of religion and was probably everywhere associated with shamanism.[8] Could it not be that the meditative response was a rational reaction by a speculative priesthood against the "irrationality" of possession trance in the evolution of the great historical religions? It must be remembered that meditation, in its fully developed form in Indian religions, meets the challenge of possession trance by producing its own forms of trance, in which visions, states of contemplative bliss, or mystical union with the godhead are achieved. Yet these trances maintain the rationality, serenity, and calm associated with meditation. Contemplative trance is the meditator's answer to possession trance.[9]

I have noted that the clerical literati of the great historical religions have been, in general, repelled by spirit possession. I think that a similar repulsion may be postulated of those whose life-styles have been influenced by the ethics and the doctrinal rationality of the great traditions, such as the literati in general and the bourgeoisie. In contrast, spirit possession has been predominantly the religion of the tribal and peasant peoples. For example, in India it is not only monks who are critical of spirit possesion, but also brahmans and all those communities that have come under the influence of brahman values. These distinctions persist everywhere even today: contemplation is positively valued by the professional and educated classes, and even the vast bourgeoisie in modern societies are not hostile to it. The opposite is true of spirit possession. Possession, in today's urban societies, is almost exclusively confined to the lower classes and the poor, and it has undergone an enormous resurgence among the sprawling working-class and slum districts of modern cities. It is a reaction to despair by the poor and dispossessed in the grim overcrowded cities where urban proletarians are segregated. Do we dare say that it too is a form of stating "I can"?[10]

Notes

1. P. Vajirāñāna, *Buddhist Meditation in Theory and Practice* (Colombo, Sri Lanka, 1962), pp. 166–182.
2. See Walter Kaufmann, *A Critique of Religion and Philosophy* (New York, 1961), pp. 396–405, for a good discussion of a related text.
3. Sigmund Freud, *Civilization and Its Discontents*, trans. Joan Riviere (1930: reprint, London, 1949).
4. For an account of the generalization of despair, see George W. Brown and Tirril Harris, *The Social Origins of Depression* (New York, 1978).
5. Victor Turner, "Muchona the Hornet, Interpreter of Religion," in *The Forest of Symbols* (Ithaca, NY, 1967), pp. 131–150.
6. Gananath Obeyesekere, *Medusa's Hair: An Essay on Personal Symbols and Religious Experience* (Chicago, 1981), pp. 53–83.
7. See my paper, "The Karmic Eschatology and Its Transformation: A Contribution to the Sociology of Early Buddhism," in *Karma and Rebirth in Classical Indian Traditions*, ed. Wendy D. O'Flaherty (Berkeley, 1980), pp. 137–164.
8. I use the term "shaman" for a religious specialist who gets into a trance as a consequence of either spirit intrusion or spirit extrusion. The latter is of course Mircea Eliade's definition of classic shamanism; this form hardly exists in South Asia.
9. I believe we got a glimpse of this contrast in early Indian religious history, when the Rigvedic *muni*s were closer to shamans and spirit mediums while the ascetics were in the opposite camp. The later takeover of the term *muni* by ascetic orders indicated the triumph of the latter.
10. The discussion of meditation in this paper is based on an earlier article, "Depression, Buddhism and the Work of Culture in Sri Lanka," in *Depression and Culture*, ed. Arthur Kleinman and Byron Good (Berkeley, 1985); the data on spirit possession is discussed in *Buddhism Transformed* by Richard Gombrich and myself (forthcoming). The reader is urged to look at these two publications for detail and context.

CHAPTER 7

Islam and

Health/Medicine:

A Historical

Perspective

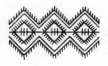

FAZLUR RAHMAN

Islam, as a religion, has played a fundamental role in the creation of a culture that has nurtured the cultivation and development of medicine. The Qur'ān stresses that socioeconomic justice is the pillar of its teaching on monotheism (the two teachings are organically related in the Qur'ān), and the literature of *ḥadīth*, or reports of the words and deeds of Muhammad, strongly underline mercy toward all creatures, particularly humans, and even enjoin the Muslim community actively to exercise good will. These potent moral-spiritual factors prepared the ground for the widespread reception and astonishing evolution of medicine in Islam. Felix

149

Klein-Franke describes the pervasiveness of the medical perspective in Arabo-Islamic literature and culture in the following words:

> Medical issues in Islam are not discussed by Arabs just in an isolated medical professional literature; medical problems also claim a significant portion of theological and juristic literature and even of belles lettres. More than among the Greeks or the Romans, medicine in Islam comprehends a part of general literature. A comprehensive treatment of medicine in Islam must, therefore, take into account the just-mentioned fields as well. Whoever undertakes to deal with medicine in Islam does not take on a slender lateral path on the side of Arabic literature—his way, rather, leads him to the very heart of Islamic culture. None of the non-Arab sciences has provoked such rich response from within Islam as has medicine.[1]

Islamic Concepts of Wellness and Illness

Before the manifestation of Islam at the hands of the prophet Muhammad during the first third of the seventh century, Arabs had a tradition of medicine that consisted for the most part of magical rituals and amulets but partly also of a more scientifically rooted medicine involving the use of seeds, herbs, and surgical practices like cupping and cauterization. According to reports, the Prophet had at first forbidden amulets along with other magical practices, but when his followers insisted that they had been using amulets with healing benefit, he reluctantly allowed the practice, with the proviso that writings on amulets consist only of verses from the Qur'ān. He did this to safeguard against the possibility that some amulets might invoke powers to achieve healing other than the one unique God of Islam.

Contemporary with the Prophet were certain medical men who were acquainted with Greek medicine—the best known being al-Ḥārith ibn Kalada, who is reported to have learned medicine at the medical school of Gundai Shāpūr. This school had been established by the earlier Iranian rulers and developed to its glory under the Sassanian emperor Anūshra-wān, who died in 579 CE, nine years after the Prophet's birth. It was this school that supplied medical knowledge and resources to the Arab Muslims in Baghdad.

The Qur'ān, the basic scripture of Islam, was revealed piecemeal to the prophet Muhammad over a period of about twenty-three years, from 610 to 632. It provides the essential elements of its worldview, for which traditions (ḥadīth) from the Prophet have historically supplied the super-structure. According to the Qur'ān, God, although infinite and transcen-dent, is nevertheless "present" everywhere in the universe; he is, indeed, "nearer to man than his jugular vein" (sura 50, verse 16); he "intervenes between a man and his heart" (8.24); and, finally, he intervenes between man and men. God created the universe and everything therein as an act of primordial mercy, for there was no obligation on his part to create. Mercy and power are, therefore, his ultimate attributes.[2]

The nature of the universe he has created is that of one firmly knit and well-ordered whole wherein there are no jumps, gaps, ruptures, or dislocations. Whenever God creates (*khalq*) something, he places the laws of its behavior (*amr*) within it as well; this is why there is a cosmos rather than chaos. God presides over and directs the whole. Although the Qur'ān accepts the miracles performed by earlier prophets or, rather, produced by God at their hands, with the coming of Muhammad these miracles ceased (17.59). The Qur'ān frequently refers not only to an orderly working of nature, but also to its plenitude, and insists upon its subjugation and serviceability to human beings. Everything in nature has been created for human beings, and humans have been created to serve God.

Humanity is God's vicegerent on earth and in this capacity has to manage its affairs well and constructively regarding the earth—not waste it, destroy it, or "sow corruption upon it." Just as nature is *muslim* (in fealty to God) because it accepts God's laws unquestioningly, so is an individual required to be *muslim:* the *is* of nature is to be replaced by *ought* in the case of humans, for whereas nature is automatic in its conduct, people have to be *muslim* by choice. Because of their responsible nature, human beings must be prepared for a judgment upon their performance in this life. Judgment upon individuals will be on the Last Day, when their "deeds will be weighed," and on this basis their future career and form of life assigned. But there is also "judgment in history," which is visited not on individuals but on peoples, collectivities, nations, and communities.

Human beings' weakness, out of which all their ills spring, both individual and social, lies in their pettiness of mind and their narrow vision. Idolatry or worship of local, tribal, or national gods is a manifestation of this pettiness. Only belief in transcendence creates the necessary spiritual space that enables people to transcend both their own narrow vision and their worship of local gods. Unless this pettiness is transcended they become the victims of selfishness and greed, refusing to share their wealth with others even though God "promises forgiveness (of sins) and prosperity" for such investment in the welfare of society (2.270). Criticizing the greed of the rich Meccan merchants, the Qur'ān says: "If you were to possess all the treasures of the mercy of thy Lord, you would still sit on them out of fear of spending them" (17.100).

Contrasts like pride and despair, absolute power and freedom, total helplessness and determinism, hope and fear are not so much philosophical problems to be resolved intellectually as moral tensions or "limits of God" within whose framework humans must live in order to assure their well-being through maximization of their moral energy. To violate either side of this tension by affirming one side and negating the other produces the same satanic state—moral nihilism. To be squarely anchored within these tensions is to keep oneself safe, whole, and integral; and to violate them is to "lose" oneself, to disintegrate the self.

This attitude and conduct constitute *taqwā*, that is, guarding and developing one's integrity and avoiding self-destruction. It is of salient interest to note that the three most basic terms in the Qur'ān have practically identical meaning. *Taqwā* comes from the root *wqy*, which means "to protect against loss," "to safeguard against wastage." The term *islām* comes from the root *slm*, which means "to be in peace," "to be safe and integral," "to be whole." *Imān*, usually translated as "faith" in English, comes from the root *amn*, which means to be "free from danger," "to be at peace—both internally and externally."

From this analysis some idea can be gained of the most basic élan of the Qur'ān—guidance for humanity. It demands of individuals a conduct that will keep them—both in their individual and collective existence and in their body and mind—sound, integral, whole, and at peace. *Taqwā*, commonly mistranslated as "piety" in English, is primarily the attribute of an individual person, but is essentially manifested in one's relation and attitude toward other people. Thus, for example, the Qur'ān says: "Be fair (to others) for this is nearest to *taqwā*"(5.8).

Although the Qur'ān's emphasis on the moral righteousness of the individual is great, individuals by themselves are not sufficient to carry out God's purposes for humanity as set forth in the Qur'ān. The Qur'ān requires the establishment on this earth of a social (and consequently a political) order that shall be ethically based and shall "remove corruption from the earth and reform it." This is not the task of individual human beings; it requires a community. To this end, the Qur'ān consciously and deliberately established a community that it called "the best community brought out for mankind" (3.110), that is, established for the benefit of all people.

This is not the place to assess whether or, if so, how far the historic Muslim community has been able to fulfill the purposes of the Qur'ān. From our present perspective, the important thing to note is that the community, thanks to the tight-knit bonds among its members established by the Qur'ān and the practice of the prophet Muhammad, developed an extraordinary cohesiveness and intense mutual feeling within its parameters. There is little doubt that it was this bond and the heavy stress of the Qur'ān on justice that produced, quite early in the history of Islam, a strong impulse to erect institutions for general welfare, including health care. The great number and size of those institutions were inspired by the teaching of the Qur'ān concerning the community and its egalitarian character. This mutual help and "outreach" to the less-fortunate segments of

Muslim society did not remain entirely confined to the limits of the Muslim community but overflowed its boundaries. Many of the larger health institutions were open to people of all races and of different faiths.

PROPHETIC TRADITIONS ON WELFARE

While the Qur'ān gave strong and general directives for mutual help and solidarity, the Prophet's own actions gave practical proof of this. Immediately after he and his Meccan followers emigrated to Medina (in 622), he created a bond of "brotherhood" *(mu'ākhāt)* between the emigrants *(muhājirūn)* and the local Medinese Muslims (Anṣār, "the Helpers"), whereby one of the Anṣār was assigned to each emigrant as the latter's "brother," providing him with a home and sharing his land and wealth with him. Also, Muhammad levied a tax called *zakāt* on the well-to-do members of the community, to be spent on the poor, orphans, widows, and others in need. This is, in fact, the only tax levied by the Qur'ān: "*Zakāt* funds are only for the poor and the needy and those who collect it [i.e., the civil service], those whose hearts are to be won for Islam [i.e., diplomatic service], for the release of war-captives, for the relief of those who are in chronic and incurable debts, for *jihād* [i.e., defense] and social services and for the welfare of the traveler [i.e., communications]—this is a duty cast by God upon Muslims—God is Knowing and Wise" (9.60).

The vast number of traditions attributed to the Prophet *(ḥadīth)* that enjoin and encourage general humanitarianism and mercy, and particularly intra-Muslim sympathies, largely constitute the source of Islamic humanism. However, it should be noted that much if not all of this literature is apocryphal and does not date back historically to the Prophet. Nevertheless, as it dates mostly from the first and second centuries of the Islamic Era (which is lunar and begins with June 622 CE), that is, the seventh and eighth centuries, and has been regarded as authoritative by Muslims since then, its general lack or deficiency of historical authenticity is irrelevant from our present perspective.

According to one tradition the Prophet said: "The Merciful has mercy on those who have mercy (on people)—have mercy on those on earth that He Who is in the heaven have mercy on you."[3] There are a great many *ḥadīth* inciting Muslims to be sincere and to have active goodwill toward the Muslim community. For example: "Muslims are like members of one body; if one member is hurt and feels pain, the whole body feels pain."[4] There are numerous other *ḥadīth* exhorting the faithful to sacrifice themselves for others, particularly for Muslims. Helping people who are in distress of any kind is particularly emphasized. "A person cannot have faith if he satiates himself while his neighbor goes without food."[5] There is a well-known *ḥadīth* that tells of a prostitute who encountered a dog that was gasping for breath and dying of thirst. There was no water around except a well. Using her shoe as a bucket, and tying it to her scarf like a rope, she drew up water and quenched the dog's thirst. God forgave her sins.[6]

THE "PROPHETIC MEDICINE"

All collections of traditions relating to Muhammad (Sunni collections dating from the ninth century to those of the Shī'a from the tenth) contain fairly lengthy sections on medicine. While it is plausible that the prophet made statements of a medical nature on several occasions and—since Arabs had an ancient tradition of medical prescriptions—that he gave informal medical advice to his family or his companions, it is certain that this entire body of traditions does not extend back to him. Ibn Khaldūn (d. 1405), the celebrated pioneer of cultural history, says in the prolegomenon to his work on history that the medicine attributed to the Prophet is actually the old Arab medicine, which is based on experience but not on scientific experimentation and hence is not founded on scientific principles. He admits, nevertheless, that such treatments can prove useful, particularly if their user "has strong faith." Even when genuinely attributed to the Prophet, however, these prescriptions belong not to his religious mission (nubūwa) but to mundane affairs in which he had no specially privileged position over others.[7]

From our perspective, the important point to note is that a body of medical knowledge has come to be universally attributed by Islamic religious authorities to the prophet Muhammad himself. The Qur'ān does not speak explicitly of medical treatment, although it sets high value on health and its restoration. It emphasizes cleanliness, both physical and spiritual, and calls itself "a cure" (10.57; 17.82; 41.44). While the Qur'ān presumably meant that it is a "medicine for the spirit," Muslims later produced a large literature elaborating its physically curative and miraculous qualities.

Beginning roughly with the tenth century and continuing through the fourteenth and fifteenth centuries, a series of works was written—a dozen and a half or more—entitled Prophetic Medicine or The Prophet's Medicine. The authors were orthodox scholars and pious men who had learned both the ancient Arabian medicine and the Greek tradition of scientific medicine. The Shī'a wrote parallel works, mostly entitled The Imans' Medicine. These men did not practice medicine, at least not professionally. What was their motivation? Although most of the literature is still unpublished, what is published leaves one with the impression that their basic motivations were to provide the public with an easy guide to health and to confer a high religious value on the art of healing. In fact, several writers of both so-called Prophetic and scientific medical works state that after the performance of basic religious duties, there is no greater service to God than to heal people.[8]

The religious justification for medical treatment of disease is found in the oft-narrated *hadīth*s, wherein the Prophet said: "Get yourself treated when you are sick, for every disease God has sent a remedy as well" and wherein he advised a sick companion to consult al-Ḥārith ibn Kalada, who, according to Muslim historians of medicine, had studied medicine at Gundai Shāpūr.[9] According to another tradition, when asked about the advisibility of medical treatment the Prophet replied affirmatively. And when asked: "What about God's pre-written decrees?" he answered: "Medications are part of God's pre-written decree."[10]

The well-known religious scholar and theologian al-Dhahabī (d. 1346), like other writers of *Prophetic Medicine* literature, states that medicines are a natural extension of foods, and, like foods, their discovery is based upon instinct followed by empirical study: just as human beings when they felt hungry continued to discover various foods, so when they felt ill, continued to discover medications. In fact, he claims that several animals have also managed to find certain instinctive cures. Snakes, for example, when their eyesight becomes weak after winter, eat a substance called *vazfang* in order to recover their sight (this substance, al-Dhahabī says, is also recommended by doctors for weak-sighted humans). The author gives several other instances of such animal behavior. For example, if a female vulture experiences difficulty in laying eggs, its male brings her a certain stone from India called *lunduga*. When the female moves it, she hears something move inside which facilitates her egg-laying. A fox, when it is taken ill in spring, eats a certain grass which works as a laxative for it; cats use the same grass as an emetic.[11]

Whatever the scientific truth in these statements, the point the Prophetic Medicine writers sought to make is that medical cures are something as natural and instinctive as is food for hunger and drink for thirst, and that deliberate empirical study follows instinctive cures. For this reason, Muslims, following ancient writers, believed that the medical art, like all other arts, sciences, and cultural amenities, was first "revealed" to certain prophets and subsequently developed by human experience and reason.[12] Therefore, most jurists hold that medical treatment is, from a religious perspective, "obligatory" upon patients, and that parents and guardians must obtain due treatment for their children. Al-Dhahabī bases the obligatoriness of treatment on the Qur'anic verse that commands Muslims: "Guard yourself" (i.e., against danger, 4.71).[13]

It is necessary to consider the problem of divine determination and human freedom in relation to treatment. As mentioned above, in reply to a question about the advisability of medical treatment in view of God's predeterminism, the Prophet said that medicine was also a part of divine determinism. Islam has no sects corresponding to those in Christianity that, in principle, are against medication. There have been individuals of this opinion, particularly among Sufi ascetics, although the vast majority of Sufis believed in healing and medical treatment.

Although determinism—theistic or physical—versus human free will has been a problem for humanity in general and religions in particular, theistic determinism has historically been at the center of Islamic theology. The reason seems to be that, in the Qur'ān, the same phenomena are mentioned as produced by God and by the human will or by God and natural causation.[14] Sometimes one finds both these causes stated in the same verse of the Qur'ān. This in itself should have warned Muslims that, since such blatant contradictions are impossible, different aspects or meanings of causation must be meant in each case. However, Muslim theological schools took opposing positions, particularly on acts of human volition: the Mu'tazilite School taught that humans had absolute free will, producing acts wherein God had no role to play and for which, therefore, they alone were responsible. The Ash'arite School, on the other hand— the school that until recently had exercised hegemony over Sunni Islam for a millennium—taught that God alone was "actor," that neither nature nor human beings had any inherent powers to produce real effects, that human volition was vacuous without God, and, finally, that causation was a meaningless word. This orthodox doctrine, when combined with the Sufi worldview that taught human beings total passivity vis-à-vis God, led several Sufis to put their whole "trust" in God and deny "secondary causes." In the debate that followed on this issue, the Mu'tazilite School, which affirmed natural causation or "the world of causes," ('ālam al-asbāb) won out,[15] but there were still some for whom natural causation and the exercise of human will were contrary to "trust in God." However, from the orthodox and Sufi doctrines of denial of natural causation and "total trust in God" no valid generalizations can be made about the efficacy of natural causes or human will—not regarding the general body of the Muslim community and not even regarding the orthodox or the Sufis themselves, about whom Klein-Franke theorizes rather broadly.[16] As for the problem of the denial of natural causation, causation is rehabilitated by the orthodoxy affirming that "it is the habit of God to make certain events succeed certain other events, a habit that is unchangeable."[17] As for the doctrine of "trust in God," in its most widely accepted form humans must first utilize the natural means God has created for certain purposes and then trust in God, for the world of nature has not been created in vain. Klein-Franke, however, cites an extreme case of the eighth-century Sufi lady Rābi'a al-'Adawīya who, during an illness, refused even to pray to God for her recovery, let alone use medicines, saying: "Who has willed illness—is it not God?" He comments that this illustrates the mental attitude of the pious in Islam.[18]

It is important to consider the etiology of illness. The *ḥadīth* literature, while emphasizing health as the greatest blessing of God after faith (*īmān*),[19] at the same time stresses that illness has certain important spiritual functions. These functions are of three kinds: (1) illness has a purgative role, (2) it may be a punishment for sins, and (3) it may entail positive reward. In all these forms or, rather, nuances, illness is to be regarded as a blessing. According to some traditions, if a person does not become a true man or woman of faith because of certain shortcomings, God sends illness in order to perfect him or her. God also makes people ill in order to compensate them with a reward in future life. According to *ḥadīth*, those who suffer from plagues and certain other illnesses, including childbirth, are martyrs.[20] On the whole, Shī'a *ḥadīth* stress this theology much more than Sunni, although much less Shī'a *ḥadīth* on medicine has been published. For example, according to some Shī'a *ḥadīth*, one night's pain and sickness is better than forty years of worship. And, one should not seek medical treatment for an illness unless it has become unbearable.[21] No parallel to these two Shī'a examples exists in Sunni *ḥadīth*. There is no doubt that this kind of attitude has been encouraged in Shī'ism by the doctrine of martyrdom and the passion motive built upon the death of Husain, the Prophet's grandson, at the hands of Umayyad government troops in 680. Sunni Islam is completely clear of the passion motive, despite the martyrdom ideal—inculcated not so much by Husain's death as by the Qur'ān's teaching on *jihād*. Although the Shī'a *ḥadīth*s quoted above reveal a certain positive evaluation of suffering, the Shī'a rulers, the *'ulumā'* (religious scholars), and the masses value medication highly.

Care and Healing of the Sick

ḤADĪTH ON CARING AND CURING

The spiritual merits of visiting the sick are greatly emphasized in *ḥadīth* literature. In a well-known *ḥadīth* the Prophet said: "Visit the sick and free the slave."[22] According to one *ḥadīth* the Prophet ordered Muslims to do seven things, according to other versions five or six, but all include visiting the sick (implying doing whatever one can to ameliorate their condition).[23] Traditions emphasize that when visiting a patient, one should make the visit brief and not tire the patient.[24] One should say things that are encouraging and inspire confidence.[25] The Prophet usually visited a sick person after three days, for it is usually only then that illness is regarded as something serious.[26] The patient should also try to respond with good cheer. It is even recommended in *ḥadīth* that, since the suffering patient is in such a pure state that his or her prayers are likely to be granted, others should ask the patient to pray for them.

Despite the gravity of illness, one must not wish for death. This subject, although broached in the Qur'ān in general terms, is made explicit in *ḥadīth*. The Qur'ān, for example, says: "Do not cast yourselves into perdition" (2.195), but the *ḥadīth* explicitly forbids a Muslim from praying for death. According to one *ḥadīth*, the Prophet said: "Let none of you (Muslims) desire death, for, if one is a good person, perchance one's goodness will increase and if one is evil, perchance they will get the opportunity to turn around." Even when one is sick of one's life, one should say: "My Lord! Keep me alive so long as life is good for me and end my life if the end is good for me,"[27] that is, one must not take the decision into one's own hands. Suicide is, therefore, forbidden in Islam.

HEALTH CARE INSTITUTIONS

In the Prophet's lifetime Arabia had no hospitals; this institution began on the large scale, during the Abbasid regime in Baghdad.

In the sixth century, the Persian emperor Anūshrawān established at Gundai Shāpūr in southwestern Iran an academy of sciences where philosophers and scientists from Athens gathered after the closure of the Platonic Academy by the Emperor Justinian in 529. Anūshrawān also invited some medical men from India. It was this medical school that enabled the Abbasids to begin their brilliant cultivation of medical sciences after the Arab Muslims' initial acquaintance with Greek medicine in Egypt. Prior to this, the Umayyad caliph al-Walīd I had established "houses" for lepers and for the blind, but these could hardly be called hospitals. In fact, the first regular hospital was founded in Baghdad by Harūn al-Rashīd (d. 809) and was directed by a Christian doctor from Gundai Shāpūr.

After al-Rashīd's, four other hospitals were founded in quick succession in Baghdad during the tenth century. Those in charge of hospitals in the early centuries were often Christians. Abū Bakr al-Rāzī (his date of death is usually given as 925) was the first Muslim director of a major hospital in Baghdad, built in the early tenth century. It is reported that he hung pieces of meat in different places in the city and examined the pieces after some days, building the hospital where the meat was found to be least infected. It was the same al-Rāzī (latinized as Rhazes) who first established clinically the distinction between measles and smallpox.

Besides regular hospitals, mobile hospitals were also instituted. 'Alī ibn 'Īsā, called the Good Vizier, wrote to Sinān ibn Thābit (d. 942), who was the official head of doctors in Baghdad:

I have been thinking concerning the people of Sawād [the countryside of southern Iraq]. There must be people there who have no access to a doctor because doctors are not to be found in the countryside. So, go ahead—may God give you long life—and send doctors along with a store of medicines and potions and let them go around in the countryside, halting in each place for as long as is necessary. Having treated patients there, let them then move further.[28]

Sinān sent a medical task force, and after a while wrote to the vizier that since diseases were rampant that year, people wanted the doctors to stay on longer. He added that most of the inhabitants there were Jewish, but that the policy in Baghdad hospitals was to treat Muslims and non-Muslims alike, though he would await the vizier's orders in this case. The vizier replied that even the animals have to be medically treated, so Jews and Christians must be treated, but that an order should be observed: first Muslims must be treated, then non-Muslims, and lastly, animals. The same vizier ordered Sinān ibn Thābit to organize medical service for the inmates of prisons:

> I have been thinking—may God prolong your life—concerning the inmates of prisons that, because of their congestion and their oppressive surroundings, they cannot fail to fall sick. Yet, they are not free to pursue measures that will be beneficial to them and contact doctors whom they can consult about their illnesses. It, therefore, behooves that you set apart for them doctors who shall visit them daily and medicines and potions be carried to them. Let these doctors visit all the prisons, treat patients therein and repel their illnesses by whatever they need of medicine and drugs. Let also [paramedical] women visit such of them as have need for them.[29]

In these hospitals there was usually a special wing for the treatment of mental patients, which Muslims took seriously. In the Mansūrī Hospital, built in Cairo in 1283—probably the largest in the medieval Muslim world—there was, as in other large hospitals, a wing for mental patients including the insane. The endowment document of this hospital laid special emphasis on the treatment of all patients irrespective of creed, class, or sex (it had a mosque for Muslims and a chapel for Christians) and on the treatment of the mentally ill. Its intent was to treat

> . . . [all] men, women, rich or poor who live in Cairo and its surroundings, or who come there from outside from other countries and provinces, no matter belonging to what race or of what description, suffering from physical illnesses, big or small . . . and from illnesses of the perceptual organs . . . and those who are disturbed in their mind and reason, the preservation of which is the greatest and most important purpose [of the hospital] since frequent attention must be paid to those whose minds have become deranged and disrupted.[30]

The use of music therapy appears to have been quite common in all important hospitals, whether Arab or Ottoman. Regular bands of musicians were kept.[31] We are told that three types of musicotherapy were developed: one for general patients in order to soothe them, a second for depressed patients, and a third for mad patients. This music was developed through experimentation with its effect upon the rhythm of the pulse and emotional response.[32] The famous philosopher al-Fārābī (d. 950), who was at the Ḥamdānid Saif al-Daula's court at Damascus, developed a special musical instrument whose various tunes produced different emotions on the part of listeners.[33] In his history of Turkish medicine Dr. Uthmān Shawqī states that musicotherapy was "first developed by Arabs in al-Madā'in" (in Iran). It is highly probable that this therapy was originally brought by doctors from India, who were invited by Anūshrawān to Gundai Shāpūr, since the science of music *(ragas)* and its effect in producing different emotions appears to have been highly developed there.

In India there were some hospitals, such as that founded by Fīrūz Shāh Tuglaq (r. 1339–1388), where the king himself, a specialist in ophthalmology, prepared a special collyrium (said to be still in use in India), and treated patients on a regular basis.[34] There was, however, a large number of clinics, as almost every king and most petty rulers and nobles founded clinics. All treatment and medication was free in these clinics and medical centers. In India, too, the Islamic medicine (called Yūnāni, i.e., Greek medicine) absorbed a great deal of the original Indian Ayurvedic system of medicines that was based on plants, herbs, and metals.

Medical education took place in the clinics and hospitals, and experimentation with treatments and diseases was conducted in the clinics. Ibn Abī Uṣaibi'a (d. 1270), the most important medical historian of Islam, has described his own medical education at the Nūrī Hospital in Aleppo (established in the mid-twelfth century):

> When Shaikh Muhazzab al-Dīn took up his residence in Damascus, he began to teach the art of medicine and a large number of prominent doctors there started learning from him. I also stayed on in Damascus in order to study with him . . . I started to study the works of Galen: He had great expertise in Galen's works and others that we read with him. He greatly admired Galen's works and when he heard anything from Galen being read of description of ailments and their treatment or principles of medicine, he would say, "That *is* medicine." I also accompanied him [as a student] when he treated patients in the [Nūrī] hospital. There I learned the practice of medicine and was directly connected with the medical art [i.e., not just the theory]. At that time, there was also with him for the treatment of patients in the hospital Doctor 'Imrān who was one of the prominent and foremost medical men, particularly in practical medicine. Thus, benefits [for me] from learning from the two of them together increased manifold because both of them used to discuss between themselves patients, their ailments and their treatment.

After describing Dr. Muhazzab al-Dīn's spectacular treatment (he calls it "magic") of certain patients, one suffering from extreme fever and another from mania (the latter he cured by administering barley water with large doses of opium), ibn Abī Uṣaibi'a continues:

> At that time, too, there served in the hospital Shaikh Raḍīy al-Dīn al-Raḥbī who was the most senior of all doctors in age, most honored and most famous. He used to sit on a raised (and carpeted) platform writing prescriptions for out-patients who took his prescriptions to the hospital dispensary where they got free medicines. After Doctor Muhazzab al-Dīn and 'Imrān finished with the lying-in patients, where I accompanied them, I used to sit with Doctor Raḍīy al-Dīn al-Raḥbī and watch his argumentation concerning ailments of out-patients, what he told the latter and the prescriptions he wrote for them. I used to discuss with him ailments and their treatments. Never did such illustrious doctors come together in this hospital ever since it was built, nor, indeed, after-wards as these three did at that time, and they remained there for quite some time:
>
>> Those years and those who lived them have gone,
>> And both are nothing more now than mere dreams.[35]

The author tells us that after returning to his house, Muhazzab al-Dīn had his meal, then transcribed works of medicine—he had transcribed for himself at least one hundred volumes—and after that various classes of students entered in succession to study with him. He endowed his own house in Damascus as a school of medicine.[36]

ETHICS AND JUSTICE

In 931, the sensational death of a patient in Baghdad led the caliph al-Muqtadir to order "the chief doctor" of Baghdad, Sinān ibn Thābit, to undertake the examination and certification (or registration) of all doctors in Baghdad. The number of doctors in that city (including court physicians who were exempted from this procedure) was found to be 860. Some were disqualified from practicing medicine, but most were allowed to continue: the testing seems to have been fairly lenient.[37] The testing of pharmacists was also instituted. However, this procedure of examination was neither universal nor uniform. While Baghdad, Damascus, and Cairo had frequent certification exams, in most other places like Antioch and the Eastern Islamic lands this institution did not exist. Where it did exist, it became a function of the department of *ḥisba*, whose task was to supervise "public morality."

To compensate for the relative lack of supervision of medical ethics, many works were written to guide the average educated person as to how to distinguish a genuine doctor from a quack. This genre of literature is known as *Miḥnat al-Ṭabīb*, that is, testing of a doctor. *Imtiḥān al-Alibbā' li-Kāffat al-Aṭibbā'* (How wise men can examine all doctors) was written by a certain 'Abd al-Aziz not long before the year 1289. It consists of ten chapters on medicine and pharmacy, each comprising twenty questions.[38]

The author of an important work written in Persian, titled *Hidāġat al-Muta 'allimīn* (Guidance for those who want to learn medicine), specialized in the treatment of mental disorders. He wrote the book for his son, and it contains many of his own experiences. In its brief introduction he says that everyone should know enough about medicine to save themselves from falling prey to quacks.[39]

There are also several works written on medical ethics. The question of whether a doctor should charge fees for his services and, if so, how much, is discussed by a doctor in a treatise titled, "In Denunciation of One Who Tries to Become Rich through Medicine."[40] Al-Dhahabī quotes a *hadīth* in justification of charging a fee for one's medical service.[41] But the most comprehensive statement published so far on the subject is *Adab al-Ṭabīb* by Isḥāq ibn 'Alī al-Ruhāwī. It belongs to the category of *adab* literature, a Persian-inspired genre concerning professional ethics.[42]

The Hippocratic oath was commonly administered to a doctor embarking on his profession. Following the tradition of Hippocrates and Galen, al-Ruhāwī insists that the medical doctor must look after the soul as well as the body. This is underlined in Islam by the name *hakīm*, which means "the wise person" and is applied both to a medical doctor and a philosopher. All great personages in the field of philosophy were also medical men and vice versa. Al-Ruhāwī holds that a medical doctor must not covet wealth for its own sake, but should earn enough to live comfortably and to educate his children. He also advises men of wealth to reward the services of doctors generously so they can look after the needs of those who cannot pay, lest the medical profession die out. It should be noted that this practice has, by and large, continued down to the present day in the traditional system of Islamic medicine, as distinguished from modern medicine, which has been implanted from the West and which has still to strike cultural roots in Islam.[43]

Turning to bioethical questions, the only issue which has had a history is that of birth control. In pre-Islamic Arabia there was a custom of infanticide of girls which was motivated by economic reasons and a sense of honor (*'irḍ*). According to Qur'ān 6.138, many pagan Arabs had come to regard the practice as sanctioned by their gods. The Qur'ān ended this. The practice of *coitus interruptus* was also very common in pre-Islamic Arabia. The Qur'ān is silent on this subject, which means that it did not regard the practice as morally objectionable. However, the *hadīth* on this issue is contradictory.[44] Because of contradictory *hadīth* and because of another *hadīth* in which the Prophet exhorted his community to reproduce and multiply in numbers, many classical lawyers in Islam were against contraception as well as abortion. But many others, including some notable figures, allowed birth control, and several also allowed abortion within 120 days of conception, before the fetus is "ensouled."[45] Abortion after this period is strictly forbidden, as the fetus after "ensoulment" comes to acquire certain rights of a living person.

According to the Shāfiʿī school of law, a husband may exercise *coitus interruptus* without the wife's consent, but according to all other schools the consent of both partners is necessary for the practice of birth control.[46] A slave wife's consent is not necessary according to all schools, for while she is entitled to orgasm, she is not necessarily entitled to children.[47] The most interesting opinion is that of the famous Sufi-theologian-jurist al-Ghazālī (d. 1111), who says that for a person who has attained to complete "trust" (*tawakkul*, one of the high Sufi spiritual "stations") in God, it is forbidden to practice birth control because he or she knows that God *will* provide for any children born. But very few people can develop such spiritual strength: the average person is always haunted by fears of economic jeopardy. An average person is, therefore, not only allowed to exercise birth control but is advised to do so. Al-Ghazālī goes so far as to state that if a husband fears that bearing children would affect his wife's good looks and that therefore he might come to dislike her, he should desist from having children.[48]

For the past two decades, most Muslim governments have launched family planning programs in view of the tremendous population growth in these (like most third world) countries. The rate of success is doubtful, although, according to the United Nations reports, Indonesia might be on the verge of a breakthrough. The success or failure of such programs depends on certain important factors—first of all on the vigor or laxity of the governments concerned. In Pakistan, for example, the family planning drive was, according to the U.N. evaluation report of 1969, effective during the regime of Muhammad Ayub Khan. However, during the regime of Zia ul-Haq, who did not appear to believe in the wisdom of family planning, the program fell into neglect. While most of the *'ulumā'* (religious scholars) would not oppose voluntary family planning on the part of individual families, most strongly oppose it when pushed as official policy. In other words, while "family planning" is regarded as all right, "population control" is largely condemned, primarily because it is seen as a Western bid to stop third world population growth.[49]

The traditionalist *'ulumā'* do not approve of organ transplants on the same ground that most of them opposed human dissection: it resembles *muthla*. *Muthla* was a pagan Arab practice of mutilating ("making an example"—*mithāl*—of) archenemies who fell in battle. However, organ transplants and dissection are easily distinguishable from *muthla* in terms of motivation and purpose, and there is an important countervailing principle in Islamic jurisprudence according to which "the needs of the living have priority over those of the dead."[50] The question here is not so much one of doctrine as of social ethos. Undoubtedly, provided the necessary medical skill and available donors, the transplanting of organs would face little difficulty in Muslim societies.

With the issue of artificial insemination, we are entering a complex territory, so far as the Islamic perspective is concerned. There is no prob-

lem in producing a test-tube baby from the reproductive materials of a
male and a female, provided they are spouses. But to inject a male's sperm
into the womb of a woman who is not his wife creates a difficulty in
Islamic law, which would consider such a procedure as adultery. For adultery in Islam is defined not only in terms of physical sexual intercourse,
but also as an admixture of foreign sperm. Indeed, the law on adultery is
quite severe in Islam. The Qur'ān prescribes one hundred lashes for both
partners in cases of adultery or fornication (24.2). The *hadīth*, and consequently the Islamic law, distinguish between the two, prescribing a
hundred lashes for fornicators and death by lapidation for adultery. It
seems certain that the latter punishment was introduced by the caliph
Umar I (d. 644) because of sexual laxity resulting from rapid large-scale
conquests and the influx of a large number of slaves and slave women.

Islamic law is anxious to keep the pedigree of parenthood "pure," and
for this reason has ruled that a divorcee or a widow must wait for a specified period of time (*'idda*) before remarrying, in order that her pregnancy,
if any, from her previous husband may be established (Qur'ān 2.228,
234). The Qur'ān even declared adoption unlawful since it creates a false
situation abusive of natural relationships: "God has not put two hearts in
any man's breast" (33.4). There are, however, certain countervailing pro-
visions in Islamic law that might be invoked to legalize artificial insemination, even though it would still be considered "reprehensible" (*makrūh*),
albeit not unlawful (*harām*). One is the legal maxim accepted universally
by Muslim lawyers that "the child belongs to the matrimonial bed."[51]
According to several well-known traditions, the Prophet prohibited the
disowning of a child by a father even when strong empirical evidence in
terms of color and features pointed to the child's not being from the putative father.[52] The other relevant principle of Islamic law is "acknowledgment of parenthood." According to this principle, if a man or a woman
(even an unmarried woman) goes to court with a child claiming it to be
his or hers, and the child has no other known parenthood, the court must
give the child to the claimant. In this case, the law holds that the welfare
(*maslaha*) of the child is paramount, and the question as to whether the
child was the result of illicit union will not be raised.[53]

As mentioned above, suicide is condemned in Islam. In fact, concepts
of safety, peace, integrity, and the like are so deeply rooted and persistent
in the Qur'ān that they can be termed the "unconscious" of the Qur'ān.
God, who has given life, is alone entitled to take it. There is only one
situation in Islamic law wherein life may be taken freely and merito-
riously: in *jihād* or "the cause of Allah." Outside of *jihād*, all fighting—
for example, wars of territorial expansion—and killing are strictly forbidden: "For this reason (Cain's murder of Abel), We laid it down upon the
Children of Israel that whosoever kill a person without a right or a war,
it is as though he has killed all humanity"(5.32).

The prolongation of life, therefore, is highly desirable. "May God give you long life" is a standard saying commonly found in Muslim correspondence, usually at the beginning of letters but also at the end of books written by scribes in reference to the living authors of these books. The *ḥadīth* forbidding Muslims to pray for death is unequivocal on this subject: the more one lives, the more one has the opportunity to do good; this opportunity in itself is a priceless and unique gift vouchsafed to human beings. But there is the other side of the picture as well. In several passages (16.7; 36.68; and others), the Qur'ān laments that old age renders humans senile and silly—one becomes like a child once again. To prolong "life" in the sense of breathing by artificial means is to make a cruel joke of human life. The question of the value of human life is certainly not unrelated to what that life can perform or yield. Otherwise, there should be no difference between the life of a man and, say, that of an earwig.

Passages

The Qur'ān describes the development of the fetus in terms of "different levels of creation" *(nasha'āt)* as follows:

> We have created man out of an extraction of clay [i.e., semen]. Then We cause it to settle firmly as a sperm-drop in the womb. Then we create this sperm-drop into a germ-cell [literally, something "hanging from" the womb], then We turn this germ-cell into a lump. Then We create bones within this lump, and, then, We clothe these bones with flesh. Finally, We transmute it into a new creature (independent of its mother)—so hallowed be God, the best of all artisans (23.14).

Thus, for the Qur'ān, each one of the stages of evolution of the fetus is a "creation," or something new. Even so, as we shall presently see, is the transformation of the person in the "hereafter." In Islamic law, once the fetus is "ensouled," it becomes a legal person and has rights: to kill it is a form of homicide, and it has rights of inheritance. The importance of the child in Islam may be gathered from the fact that, under classical Islamic law, once a slave woman bore a child and gained the status of the "Mother of the Child," she could not be sold or gifted by her master, and after the latter's death, became automatically free as did her children.

On attaining puberty (or coming of age) boys or girls, if named, are legally possessed of *rushd* (i.e., the capability of telling right from wrong) provided they have had the "right upbringing." This "right upbringing" determines the law on the custody of children in cases where parents are divorced.[54] According to the general classical Islamic law, a male child was given to the mother until the age of nine "in order to get love from the mother." At nine, however, he was given to his father because he then needed direction and "moral training" *(adab)*, which the father could better supply. A girl remained with her mother up until the age of fourteen or fifteen in order to get not only love but training in the household tasks. After that, she needed "protection" and went to her father, who could better provide such protection. The actual decisions of courts vary greatly according to different circumstances of cases, particularly the character of the mother and father. In 1979 a law was enacted in Egypt (known as the Jihan Sadat Law) which raised the age up to which children could stay with their mother. However, this was repealed in May 1985 under pressure from rightist religious forces, the *'ulumā'* and the Muslim Brotherhood.

Classical Islamic law allowed polygamy up to four wives.[55] The entire discussion of the Qur'ān on this subject (4.2–3, 127, 129) takes place with regard to the context of orphaned girls. The Qur'ān accuses the custodians of the orphan girls of mishandling them and embezzling their properties and of wanting to marry them rather than returning these properties to them when the girls came of age. The Qur'ān then says: "If you fear you will not be able to do justice to these orphans then you may marry from (these) women such as you like—two, three, or four. But if you fear you cannot do justice among co-wives then marry only one" (4.3). But in verse 129 of the same sura the Qur'ān says: "You will never be able to do justice among women no matter how desirous you may be of doing so." Despite its specific context, the classical lawyers of Islam made the permission for polygamy clause general and regarded it as having legal force. But they regarded the clause concerning the incumbency of justice among cowives to be a recommendation to the conscience of the husband, albeit a solemn recommendation. Of course, a wife whose rights were grossly violated could go to court to have her wrongs redressed and, indeed, could obtain a divorce (this divorce is called *khul'*).[56] Modern legislation on the issue, enacted in all major Muslim countries except Saudi Arabia, on the other hand, takes the justice clause as being of primary force and, in view of the Qur'ān's categorical statement of the impossibility of such justice, has either abolished polygamy or restricted it.[57]

While a woman had to go to court to get a divorce, the husband had the right to repudiate his wife unilaterally without going to court. This was a particularly heinous form of divorce, which had no root either in the Qur'ān or in any authentic precept of the Prophet. Called "triple or innovated repudiation" *(talāq al-thabāth or talāq al-batt)*, it was effective upon the husband's thrice uttering in the same sitting: "I repudiate you three times." In all major Muslim countries the right of divorce is now vested in courts or other judicial bodies, which first try reconciliation between the couple in accordance with the Qur'ānic injunction (4.128). If reconciliation is not achieved within three months, divorce takes effect, after which, however, the couple can remarry—indeed, the Qur'ān is emphatic on remarriage, if at all possible. After a divorce the three-month "waiting period" (*'idda*) is imposed on the woman by the Qur'ān, both for the purpose of reconciliation and to clearly establish the parenthood of the child in case of a possible pregnancy.

In pre-Islamic Arabia daughters were barred from inheritance: the only persons who inherited were those who could fight on the battlefield, which meant sons or, in the absence of sons, agnate male relations. The Qur'ān granted shares to daughters, but placed their shares at half of the sons'. In the present century some suggestions have been made, notably by Zia Gākalp, the Turkish sociologist (d. 1926), that a daughter's share should be made equal to a son's. So far no Muslim country has passed such legislation except Turkey, which, in any case, secularized its polity under Atatürk and substituted civil codes for the Sharī'a law. Muhammad Iqbal, the philsopher-poet of Pakistan (d. 1938), argued in his *Reconstruction of Religious Thought in Islam* (chapter 5) that since the girl received a dowry from her husband at marriage, her allotment of one half of that of her brother's share in inheritance is justified, for if she were to receive equal to his share it would be tantamount to discrimination against him. The question is obviously a complex one, and more empirical investigation into the comparative values of an average dowry with average inheritance value is needed.[58]

On the subject of death, the first thing to notice is that for Muslims death is passage to another life and not the end of life. The hereafter is literally true. At the beginning of this essay the importance of the meaning of action in and for human life was underlined: a human is not like an animal, the meaning of whose action is exhausted at the moment of action for the animal itself. Thanks to the fact that human beings possess reason and feelings of moral obligation, human actions are qualitatively different from those of animals. The element of future orientation, in view of these two faculties, becomes intrinsic to the evaluation of human action. This is the whole meaning of the idea of the "weighing of deeds" on the Day of Judgment so frequently repeated in the Qur'ān. "Say (O Muhammad!), Shall we inform you of those who are the greatest losers in terms of their deeds? It is those whose whole effort is lost in [pursuit of] this wordly [i.e., lower] values and ends, but they imagine they have performed prodigies" (18.103–104). Again: "Whenever they are asked not to sow corruption on the earth, they reply, we are only reforming [the earth]. Beware! These *are* the corruptors, but they realize it not" (2.12).

It is on that day, that hour of truth, that persons will really face themselves starkly for, throughout this life, they can and do form layers upon layers of self-deception, and resurrection will, therefore, primarily mean resurrecting the real human personality shorn of all facade: "You were in heedlessness of this, but now that We have shorn off your veils, your sight today is keen!" (50.22). Although the Qur'ān often speaks of resurrecting the dead and dry "bones from the grave," this is essentially in reply to the objection of the Meccans as to how God will reconstitute a living person from rotten and decayed bones: "Did We not constitute you in the first place, when you were nothing?" (36.77–79). The real answer to the question of the afterlife is given in verses such as 56.60–62: "We have appointed the death of you and We cannot be excelled [by any of your false gods] in that We shall transmute your models and re-create you in [forms] you do not know. You already know your present form of creation, so why do you not take a lesson?" The Qur'ān also calls the hereafter "a new creation," "a new level of creation." In all such passages it is implied that the next life will be a transmutation of life-models, a rearrangement of the factors (based primarily on achievement in the present life) and not a mere repetition of the present mode of life.

Because death is a passage and a link between two periods of life, it is sometimes likened by the Qur'ān to sleep, which is a passage between two waking periods (e.g., 39.42). In the ḥadīth, as distinct from the Qur'ān, there appears the doctrine of the barzakh, or the state between death and resurrection. This doctrine, which appears to have come in all its concreteness from ancient Iran (although there is a vague mention in the Qur'ān that Pharaoh and his followers are "exposed to fire" every morning and evening even before the Day of Judgment—40.46) is known as the "Chastisement of the Grave," and it states that sinners will already begin to be punished "in the grave" and likewise good people will begin to be rewarded. In some ḥadīths, even high fever is described as a "breath of Hell" which comes to such people as a punishment, as expiation, or in order to increase their goodness.[59]

Since Islam regards every individual as directly responsible before God and capable of directly communicating with him, without any intermediaries, there is no "priest" present when a person dies, and no "sacraments" are administered. The person is normally attended by his or her relatives, neighbors, and friends, who usually recite Qur'ānic verses or say prayers, as does the dying person. At death, a Muslim is expected to recite the profession of the faith: "There is no god but Allah and Muhammad is His Messenger." The sacred law demands that a dead person be buried as soon as possible, usually within hours after death. Loud wailing is not allowed, and formal observation of death (ma'tam) is disallowed after three days.

In practice, however, this picture of stark simplicity and directness is seriously modified by several beliefs and practices, particularly at the folk level. First of all, the picture of direct communication and responsibility before God—"You shall come to Us alone even as We created you first" (6.94)—is drastically changed by the doctrine of successful intercession by Muhammad on behalf of the sinners of his community, which the Qur'ān appears to reject but which figures prominently in the *ḥadīth*. And although the practice of burying a person soon after death continues, the "remembrance" of the dead is usually quite an elaborate ritual. One of these rituals is held on the third day after death, but an important one is observed on the fortieth day, and is almost universal among the Muslim masses. The gathering is large, the Qur'ān is recited, usually in its entirety, meals are served, and the entire "spiritual reward" is "made over" to the dead person. There is little doubt that these practices are survivals from the pre-Islamic past. The orthodox have kept up pressure over the centuries to discourage and, if possible, to eradicate them, but change is slow in the most outlying regions of the Muslim world, particularly in South and Southeast Asia.

Doctrinally and ideally, a Muslim must be forward-looking at death in view of his or her return to the creator, who can punish but whose mercy and forgiveness are also all-encompassing and infinite. This is, indeed, the picture that emerges from the Qur'ān and much of the *ḥadīth*. The Qur'ān belittles all the "natural relationships" one builds up in this world in terms of blood relationships, friends, and wealth, all of which it calls the "tinsel of this life" (18.46, for example) in opposition to the "abiding good deeds" (18.46; 19.76, for example). It was on these grounds that Muhammad Iqbāl said: "What else can I tell you of the sign of a man of faith / When death comes to him, it finds him smiling."[60]

Although this forward-lookingness is probably not entirely lacking in an average Muslim, the fears and anxieties that are the lot of an average human are not entirely absent either. The following lines of admonition often attributed to the great Persian poet Saʿdī of Shīrāz (d. 1292) must remain the ideal:

When you were born, everybody was smiling but you were crying. Live such a life that, when you depart, everyone is weeping but you are smiling.[61]

Notes

1. Felix Klein-Franke, *Volesungen uber die Medizin im Islam* (Wiesbaden, 1982), pp. 120 ff.
2. This introductory section is based on the first two chapters of my *Major Themes of the Qur'an* (Minneapolis, 1980) and on the second chapter of my *Islam* (Chicago, 1979).
3. *Mishkāt al-Maṣabīḥ*, a famous and authoritative anthology of *ḥadīth* (Delhi, 1955), p. 423; English translation by James Robson (Lahore, 1963), p. 1034.
4. Ibid., p. 422 (Robson, p. 1032).
5. Ibid., p. 424 (Robson, p. 1038).

6. *The Ṣaḥīḥ* of Muslim, vol. 4 (Beirut, 1972), p. 1761.

7. Ibn Khaldūn, *al-Muqaddima* (Cairo, 1867), p. 412.

8. See my article "Islam and Health," *Hamdard Islamicus* 5, no.4 (1982):79. It is not, therefore, correct to say, as Manfred Ullmann does, that the motivation behind the *Prophetic Medicine* literature was to assert the authority of the Prophet and rob a "pagan Zalen" of his merit. In fact, these works freely combine Arab or "Prophetic" medicine with principles and prescriptions of the Greek scientific medical tradition. See my article "Islam and Medicine: A General Overview," *Perspectives in Biology and Medicine* 27, no. 4 (1983/84): 588–589.

9. *Mishkāt*, p. 387 (Robson, p. 945); on the report about al-Ḥārith ibn Kalada, see (Ibn) al-Qifṭī, *Akhbār al-Hukamā'*, p. 112; Ibn Qayyim al-Jauzīya, *al-Ṭibb al-Nabawī* (Prophetic medicine) (Cairo, 1978), p. 164.

10. Ibn Qayyim al-Jauzīya, p. 76.

11. al-Dhahabī, *Al-Ṭibb al-Nabawī* (Prophetic medicine) (Cairo, 1961), p. 108.

12. All works on *Prophetic Medicine* discuss this question, but the most detailed discussion is to be found in *'Uyūn al-Anbā' fi Ṭabaqāt al-Aṭibbā'* by Ibn Abī Uṣaibi'a (Beirut, 1965), pp. 11ff.

13. Some jurists, however, like Ahmad ibn Hanbal (d. 855)—according to one recension of his opinion—recorded medical treatment as religiously allowed but not obligatory; indeed, in this opinion it is better to trust in God than to trust the efficacy of drugs. But, according to another recension of ibn Hanbal's opinion quoted by ibn Taimiya (d. 1328), medical treatment is obligatory. See al-Dhahabī, 103–104.

14. For a more detailed discussion of this question, see my *Major Themes of the Qur'ān*, chaps. 1 and 2 and *passim*.

15. See *Health and Medicine in the Islamic Tradition* (New York, 1987), chap. 1, sec. 1C.

16. Klein-Franke, pp. 120 ff.; see my brief review of this book in the *Johns Hopkins University Bulletin for the History of Medicine* 58, no. 2 (Summer 1984): 258, and also my critique referenced in the preceeding note.

17. See the chapter "Natural Causation" in al-Ghazālī, *Tahāfut al-Falāsifa* (Incoherence of the philosophers), trans. S. A. Kamali (Lahore, 1958). It is interesting that while al-Ghazālī explains natural causation as "the habit of God," Hume explains it as habit of the human mind formed by witnessing similar successions of events.

18. Klein-Franke, pp. 120 ff.

19. See *Mishkāt*, pp. 133 ff. (Robson, 321 ff.); al-Dhahabī, pp. 6–7, 143 ff.

20. *Mishkāt*, pp. 133 ff.

21. Rahman, "Islam and Medicine," pp. 589 ff; Rahman, "Islam and Health," p. 84.

22. al-Dhahabī, p. 145.

23. *Mishkāt*, p. 133 (Robson, p. 321).

24. Ibid., p. 138 (Robson, p. 331).

25. Ibid., p. 137 (Robson, p. 330).

26. Ibid., p. 138 (Robson, p. 331).

27. Ibid., p. 139 (Robson, p. 333).

28. Ibn Abī Uṣaibi'a, p. 301.

29. Ibid.

30. Aḥmad 'Isa Bib, *Ta'rīkh al-Bīmaristānāt fi'l-Islām* (History of hospitals in Islam) (Damascus, 1939), p. 138.

31. *Encyclopedia of Islam*, new ed., s.v. "Māristān."

32. 'Uthman Shevqi, *Türk Tebabetin Bej Bucuk Asirlik Tarihi* (History of Turkish medicine during five and a half centuries) (Istanbul, 1925), pp. 118–119.

33. Ibn Abī Usaibi'a, p. 604.

34. Muḥammad Zubayr Siddiqi, *Studies in Arabic and Persian Medical Literature* (Calcutta, 1959), pp. xxxii–xxxiii.

35. Ibn Abī Uṣaib'a, pp. 731–732.

36. Ibid., p. 733.

37. Ibid., p. 302; Ullmann, 225 ff. However, Ibn Abī Uṣaibi'a also says (p. 351) that Amīn al-Daula ibn al-Tilmīdh (d. 1165) was authorized by the caliph (al-Mustaḍī' seems to be a mistake for al-Muqtafī) to examine (or register) all the doctors. Each of the two events may well be true in itself, but modern historians appear to have mixed up the two. 'Alī ibn Aḥmed Nayyir Wāsiṭī, in his *Ṭibb al-'Arab* (Lahore, 1969), an Urdu translation and commentary on E. G. Broowne's *Arabian Medicine*, discusses this problem, but in a rather apologetic tone.

38. Nayyir Wāsiṭī, p. 260.

39. Abū Bakr Rabī' ibn Aḥmad al-Akhawainī al-Bukhārī, *Guidance for Those Who Want to Learn Medicine* (Maskhed, Iran, 1965), p. 246, no. 6.

40. This work is *Fī Dhamm al-Takassub bī-Ṣināı 'at al-Tibb* by 'Abd al-Wadūd ibn 'Abd al-Mālik. There are several other such works mentioned by M. Ullmann, pp. 226 ff.

41. Al-Dhahabī, p. 110.

42. English trans. Martin Levy (Philadelphia, 1967).

43. See my article in *Hamdard Islamicus* (cited in n. 8) for a summary both of al-Ruhāwī's views and of traditional medical ethics in Islam.

44. See my article in *Perspectives in Biology and Medicine* (n. 8).

45. B. P. Musallam, *Sex and Society in Islam* (Cambridge, 1983), pp. 39 ff.

46. Donna Lee Bowen, "Religious Attitudes to Family Planning in Morocco" (Ph.D. dissertation, University of Chicago, 1980); see especially the chapter "Law and Contraception."

47. Ibid.

48. See n. 8.

49. Ibid.

50. Ibn Qudāma, *Kitāb al-Mughnī* (Cairo, 1968), pp. 410–411, 525, and the *ḥadīth*s quoted there.

51. See my monograph, *Health and Medicine in the Islamic Tradition* (New York, 1987), chap. 4.

52. *Mishkāt*, pp. 286–287 (Robson, pp. 606–607).

53. *Health and Medicine in the Islamic Tradition*.

54. See any work of Islamic law for a discussion on custody (*ḥaḍāna*).

55. For a detailed discussion of family law, see my chapter entitled "Status of Women in Islam," in *Separate Worlds—A Study of Purda in South Asia*, ed. H. Papanek and G. Minault (Delhi, 1982); see also my article entitled "A Survey of Modernization of Muslim Family Law," *International Journal of Middle Eastern Studies* 14 (1982).

56. Ibid. The word *khul'* literally means "to cast off undesirable clothes."

57. Ibid.; see sections on modern family reform laws of Pakistan (1961), of Indonesia (1974), etc. The only country that has abolished polygamy on an Islamic basis is Tunisia (Turkey abolished it on a secular basis), while all other major Muslim countries have restricted it: a man wishing to marry a second wife has to petition a court/judicial authority stating the

grounds by which he deems a second marriage necessary. Such permission is granted if the first wife is an invalid or barren and in some cases if there is no male issue. In Iran, however, where such a law was enacted in 1967, the present-day Khomeini regime has abrogated that law; indeed, this government has undertaken a systematic campaign to "educate the public in *mut'a* (temporary) marriage," which had fallen into benign neglect during the late Shah's regime. See Shahla Haeri, "The Institution of Mut'a Marriage in Iran," in *Women and Revolution in Iran*, ed. Guity M. Mash'at (Boulder, 1983).

58. See the references in n. 5.
59. *Mishkāt*, pp. 133–139 (Robson, pp. 320ff.); on *barzakh*, see the *Encyclopedia of Islam*, new ed.
60. *Kulliyāt-i-Iqbāl* (Lahore, 1973), p. 998.
61. See Ali A. Dezzhudā, *Amthāl wa Hibam* (Proverbs and wise sayings), vol. 4, 2nd ed. (Tehran, 1960), p. 2025.

CHAPTER 8

Medicine and the Living Tradition of Islam

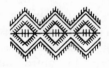

PETER ANTES

The Islamic world has been strongly influenced by European ways of thinking in the nineteenth and twentieth centuries. Moreover, in recent decades it has been influenced by the American way of life. This gradually noticeable westernization has led to numerous reactions among Muslims. The two extreme responses have been a warm support of all aspects of westernization, making a clear distinction between the private practice of religion and a public morality separate from any religious influence, and a total rejection of westernization as far as the value system and behavior patterns of the West are concerned. Consequently, westernization has become the most crucial question in the acceptance or denial of the Islamic tradition.

In an excellent study tracing the portrayal of Europeans through modern Arabic narrative and dramatic literature, Rotraud Wielandt came to the conclusion that from the beginning of westernization, "self-under-

standing of the Arab World has widely been shaped by the evaluation of
European patterns of behaviour. Thus, talking about Europeans very
often became a way of defining one's own cultural identity and values."[1]
The definition of Islam itself often implied the answer to the question of
westernization and tried to show, as in Āl-i Aḥmad's book on westernization,[2] that all negative phenomena (for example, evils found in Iran
under the Shah) are but the consequence of evils imported from the West
to the Muslim world. The argument of the author is that were Islam still
being practiced as it was taught in the classical handbooks of the past,
people would live in sane communities free from the diseases of the West.
These evils include disorderly sexual relations, drug problems, and alcoholism, among other problems.[3]

The Muslim world today faces the challenge of both the necessity of
fulfilling Islamic duties and of a certain open-mindedness to go in new
directions. Tradition and change, religion and modernity all seem to be
imperative for Muslims if they are to seek the means by which to preserve
their cultural identity and to improve the quality of life for individuals as
well as for the community.

The living tradition of Islam must therefore consider both the ethnomedical tradition—that is, the indigenous medical system—and modern methods and techniques in order to determine to what extent notions
of wellness and illness, caring and curing, ethics and justice, and the life
passages are influenced by and in confrontation with Islamic thoughts.
Indeed, all aspects of life are deeply affected by Islam as understood in a
very specific sense. A Muslim's daily life is regulated by Islamic guidelines. It is necessary to begin by considering the effect of Islam on daily
living, and to show how behavioral patterns are thus informed. The medical practitioner must work within the Muslim worldview, which sees all
particular actions as part of the whole religious world. In this way it is
possible to see that in the eyes of the pious Muslim, medicine is closely
linked to the living tradition of Islam.

The Islamic Worldview

In many modern portrayals of Islam, Muslim writers emphasize the
uniqueness of God's revelation to Muhammad, in which religion and
morality are seen as inextricably linked. In *Islamic Ideology* Khalifa Abdul
Hakim states:

> Islam found religion and morality divorced from life and its greatest contri-
> bution to the advancement of humanity is the conception of religion as well-
> being, as life well-lived with love and justice, fulfilling all the demands of
> human nature within the limits prescribed by reason and social well-being.

With Islam, the purpose of life is better and richer life, intensely and completely lived, and harmoniously developed.[4]

Thus Islam is not only a religion of dogma and theological statements, but it also influences deeply the behavior of every believer in all areas of his or her life. The Islamic way of life embraces the totality of what one should or should not do. 'Abd al-Kādir, a representative of the conservative Muslim Brothers movement in Egypt, summarizes how it is that actions in daily life are connected to reality:

> Islam as a system has an influence on the Muslim in peace and in quiet; it has an influence on him in thoughts and in intentions, in speech and in work; it has an influence on him in secret and in public, in the hidden and in the unveiled; it has an influence on him standing and sitting, sleeping and awake; it has an influence on him in eating and in drinking, in dressing and in adornment; it has an influence on him in buying and in selling, in money change and in business transaction; it has an influence on him in effort and in relaxation, in joy and in sadness, in content and in rage; it has an influence on him in bad and in good luck, in illness and in health, in weakness and in strength; it has an influence on him rich and poor, young and old, great and despised; it has an influence on him with regard to his sons and his family, with regard to his friendship and his hostility, with regard to peace and war; it has an influence on him as an individual and in community, as a governor and a subject, as an owner and a beggar. Consequently, there is no imaginable behavior nor a situation for man where Islam has no influence on the Muslim.
>
> Whoever thinks, therefore, that Islam is a belief and not a system as well, is foolish and doesn't know anything of Islam.[5]

The Arabic word for "system" used in al-Kādir's text is *nizām. Nizām* and *nizāmiyya* (both are neologisms in this technical use of the terms) stand for a modern understanding of Islam. The meaning of *nizām* stresses the unity between religious practices in the Western sense *(dīn)* and legal institutions, which together regulate everything concerning the behavior of the individual and the community *(dawla)*. Islam is directly opposed to the Western type of society which renders "to Caesar what is Caesar's and to God what is God's" (Mt. 22:21). This distinction is not accepted in Islam and is explicitly rejected by the majority of Muslims today. They insist on declaring that there is only one reality, which is wholly submitted to God's rule. This is in contrast to the Western dichotomy that exhibits a separation between moral principles as preached by Christian denominations and the principles of conduct as formulated by the secularized Western society. Islam does not recognize the existence of any realm separate from God's rule and declares instead that each sector of life must be guided by divine principles. No autonomous decision in the field of conduct is accorded to humans.

Islam as *niẓām* suggests that a well-established system was laid down in the Qur'ān and was then handed down from generation to generation without any changes. Consequently, everything in the system should be in the Qur'ān, from the very beginnings of Islam. This presumption is, however, in reality incorrect. A close look at the Qur'ān and the Muslim tradition reveals that the Qur'ān alone was not sufficient to answer all the questions of Muslims of later periods. Shortly after Muhammad's death (632 CE) Muslims enlarged their corpus of authoritative references by adding the *sunna* of the Prophet, a collection of writings on the sayings and doings of Muhammad. Further, they felt the need to add two more sources of authority, the consensus of specialists *(idjmāʿ)*[6] and analogy *(ḳiyās)*,[7] so that not only the Qur'ān but all four sources together serve as principles of reference for new decisions made by the representatives of the Islamic law schools.[8] On the basis of these four principles (even more in certain law schools) new problems are settled in an Islamic way. Thus, what in retrospect appears to be a well-established system formulated in classical handbooks of the past is in fact the result of historical developments. For rarely does the Qur'ān contain a verse giving an appropriate answer to a problem; in most cases a concrete solution to a problem has been found only by employing a combination of Qur'ānic and non-Qur'ānic sources.

Fazlur Rahman makes this process clear in his article in this volume. In regard to each problem he shows what the Qur'ān, the *sunna*, and finally the tradition have to say in a particular case. He retraces the stages of making the final decision *(fatwā)*,[9] and he indicates that new problems have required and indeed have been given new answers. When confronted with ancient Greek knowledge of medicine and philosophy, Muslims answered the challenge positively and picked up the main lines of thinking by integrating it into their own system of thought and belief. When modern writers who oppose Muslim attitudes of the past assert that the present system stems as such from the Qur'ān, and on that basis reject any adaption of Islamic daily living to present-day circumstances, they are not arguing historically, and they overlook the fact that Islamic tradition itself is a complex phenomenon molded by historically conditioned circumstances that are founded on an initial divine inspiration.

A detailed and critically historical survey of the past should open possibilities for ways to resolve future conflicts between modernity and Islam. Moreover, it would reveal that many pre- and non-Islamic elements were absorbed by Muslims of the past (for example, aspects of Greek medicine) and so perfectly integrated into Islam that later generations had the impression that these elements were a part of Muslim heritage. Knowledge of the ways in which Muslims of the past came to terms with difficult problems could have the effect of enabling and encouraging Muslims today to use similar methods in regard to present-day problems.

It is therefore necessary to incorporate both Qur'ānic data and modern challenges into a discussion of medicine and the Islamic way of life so as to make clear the problems for Muslims today and the ways in which they envisage eventual solutions.

Thus, Islam functions as a system that covers all aspects of everyday life. It lays down the rules that Muslims must accept as long as they are trying to obey God's will. These rules concretely address the concerns of wellness and illness, caring and curing, ethics and justice, and life passages, just to mention some of the more striking aspects of Muslim life.

Islamic Concepts of Wellness and Illness

Salīm and *ṣaḥīḥ* are two Arabic words often translated as "healthy" in English. The basic root of *salīm (s-l-m)*, found also in the word "*islām*," evokes well-being, intactness, peace, safety, and security. *Ṣaḥīḥ* is derived from the Arabic root *ṣ-ḥ-ḥ* and conveys the idea of faultlessness, rightness, correctness, genuineness, truth, and credibility. Both words indicate that health should be seen in a broader context of general well-being.

Different types of health can therefore be distinguished. In a doctoral thesis on the ethical education in Islam, Miḳdād Yāldjin writes of Islam as "aiming at the education toward the realization of corporal, mental, intellectual, spiritual and emotional health all together."[10] Such an understanding obviously refers to various categories of human conduct, both of the individual and the community. Health and wellness are described not simply as the absence of disturbing factors such as illness, but as embracing the wholeness of human well-being.

According to the fundamental principles of Islam, wholeness is more than an expression of human will, and it cannot be realized by human work alone. It is granted by God, who is the cause of all human well-being and therefore of all wholeness, for God gives food and drink, heals the sick, and makes persons die and live again. (See Qur'ān 26.79–81.)

Since God is the creator of everything (6.102), all evil is related to him insofar as it is caused in order to remind humans of misdoings in order to better the wrongdoer's attitude. Satan is sometimes mentioned as the one who produces pain and suffering (38.41). In any case, the Muslim knows that God's will is somehow involved, either by directly causing suffering or by allowing it to happen. Surrender (the literal translation of the Arabic word *islām*) to God's will is thus the only wide and practical attitude for every person who understands how the world really is. God's will is the answer to all human questioning. Suffering and illness clearly show that the originally intended wholeness has been disturbed either because God is punishing the wrongdoer or because humans must directly suffer the consequences of human sins. The Qur'ān thus describes the unbeliever and the hypocrite as the sick or the ill (2.9; 33.60). In his list of illnesses Yāldjin includes "moral illnesses" as the origin of delinquency.[11]

In terms of modern Western psychology one could say that the Islamic concepts of wellness and illness cover the whole range of psychosomatic phenomena. Illness is not only a physical (or somatic) reality, but it often has psychological causes as well.[12] Moreover, what is true for the individual is even truer for the society as a whole.

Moral education is therefore an important preventive measure to preserve a sane community and to guarantee the individual's happiness within that community. Medicine, hygiene, and regulations for healthy living together form the guidelines for good living according to God's will. It is not surprising that these forms are described under the general theme of "medicine in the Koran" as found in Karl Opitz's famous book on the subject.[13] General medical advice is given in the first chapter, but the second chapter already widens the book's perspective by adding personal health concerns such as rest, skin care, nutrition, and drinking, and general health care problems such as housing and contagious and epidemic diseases. Finally, health regulations are mentioned in the third part of the book, giving orientation in the fields of alimentation (for example, alcoholism), sexual conduct (e.g., matrimonial and extramarital sexual intercourse and procreation), ritual practices such as circumcision and fasting as a form of purity, and social hygienic principles with regard to killing and retaliation. Opitz clearly shows that medicine and health are not separate realities capable of analysis from the fragmentary point of view of the specialist. On the contrary, medicine and health must be seen as integral parts of wellness in general. The wholeness of sane and healthy behavior or conduct cannot be divided into sectors that are completely separated from one another.

Muslims in the "Muslim countries" feel themselves psychologically at home. Their way of life is deeply influenced by Islam and Islamic traditions, and they see themselves as embedded in a cultural setting that gives them a feeling of wholeness and thus provides the conditions for healthy living. This feeling of wholeness faces a double challenge from the modern world: not only do Muslims leave their native countries for work opportunities in foreign countries where Islam is not the dominant religion, but Muslim societies themselves, as a whole, aim at westernization, so that the distinctive character of an Islamic society seems to be slowly but perceptibly disappearing.

When people leave their native countries for economic reasons, as hundreds of thousands of Turks, Pakistanis, and North Africans have done and continue to try to do, seeking work in the countries of the Western community—in particular, the United Kingdom, France, and the United States—they encounter living conditions wherein their Islamic concepts of wholeness are no longer shared by the majority of people in the country. Religion and society are distinct in Western countries because religious practices and convictions are largely private matters with little direct influence on the public level of state affairs or ideal behavioral patterns. This dichotomy between the Islamic expectation of wholeness as the most important principle of the Islamic way of life and the Western secularized life-style is capable of causing unhappiness among the Muslims and of resulting in psychosomatic illnesses; it is worth paying attention to and studying in great detail.

In contrast, when societies in the Muslim world change by introducing Western forms of life, the whole culture is involved in the change. The transition is seldom without problems for the individuals involved, but unlike their fellow believers in non-Muslim countries, they do not lose their sense of identity and belonging. Many of the changes that occurred in the 1970s and 1980s were blamed for having contributed to the rise in the number of delinquent acts. Lari's book states that all evil has been imported from the West and that, to use Yāldjin's terminology, the increasing instances of deviant acts are expressions of "moral illnesses" existing within society.[14] These accusations, often generated by and repeated in conservative Muslim circles, make little distinction between the traditional life-style of a particular country as a cultural entity and Islam as the revelation of unchangeable guidelines for human conduct.

In all these accusations, one thing is clear: humans have the responsibility to put the divine principles into practice. Every human being is expected to act according to God's will. All actions, good and bad, are carefully recorded and will weight the balance on the Day of Judgment (99.6–8). All human beings are given the privilege to act as "God's vicegerents" on earth (2.30) and therefore have great responsibility in assuming the duties of this highly prestigious task. They must fulfill God's plans but are capable of acting against God's will. Indeed, all human planning is seen as subject to the condition *in shā' Allāh* ("if God wills"), to which all Muslims frequently refer. This type of speech indicates as well that God's omnipotence is not the only reason for the course of events; human activity also plays a role within the framework set by the Almighty. In fact, no dominant school of contemporary Islam claims that human action is purely the result of God's unknowable predestination, to the extent that there is no human responsibility involved in action.

Therefore, in the past, Muslims did not merely wait for God to act but encouraged their scholars to accumulate as much knowledge as they could, even if they had to go "as far as China" in order to work effectively. With regard to medicine they were prepared to integrate Greek and other foreign medical techniques in order to cure the sick—at least as far as God allows for success in curing, as no one dies unless it is God's decision (3.45). According to the Qur'ān (5.32), saving and preserving life are among the highly regarded tasks. In practice, Muslims have taken this responsibility very seriously. They were among the first in the world to build hospitals for more effective cure of the sick. Operations were performed and sophisticated lists of plant effects were recorded that made it possible to prepare a variety of medicines for both corporal and mental illnesses.

Mental illness merits special mention here. For Muslims, mental illness generally implies no control over the body and its actions and relieves one of responsibility or guilt. This has led Muslims in the past and present to believe that madness is a special gift from God, granted to free a person from particular religious duties. Gramlich, for instance, reports that a dervish in Iran mentioned to him the case of Luḵmān-i Sarakhsī (d. about 1000 CE), who asked God for the favor of becoming mad in order to be free from his religious duties.[15] Like the lord on earth who gives freedom to the loyal slave after many years of service, God has mercy on some of his most obedient servants by according the grace of madness to them so that there is no further need to fulfill the religious duties typical of the pious Muslim. It is noteworthy that Muslims therefore have treated and still treat the mad with great respect due to the special favor God has shown to them by granting madness.

A different type of uncontrolled behavior is that of possession. Here, evil ghosts, called *djinn*s in the Qur'ān, are said to cause the disturbances and eventually to cause deviation from Islamic law. The special knowledge of certain pious men or women is needed to recognize what is going on in such situations. These kinds of uncontrolled actions coexist with a third type, a loss of consciousness that is practiced by Muslim mystics ('Ṣūfīs) and is usually known as ecstasy. It occurs when God takes full possession of the mystic so that the mystic's self disappears *(fanā')* and God alone is there to act and speak. As in the case of possession by a *djinn*, the consciousness of the visible person has been replaced with an invisible actor, but unlike the *djinn*, who has bad intentions, God himself is here at work in order to accomplish the highest form of oneness to be reached in mystical experience.[16] Phenomenologically speaking, mystical ecstasy, possession by a *djinn*, and madness have very similar forms of manifestation. Only the specialist is able to distinguish one from another. In this case the specialist is not the medical doctor but someone specializing in religious experience.

Prior to a description of the details of caring and curing it may be helpful to summarize the main aspects of wellness and illness developed thus far. Both terms refer to an understanding of wholeness that is different from the usual understanding of the West. Rules of behavior laid down in the Qur'ān and prescribed by the religion help to provide the psychological conditions of wellness and happiness. Yet, even combined with the customary patterns of behavior in each country, they alone are not adequate in guaranteeing well-being because the world is in order and free from disturbances only if God wills. Illness is thus a symptom of a break in the feeling of wholeness as a result of sin, divine punishment, or bad influence on the part of Satan or *djinn*s. But it is noteworthy that not all deviant behavior is negative, that there are positive deviances when God takes possession of the mystic or allows the obedient servant to live free from religious duties for the rest of his or her life by bestowing madness. In the context of caring and curing, therefore, we must keep this wide range of possibilities in mind in order to respond adequately to the needs of wholeness.

Islamic Approaches to Caring and Curing

Since wholeness is the guiding principle of well-being and closely related to the concepts of wellness and illness, methods of caring and curing must follow this holistic perspective. As previously stated, illness is not merely a somatic phenomenon but must be seen in the context of psychosomatic reactions; moreover, certain psychic anomalies that would be labeled in Western countries as illnesses in the medical sense are looked at in a quite different way in Muslim countries.

An inquiry into the categories of caring and curing must therefore take into account the Muslim ethnomedical vision as regards the function of the medical doctor, the importance attributed to his or her work—including the emphasis placed on the need for research and biotechnical progress—and healers other than medical doctors.

DEFINITION AND RESPONSIBILITY OF THE MEDICAL PROFESSION

In January 1981 the First International Conference on Islamic Medicine was held in Kuwait. One outcome of the conference was the publication of the *Islamic Code of Medical Ethics*, which is as yet without any parallel in the Christian world. It is a remarkable document in that it tries to account fully for the current revolutionary progress in the medical and life sciences and to respond to the challenge in a spirit of real Islamic commitment to the religious heritage of moral values and codes of behavior. This document, known to me only in its English version, is a collection of statements regarding the different problems of medical practice in Muslim countries. It is noteworthy as such, although it is not representative for all Muslim doctors. However, it shows that if elsewhere in Islam there are conservative, less open-minded positions, the type of thinking exemplified in this document exists among Muslims as well, and it shows also that this second attitude follows the adoptive practices valued by Muslims of the past. With regard to Muslim patients in Muslim countries, the document assures the observer that medical practice is not significantly hindered by the religion in terms of techniques. However, with regard to Muslim patients living outside the Muslim world, it makes clear that there is a specific ethnomedical expectation of the doctor's role. It offers a unique chance for the outside observer to take note of an Islamic answer that gives room to both tradition and change, as outlined in the introductory remarks of this article. The introduction of the document expresses its major intent:

> Every Muslim doctor will hopefully find in it the guiding light to maintain his professional behaviour within the boundaries of Islamic teachings. . . . Medical and paramedical students should find in it a window over the future, so that they enter their professional life conversant with what to do and what to avoid, well prepared to face pressures or temptations or uncertainties. . . . To medical scientists it serves the function of the rudder to the ship . . . directing their efforts to harness science and technology only to the welfare of humanity but not to its danger or destruction.[17]

The clear reference to "the boundaries of Islamic teachings" reminds the reader of the principle of wholeness. Medicine and theology are closely interrelated; therapeutics and medical knowledge are seen in direct collaboration with God's own actions:

> [Therapeutics] is a noble Profession . . . God honoured it by making it the miracle of Jesus son of Mary. Abraham enumerating his Lord's gifts upon him— included "and if I fall ill He cures me."
> Like all aspects of knowledge, medical knowledge is part of the knowledge of God "who taught man what man never knew.". . . The study of Medicine entails the revealing of God's signs in His creation. "And in yourselves . . . do you not see?" The practice of Medicine brings God's mercy unto His subjects. Medical practice is therefore an act of worship and charity on top of being a career to make a living.[18]

Like all human activity, medical practice can be both an act of worship and a pitfall, if God's mercy is misused to evil purposes. Therefore the community, and in particular the ruler, must keep an eye on medical practice in order to avoid misuse and to guarantee that the integrity of the medical profession is preserved and its position protected. Medical doctors are exhorted to work sincerely under the guidelines of the religion, to avoid all temptations of personal arrogance or richness, and to resist all kinds of social pressures, be they personal, political, or military.

The importance given to the proper use of medicine is so highly appreciated that the provision of medical practice is seen as a *farḍ kifāya*, that is, a collective duty among the religious obligations, in that medicine is a religious necessity for society.[19] Medical caring and curing should therefore be practiced "always in a climate of piety and awareness of the presence of God,"[20] hence the principles for both the patient and the doctor:

> The preservation of man's life should embrace also the utmost regard to his dignity, feelings, tenderness and the privacy of his sentiments and body parts. A patient is entitled to full attention, care and feeling of security while with his doctor. The doctor's privilege of being exempted from some general rules is only coupled with more responsibility and duty that he should carry out in conscientiousness and excellence in observing God.[21]

The understanding of medical practice as worship has an enormous impact on the physician. Describing the characteristics of the physician, the document depicts him as the one who "should be amongst those who believe in God, fulfil His rights, are aware of His greatness, obedient to His orders, refraining from His prohibitions, and observing Him in secret and in public."[22] Moreover, the physician "should firmly know that 'life' is God's . . . awarded only by Him . . . and that 'Death' is the conclusion of one life and the beginning of another."[23] Consequently:

> [The role of physician is] that of a catalyst through whom God, the Creator, works to preserve life and health. He is merely an instrument of God in alleviating people's illness. For being so designated the Physician should be grateful and forever seeking God's help. He should be modest, free from arrogance and pride and never fall into boasting or hint at self-glorification through speech, writing or direct or subtle advertisement.[24]

Since the medical profession is fundamentally "the vocation to help Man under stress and not to exploit his need,"[25] the medical profession "is unique in that the client is not denied the service even if he cannot afford the fee."[26] In any case, with regard to the doctor-patient relationship, this principle should be kept in mind:

> For the sake of the patient the Doctor was . . . and not the other way round. Health is the goal and medical care is the means . . . the "patient" is master and the "Doctor" is at his service. [It follows that] top-priority status is conferred on the patient because and as long as he is a patient . . . no matter who he is or what he is, a patient is in the sanctuary of his illness and not of his social eminence, authority or personal relations. The way a Doctor deals with his various patients is a perfect portrayal of his personal integrity.[27]

The *Islamic Code of Medical Ethics* thus insists on the personal integrity of the physician. A highly sophisticated knowledge of medical techniques is not sufficient; in addition to this and to his religious conviction, the physician must show "good example by caring for his own health. It is not befitting for him that his 'do's' and 'don'ts' are not observed primarily by himself. He should not turn his back on the lessons of medical progress, because he will never convince his patients unless they see the evidence of his own conviction."[28]

Medical education is therefore only one aspect of wholeness and gains convincing force from the living examples. Thus the document concludes:

> [Medical education,] despite being a speciality, is but one fiber in a whole mesh founded on the belief in God, His oneness and absolute ability, and that He alone is the Creator and giver of life, knowledge, death, this world and the hereafter.
>
> In planning the making of a Doctor, a principal goal is to make him or her a living example of all that God loves, free from all that God hates, well saturated with the love of God, of people and of knowledge.
>
> The *Medical* Teacher owes his students the *provision* of the good example, adequate teaching, sound guidance and continual care in and out of classes and before and after graduation.[29]

This understanding of medicine and of the role of medical practice has been observed by medical doctors in West Germany, who realize that the Muslim Turks have high expectations of them but have a rather limited confidence in medicines.[30] This is particularly important with regard to a medical practice such as that in West Germany, which gives priority to medicines and medical techniques and tends to ignore the role of the doctor as a person. To Turkish Muslims, the doctors seem to believe more in the results of machine examinations than in the descriptions of their sick patients. When the machine fails to produce any data that reveals an illness, the doctors think that their patients are not ill, despite the patients' feelings of serious illness. The basis for the healing process, namely mutual confidence, has been replaced with the doctor's belief in a machine and the patient's perception of being taken for a liar.[31]

In addition to religious background, other elements contribute to this lack of successful communication. Since most Turkish Muslims working in West Germany are not sufficiently capable of expressing themselves precisely to a well-trained specialist of modern medicine, they use cultural patterns to express their feelings. For example, they will say they have liver aches if they feel depressed or unable to work. In most cases the medical examination shows no malfunction of the liver, and the doctor usually ignores the fact that in Turkish all sadness is attributed to and located in the liver. Thus the patient's reference to liver aches is often analogous to a German's reference to heartaches under particular psychological or emotional pressures such as homesickness, work depression, bad housing conditions, and so forth. It is interesting to note that among these Turkish people a shift from liver to heart problems has taken place within the last few years. When asked why this occurred, people from

East Anatolia explained: "Ciğer [i.e., liver] is Anatolian—to say Heart is more modern."[32]

Contrasting the Muslim expectation to the German situation does not deny the value and efficacy of medicines and other measures in the healing process, but it emphasizes the patient-doctor relationship as a healing process in itself. From the Islamic point of view, the medical doctor sees his or her own activity as an act of worship by working to preserve life and health. The medical practitioner is thus an instrument of God in alleviating people's illness.

This view illustrates how intimately illness and wellness correlate with other factors of the wholeness of well-being. Somatic phenomena are only one aspect of the loss of wellness. The Western specialization of medicine with its differentiation into different fields risks losing this holistic perspective characteristic of the Muslim worldview. The introduction of psychology and psychoanalysis proves the need in the West for a broader understanding of illness and wellness, but these disciplines place circumstance-produced illnesses in too close a proximity to mental disorders in the eyes of many Muslim patients.

Therefore, more attention must be paid to wholeness in the process of caring and curing. Each medical doctor needs to be aware of both physical and emotional causes of illness and should investigate the possibility of both. Placebo experiments have convincingly proved that the results of medical treatment are often due more to the patient-doctor interaction on the basis of mutual confidence and common belief in the healing process than they are due to the chemical effects of the medicine. Such results are even more positive with traditional Muslim patients.

THE NEED FOR RESEARCH AND BIOTECHNICAL PROGRESS

Knowledge in the field of medicine is not static. Progress has constantly been made, and as new methods have become applicable Muslims have found ways to accommodate them. Some examples from dentistry may serve to show that the situation in the past was not unlike that of the present. In mid-eighteenth-century Turkey dentists began to tie up loose teeth with golden files. They obtained a *fatwā* (final decision) approval by saying that such a dental procedure was in accordance with arguments put forward by Imām Muḥammad (al-Ḥasan ash-Shaybānī, d. 805 CE). In another instance, a Turkish *fatwā* of 1960 accepted fillings and crowns as a licit dental cure in modern times.[33]

The *Islamic Code of Medical Ethics* of 1981 emphasizes the need for medical research and declares:

> There is no censorship in Islam on scientific research, be it academic to reveal the signs of God in His creation, or applied aiming at the solution of a particular problem.

Freedom of scientific research shall not entail the subjugation of Man, telling him, harming him or subjecting him to definite or probable harm, withholding his therapeutic needs, defrauding him or exploiting his material need.

Freedom of scientific research shall not entail cruelty to animals, or their torture. Suitable protocols should be laid upon for the uncruel handling of experimental animals during experimentation.[34]

The document is particularly open-minded with regard to new challenges in the field of medical research and to organ donation:

The guiding rule in unprecedented matters falling under no extant text or law, is the Islamic dictum: "Wherever welfare is found, there exists the status of God."

The individual patient is the collective responsibility of Society, that has to ensure his health needs by any means inflicting no harm on others. This comprises the donation of body fluids or organs such as blood transfusions to the bleeding or a kidney transplant to the patient with bilateral irreparable renal damage. This is another *fard kifāya*, a duty that donors fulfill on behalf of society.[35]

The document further requires that effective legal measures be taken in order to organize organ donation during the donor's life and after his or her death by a statement in the donor's will or the consent of his or her family. The document favors the establishment of tissue and organ banks for tissues amenable to storage and suggests that cooperation with similar banks abroad be established on the basis of reciprocal aid. It thus seems to go beyond a *fatwā* issued by the highly prestigious Cairo Azhar mosque and Islamic University of the early 1970s that declared a cornea transplant legal if taken from a Muslim or non-Muslim and given to a Muslim, but forbidden if taken from a Muslim and given to a non-Muslim.[36]

Central to the arguments in the document is the principle of the sanctity of human life. Literally it says:

Human Life is sacred ... and should not be willfully taken except upon the indications specified in Islamic Jurisprudence, all of which are outside the domain of the Medical Profession.

A Doctor shall not take away life even when motivated by mercy. This is prohibited because this is not one of the legitimate indications for killing.[37]

However, although the doctor is strictly excluded from active participation in the process of taking life, the curtailing of medical treatment may be accepted in certain circumstances:

[The] Doctor is well advised to realize his limit and not transgress it. If it is scientifically certain that life cannot be restored, then it is futile to diligently keep on the vegetative state of the patient by heroic means of animation or preserve him by deep-freezing or other artificial methods. It is the process of life that the Doctor aims to maintain and not the process of dying. In any case, the Doctor shall not take a positive measure to terminate the patient's life.[38]

According to this life-ensuring principle the document finally states that "the sanctity of human Life covers all its stages including intrauterine life of the embryo and fetus."[39]

Rahman and others have shown the extent to which traditional Islamic medical practice paid attention to hygienic concerns.[40] Hospitals (*bāmāristān*)[41] were usually built in healthy parts of towns, near a river and if possible in a gardenlike surrounding, so that fresh air and the pleasant smell of flowers might enhance the healing process. Music and bath therapies were also used to help restore wellness. In contrast to the welcoming atmosphere of Muslim hospitals of the past, modern Western-style hospitals often give the impression of sterility. As a result patients seldom feel helped and restored, but are more often depressed because of the completely foreign and unpleasant setting as compared to the normal one of his or her everyday life. Moreover, the professionalization of medical practice within the last one hundred years in the West has made the medical doctor almost the only officially recognized healer. In many cases midwives have been replaced by gynecologists who are very often men, and it is considered inappropriate to visit them by many traditional Turkish women living in West Germany. They usually prefer to have female doctors and midwives.[42] For mental illnesses many Muslims still turn to nonmedical (traditional) healers.

TRADITIONAL HEALERS

The efficacy of religious practices undertaken for the recovery of health, such as pilgrimage and consulting a marabout, has been brought into full relief by Crapanzano's famous study in Moroccan ethnopsychiatry, which illustrates the healing methods and results of the Hamadsha, a Moroccan sect in the tradition of Islamic mysticism.[43] A 1983 investigation in Morocco done by Zakia Ghanjaoui and a similar study made by Omar Samaoli at nearly the same time show that until recently mental illness was often seen in close connection with external causes. Different types of mental illness are distinguished, belonging mainly to two groups: madness and possession.

Two types of madness are delineated by Ghanjaoui, the smooth and the dangerous. It is typical of smooth madness that the patient is quiet and pensive, not bothersome to others, and therefore able to live in society. It is characteristic of dangerous madness that the patient beats people, throws stones, and may even kill and is therefore dangerous to the public.[44]

In Ghanjaoui's interviews persons between the ages of twenty and thirty-five ranked the following factors as primary causes of mental illness: environmental causes such as relationship problems and discontent with the family (40 percent); a consequence of events such as failure in an examination or the loss of a beloved person (22.5 percent); traditional causes such as sorcery or fate (21 percent); genetic factors (9 percent); and drugs (6.7 percent). It is worth noting that there is no significant difference in regard to the level of education of the young interviewees. For people over the age of fifty the frequencies are reversed. Here, traditional causes are ranked first (37.5 percent), followed by temperament (20 percent), no answer (17 percent), consequence of events (14 percent), environment (6 percent), and drugs (3 percent).[45]

Since madness is incurable in the eyes of many of the interviewees, the hope that the patient will get rid of his or her illness is rather limited and has a negative effect on the therapy. It is striking however, that over 50 percent of those interviewed think that medical doctors should be consulted in such cases. Rare indeed are those who favor traditional healers alone (6.6 percent). Instead, a combination of both medical and traditional help is the priority for 25 percent of the interviewees. Looked at more closely, this result reveals an important change in the views of the two age groups of the investigation. It shows that modern medicine alone is given preference by younger persons and among them by those of higher education levels, while elderly people and the less-educated young population have a tendency to rely exclusively on traditional healing methods. Younger people are in favor of the combined procedure, regardless of their education or social origin.[46]

Possession, on the contrary, is regarded in a different way. First, most consider it to be a curable illness, and second, it is caused by external factors alone, frequently belonging to the realm of religion and popular belief. The Moroccan Arabic dialect, for instance, offers numerous terms to designate and distinguish the possessed.

Mshiyer or *laryah* refers to a type of possession accompanied by spontaneous crying, trembling, or laughing or by momentary losses of consciousness and prevision of future events. It is commonly accepted that if the possessed speaks during these moments of crisis it is not he or she personally but the spirit who is acting through the possessed. These moments are often called moments of trance. Longer-lasting phenomena sometimes accompanying this type of possession are the loss of sight, paralysis, and other physical signs. Different causes of possession are mentioned: an individual's aggressive attitude toward a spirit prompts the spirit's revenge, a spirit has beaten an individual and taken possession, or more simply, the transgression of prohibitions such as beating a cat or stepping over a gutter or a puddle of blood. The last two examples are transgressions typical of a society where such prohibitions exist on a large scale.

As concerns therapies appropriate for possession, in both age-groups the dominant suggestion is that of traditional healings, though here again elderly and less-educated younger people put a slightly greater emphasis on these methods. All, nevertheless, are in favor of traditional therapies and only 1 percent of the interviewees in both age groups thinks that such an illness is suited to medical treatment.[47]

Mamlūk and *maskūn* are two other words that designate the possessed, although many interviewees do not distinguish these from the *mshiyer*. Those who do, in particular elderly people, indicate that possessed persons of this category, unlike the preceding categories, are inhabited by a spirit permanently. If the spirit is of the opposite sex, then the possessed is regarded as being married to the spirit and is not allowed to marry another person; hence great isolation results for the possessed. The normal life of the possessed is then characterized by serving the spirit and by occasional trance moments following music rhythms. Often such a possessed person finds work in healing institutions of the Islamic tradition. A woman among the interviewees reports that a man of her family had lost blood from his nose again and again and therefore went to see medical doctors and *fakīh*s (here both the specialist in religious law and the traditional healer), but none were able to help the man. Finally he was brought to Bouya Omar, a saint well-known for specializing in mental troubles. There the man had some communication with spirits who took possession of him and who in order to heal him asked that he become a *fakīh* (therapist) himself.[48]

Though there are other words to designate the possessed,[49] Ghanjaoui mentions a final type of person exhibiting deviant behavior: the *madjūb*,[50] an illuminated person who has been given the *baraka*, a special blessing bestowed because of outstanding religious qualities. The *madjūb* is quite often a mystic (Ṣūfī), good at the psalmody of the Qur'ān and fascinated by old-fashioned words of the tradition. Often the *madjūb* is a descendant of a saint and/or a member of a religious order or brotherhood. In trance the *madjūb* foresees and foretells future events and is able to cut his or her skin or to walk barefoot over burning surfaces without harm or pain. Other special abilities are eating serpents and vipers as well as drinking boiling water without being harmed or injured. Needless to say, the real *madjūb* is extremely rare and needs no cure or healing at all. Here God's special gifts are at work and should not be replaced with "normal" behavior. In practice, however, great vigilance is necessary to recognize the true *madjūb* and to distinguish him or her clearly from the charlatan.

Samaoli describes the healing practices of the Aïssaoua ('Isāwā), a Moroccan confraternity, in detail. The possessed person is brought to the members of this confraternity in order to be healed in special sessions organized on particular occasions. Dances are performed according to a thoroughly prepared choreography with namings and rhythms as well as masks representing different worshiping groups in the community. The whole dance is seen as being part of the healing process and is often quite successful.[51]

Ghanjaoui also mentions the practice of incubation, that is, sleeping in the sanctuary with the expectation of a dream that indicates what one is to do, and the so-called rite of the word, which includes, for instance, the directive that the patient swallow a piece of paper with some verses of the Qur'ān on it or drink the water in which a piece of paper with verses of the Qur'ān has been soaked. Some marabouts as well as certain tombs of saints have the reputation of possessing healing powers. These tombs attract many pilgrims on special occasions when healing ceremonies are held.[52] In the past and in some remote areas today these pilgrimages are not restricted to possession cases alone. It is reported that some places are known for curing female sterility and backaches.[53] In many rural areas this kind of curing still seems to be quite widespread, and even in towns this type of treatment is more affordable by poor people than the expense of medical advice from doctors.

Morocco is not the only country of Islamic tradition where these practices are observed. Concrete examples from Mauretania, Egypt, Pakistan, and Muslim India are also known to me, making it clear that this is part of the worldview of many Muslims without necessarily being part of the religion as such. Popular beliefs play an enormous role, as in the case of the evil eye, a tradition claiming that the glance of a person intending to inflict harm may lead to bad consequences for another. Protection measures are therefore taken for newborn children, and amulets are worn to protect against many kinds of harm that might come from the spirits or from people with bad intentions (who are working on their own or simply serving as instruments of devils or evil *djinn*s).

A peculiarity of medical diagnosis should be added here. I came across this information in discussions with medical doctors in Upper Egypt. There men will not infrequently come to the doctor as a surrogate for their wives, anticipating that the symptoms reported will result in the diagnosis of pregnancy. They report literally their wives' symptoms in reference to their own "substitute" body, that is, they do not explain that the illness they are describing is not their own. Doctors who have no experience with "substitute patients" may misunderstand this kind of situation and may not make an appropriate diagnosis.

In conclusion to this section on caring and curing one may say that the extent to which all medical action is embedded in the sociocultural framework of the understanding of wellness and illness—and in the different categories of healing procedures—is striking. This ethnomedical perspective needs to be kept in mind when medical doctors outside the countries of Islamic tradition are confronted with Muslim patients. They should then not be surprised when they notice that some of their patients, mostly the illiterate from rural areas, continue to see other healers as well.

There are cases involving Turks living in West Germany who did not consult the medical doctors at all, but only the *hodja* in the mosque, often in cases wherein the virus or microbe causing the disease was well known to medical doctors.[54] An avoidance of these incidents requires good interaction between modern medical health care and society as a whole.

Medical Aspects of Islamic Ethics and Justice

The *Islamic Code of Medical Ethics* lays down the main guidelines of medical ethics and justice from the Islamic perspective in these words:

> The Doctor is in every sense a member of Society, fully acting, interacting and caring for it. [Therefore] the Medical Profession shall take it as duty to combat such health-destructive habits as smoking, uncleanliness, etc. Apart from mass education and advertence, the Medical Profession should unrelentlessly pressurize [sic] the judiciary to issue necessary legislation.
> The combat and prevention of environment pollution falls under this category.
> The natural prophylaxis against diseases and the other complications ensuing upon sexual licence, lies in revival of the human values of chastity, purity, self-restraint and refraining from advertently or inadvertently inflicting harm on self or others. To preach these religious values is "Preventive Medicine" and therefore lies within the jurisdiction and obligation of the medical profession.[55]

Thus, preventive medicine is seen as the application and fulfillment of religious values. Indeed, it is this ethicoreligious aspect of wholeness that primarily guarantees wellness, for faith "is remedial, a healer, a conqueror of stress and a procurer of cure. The training of the Doctor should prepare him to bolster 'Faith' and avail the patient of its unlimited blessings."[56]

There is no room here to describe the entire ethical value system of the Qur'ān and of medieval and present-day Islam,[57] but it must be repeated that this value system alone sets the framework for the doctor's actions. The Kuwait document states:

> The Muslim Medical Profession should be conversant with Islam's teachings and abiding by them. It should also thoroughly study at first hand the data, facts, figures and projections of various parameters actually existent in Muslim societies. Upon this should be decided what to take and what to reject from the experiences and conclusions of other societies. Reconciliation with a policy of uncritical copying of alien experience should be stopped.[58]

Here the question of Islamic identity is again put forward, and it is suggested that when Islamic teachings are at odds with Western medical conduct or advice the Islamic dictum should be given priority. This policy may in practice hinder committed but anxious Muslims from incorporating new healing techniques. The Kuwait document, however, does not dictate this conclusion. On the contrary, it states: "Medical Education is neither passive nor authoritarian. It aims at sparking mental activity, fostering observation, analysis and reasoning, development of independent thought and the evolvement of fresh questions."[59] There is a need for an information campaign because—as shown in Ghanjaoui's investigation—there is at this point too little concrete knowledge among less-informed circles in towns and rural areas. This campaign would need to make clear what the approved orthodox religious values are. It would also serve to point out how many courses of action taken in Muslim society are not based on the Qur'ān or other Islamic teachings but are local practices that should perhaps be abandoned.

A problem of medical ethics lies in trying to determine to what extent the will of the patient is to be respected when his or her refusal of, for instance, surgical interference may result in inadequate treatment of a disease. Here again the *Islamic Code of Medical Ethics* gives clear advice:

> When fear is the obstacle preventing the patient from consent, the Doctor may help his patient with a medicine such as a tranquillizer to free his patient from fear but without abolishing or suppressing his consciousness, so that the patient is able to make his choice in calmness and tranquillity. By far the best method to achieve this is the poise of the Doctor himself and his personality, kindness, patience and the proper use of the spoken word.
>
> In situations where urgent and immediate surgical or other interference is necessary to save life, the Doctor should go ahead according to the Islamic rule "necessities override prohibitions." His position shall be safe and secure whatever the result achieved, on condition that he has followed established medical methodology in a correct way. The "bad" inherent in not saving the patient outweights the presumptive "good" in leaving him to his self destructive decision. The Islamic rule proclaims that "warding off" the "bad" takes priority over bringing about the "good."[60]

With regard to patients with incurable disease and what to say to them, the Kuwait document suggests as follows:

> The Doctor shall do his best that what remains of the life of an incurable patient will be spent under good care, moral support and freedom from pain and misery.
>
> The Doctor shall comply with the patient's right to know his illness. The Doctor's particular way of answering should be tailored to the particular patient in question. It is the Doctor's duty to thoroughly study the psychological acumen of his patient. He shall never fall short of suitable vocabulary if

the situation warrants the deletion of frightening nomenclature or coinage of new names, expressions or descriptions.[61]

Facing the concerns of those unable to afford medical treatment and their right to receive it, the document states that the "Medical Profession is unique in that the client is not denied the service even if he cannot afford the fee. Medical legislation should ensure medical help to all needy of it, by issuing and executing the necessary laws and regulations."[62] The needy must in any case be looked after, even when it is the enemy soldier in time of war, for "whatever the feelings of the Doctor and wherever they lie, he shall stick to the one and only duty of protecting life and treating ailment or casualty."[63]

The doctor's duty in wartime is summarized as follows:

> As part of the international medical family, Muslim Doctors should lend all support on a global scale to protect and support this one-track noble course of the medical profession . . . for it is a blessing to all humanity if this humanitarian role is abided by on both sides of the battle front.
>
> The Medical Profession shall not permit its technical, scientific or other resources to be utilized in any sort of harm or destruction or infliction upon man of physical, psychological, moral or other damage . . . regardless of all political or military considerations.
>
> The doings of the Doctor shall be uni-directional aiming at the offering of treatment and cure to ally and enemy, be this at the personal or general level.[64]

The attitudes of reverence and protection of life together with the standard of justice (in the sense of helping both the poor and the wealthy when in need) and the ethicoreligious values of Islam constitute the criteria for copying and incorporating alien methods and experience. They make clear that medical practice is an integral part of the Islamic way of life; therefore it must take into account concrete religious prescriptions in the context of the life-passages.

Life-Passages in Islamic Custom

With regard to problems in the category of passages, the *Islamic Code of Medical Ethics* declares:

> The Physician should be in possession of a threshold knowledge of jurisprudence, worship and essentials of *Fiqh* [Islamic Law] enabling him to give counsel to patients seeking his guidance about health and bodily conditions with a

bearing on the rites of worship. Men and women are subject to symptoms, ailments or physiological situations like pregnancy, and would wish to know the religious ruling pertaining to prayer, fasting, pilgrimage, family planning etc.

Although "necessity overrides prohibition," the Muslim Physician—nevertheless—should spare no effort in avoiding recourse to medicines or ways of therapy—be they surgical, medical or behavioural—that are prohibited by Islam.[65]

The regulation for fasting merits special mention here. During one whole month (Ramadan) adult Muslims are not allowed to drink, eat, smoke, or have sexual intercourse during the daytime, although all these things are permitted at night. As the rhythm of eating and drinking is shifted from the normal daytime schedule to the night, the whole functioning of the organism consequently undergoes a radical change. This can create numerous problems for the health care of the pious Muslim. For example, problems will arise when medicines must be taken regularly. Notwithstanding dispensations in favor of the sick, Muslims often think that they are not so ill that they need to make use of the dispensation. Instead they set aside the medicine during the daytime, only taking some during the night. Medical doctors in Islamic societies are, of course, aware of this potential for irregularities in medicinal dosage, and they also know that injections will normally be refused as well. Medical doctors in non-Muslim countries, however, are not attuned to this possibility and are thus surprised when they discover that their Muslim patients are not following the instructions or prescriptions.[66] Another matter of medical relevance is that nursing mothers must fast unless the life of the mother is in danger.

It must be pointed out that contrary to the expectations of the Western observer, Muslims generally have a positive attitude to Ramadan fasting. They do not focus on the restrictive regulations but rather are emotionally attached to the Ramadan. Like Christmas, which may be the last link many Christians maintain with the church, Ramadan is an occasion for even the skeptical Muslim to show his or her solidarity with the Muslim community. Ramadan is the annual period of excellent dishes at the evening meals and is therefore full of good reminders of the joyful days when as a child one waited for the special Ramadan food in the evenings as well as for the special gifts that mark the breaking of the fast at the end of the month.

In other religious practices, such as prayer, purity (*ṭahīra*) is very important and is paid special attention. Purity in this context refers to both physical cleanliness and mental good and right intentions. The whole educational process therefore aims at teaching purity to the child, including correct performance of the prescribed washings (*wuḍū'*).

BIRTH AND CHILDHOOD

In many societies birth is accompanied by numerous religious acts, which may be labeled "rites of passage," according to terminology introduced by van Gennep. Muslims regard birth as a difficult and dangerous passage; Ibn Ḳayyim al-Ghawziyya (c. 1292–1350) described it as the change from a well-protected warm womb existence to naked being in a world of cold and heat, hunger and pain—a world full of dangers and temptations.[67] Human life starts with the fetus. In Islamic tradition there have been disputes about when the fetus is "ensouled," in an effort to determine at what point abortion is to be considered killing (see chapter 7 in this book). Today there is a noticeable tendency to state that the fetus is a complete human being from the moment of conception and therefore deserves and needs protection; this opinion is expressed in the *Islamic Code.*

There are many Islamic practices that accompany birth to mark the entrance of the newborn into life on earth, but none of these is imperative in terms of religious duties. However, in most Muslim countries it is still customary to say the Muslim Creed ("I witness that there is no God but Allāh; I witness that Muhammad is Allāh's messenger") into the ears of the newborn in order to invite the child to accept Islam as his or her religion. A name-giving ceremony is held soon after birth. On the seventh day after birth there are other ceremonies expressing thanks to God and celebrating the existence of a new member of the community. Having children is seen as a great blessing, and taking good care of them is among the most honorable duties of the parents.

The main stages in the physical growth of the child are expressed in classical Arabic. *Walīd* is the term for the newborn, then follows the "weak" stage (*ṣadīgh*) until the seventh day. Next is the time of suckling (*rāḍiʻ*) for a child up to nearly two years old, indicating that nursing time in traditional Islam is longer than the usual Western practice. Then comes the stage of weaning (*faṭīm*); the stage of "slowly moving around" (*dāridj*), when the child begins his or her first steps alone; and the "quintuple" stage (*khumāsī*), when the child measures five spans. After the *khumāsī* comes the "tooth-loser" (*mathghūr*), when the first teeth are lost, and the stage of getting new teeth again (*muththaghir*), to mention only the most common terms.[68] The psychological development of the child is charted less distinctly. It is described as a slow process leading up to the use of the intellectual capacities at an age when children behave reasonably and know how to make distinctions (*sinn at-tamyīz*), that is, around the age of seven. It is also at this age that a role-specific education starts to prescribe significant differences for boys and girls. From this point onward the father himself or a teacher is concerned with the religious and professional instruction of the son, while the mother usually continues to look after the daughter as she has done for both the son and the daughter from birth up to this age.[69] As regards the education of girls, honor and shame, respect and obedience are typical characteristics of the well-educated Muslima.[70]

Though not prescribed by the Qur'ān, circumcision is widely practiced on the boy and is regarded by many Muslims as being imperative for him.[71] It is normally not practiced on girls, although there are some areas such as the Sudan where female circumcisions are still reported. The age of circumcision for boys varies considerably from one region to the other, ranging from the seventh day after birth to the age of fifteen years. This wide range alone indicates that its origin is not a rite of puberty marking a cause for celebration but some other tradition that apparently has several pre-Islamic prototypes. Circumcision today is performed by medical doctors in many modern town districts. Traditionally it was not the doctor's work but was executed by specialists in this ritual, who, as in Eygpt, arranged public circumcisions on the occasion of great festivities in the middle of the crowded marketplace next to other amusement booths. It is noteworthy that where circumcision is still practiced in the traditional way, results are generally good in spite of equipment that does not meet Western standards of hygiene, and cases of infection seem to be extremely rare exceptions in the rule. On the contrary; it is often said in Egypt that infections occur much more frequently in the medical practice than after the public circumcision.

MARRIAGE

Marriage is another passage that is extremely important in the eyes of the Muslim, for sexuality is seen as an integral part of the human constitution. Man and woman both find their human fulfillment in procreation and in sexual pleasure. However, sexual activity is allowed only to those who are married, for the Qur'ān states the obligation of the woman to keep her virginity until marriage (4.24).[72] Premarital sexual intercourse, consequently, is not allowed for girls nor is the use of contraceptives for this purpose. The same rules apply in theory for young men—however, the breaking of the rule by males is less often noticed and in practice is considered in the minds of many Muslims to be one of the pardonable sins. For girls, on the other hand, being untouched is seen as being so important that the bride's virginity or lack of it is a matter of honor and shame for her whole family and not a private matter pertaining only to herself. It is reported, for instance, that West German Turkish mothers who bring their daughters to see medical doctors asking whether or not the daughter suffers from appendicitis expect in reality that the doctor will examine the hymen in order to tell whether or not it is still completely intact.[73]

As a consequence of this insistence on the virginity of unmarried females, Muslims have traditionally tended to marry girls at a rather young age. In the past, the age of most girls at marriage was around twelve or thirteen, while most boys were slightly older, between thirteen and fourteen. Today most Muslim countries follow Western trends in marriage, and most couples wait until they are eighteen years old. Some girls, however, are betrothed at a much younger age.

According to Islam, sexual intercourse is allowed only if practiced between the husband and his legitimate wives (up to a maximum of four simultaneously married); in earlier times, it was permitted between the lord and his female slaves. Besides these situations, no form of sexual behavior is considered licit in the classical handbooks of Islam. Consequently, homosexuality (for both men and women), as well as masturbation and sexual intercourse with animals, is strictly forbidden,[74] though certain manuals of good behavior in Persia have included and even encouraged homosexual relations.[75] The statements concerning homosexuality clearly indicate that the social reality often was and still is different from the ideals expressed in the handbooks. This is also true for prostitution, which in theory was not allowed but in reality is well known to Muslims.

Another type of marriage, allowed by Shī'a law only, is worth mentioning here. It is the temporary marriage (*mut'a*), in which the marriage treaty clearly lays out from the very beginning its automatic expiration date and the consequences of the termination.[76] As far as family planning is concerned there is no general rule accepted by all Muslims. As with so many other problems the debate is still going on, with a certain tendency to favor contraceptive measures decided upon by the spouses themselves but to reject prescriptions put forth by the state or ruling party.

Closely related to active sexuality is the issue of nakedness. Classical handbooks of Islam insist on proper dressing for the Muslim, for indecent nakedness is considered to be terribly shameless. This concerns the medical doctor in that some Muslims do not allow their wives to undress in front of a male doctor. It seems, at least, that in West Germany only those Turkish women who have been given explicit permission by their husbands are willing to disrobe in front of a male doctor.[77] This attitude is prevalent among uneducated Turks but not among those who work in more highly skilled positions.

DEATH

The last life-passage is that from life to death. As has already been stated, the Muslim believes that death occurs in accordance with God's will. It is therefore prohibited to end one's life by committing suicide.

Medical assistance should be oriented toward saving life and doing

everything possible to protect it. Medical techniques are seen as being for
the benefit of the patient; if there is no longer any hope, only the mechanical functioning of the organism guaranteed by a machine may be dismissed. Thus, euthanasia is forbidden, and medical action may not put an
end to an otherwise unfinished life; however, the simple prolongation of
life without any lifelike quality is not seen as an end in itself. The *Islamic
Code* makes clear statements on these matters, as well as on the care to
be taken in determining that a life has ended: "To declare a person dead
is a grave responsibility that ultimately rests with the Doctor. He shall
appreciate the seriousness of his verdict and pass it in all honesty and
only when sure of it. He may dispel any trace of doubt by seeking counsel
and resorting to modern scientific gear."[78] A vigilant attitude is particularly important with regard to organ transplants. Legal regulations must
help to avoid any misuse of eventual donorship. Here Muslims, like most
people, must express their desire to ensure and protect life through laws
to guard against misuse of any kind.

The belief of Muslims in resurrection and the hereafter does not concretely affect their attitude toward the dead. Since death ends human life
on earth and God will create the world anew on the Day of Judgment
(30.27), there is no special advice with regard to the corpse except for the
obligation to respect its dignity as if the deceased person were still alive.
For instance, men who wash a male corpse must respect rules of shame,
washing under the special dress of the corpse but not removing it. The
same is true for the women who wash female corpses. Washing the dead
is only one of many actions taken at death. It would be too lengthy and
inappropriate to describe the whole procedure here in detail, but it may
be observed that in all Muslim societies burial must take place as quickly
as possible and that only men are present for the funerals of both men
and women.

Conclusion

A consideration of the ethnomedical framework is central to a successful
Islamic medical practice. Wellness and illness are embedded in a concept
of wholeness that is taught by Islam and that is seen as being granted by
God. Illness thus indicates a disturbance of this originally balanced well-
being, caused either by God, Satan, or the *djinn*s. Faith is thus an important remedy and part of healing. The medical doctor has the privilege and
the honor of worshiping God by working to preserve life through the use
of technical knowledge. Successes in medicine are not the result of human
activity alone but are always part of God's merciful acting on and in
human life.

A patient's full acceptance of the physician's opinion presupposes that doctors are aware of this religious component of medical curing. Strict personal integrity is therefore required in every medical doctor so that confidence may become the basis for a good doctor-patient relationship. Each patient who is in need should be treated justly, and medical services may not be refused if the patient is unable to afford treatment. Life is to be given priority in all actions, so long as there is a chance of restoring the patient. Euthanasia is thus forbidden, but withdrawal of care is permitted in those cases wherein there is no hope of recovery and patients are being kept alive solely by artificial means. Because life is sacred and everything possible is done to maintain it, the First International Conference on Islamic Medicine issued a statement favoring organ transplants as a way of helping the living.

Medical research is highly regarded and encouraged, and since medical practice is seen as an act of worship, the doctor's sense of responsibility is particularly emphasized. It is said that the medical doctor, being merely an instrument of God in alleviating human illness, should be grateful and forever seeking God's help. It follows that the medical doctor should be modest, that is, free from arrogance and pride, and should never fall into boasting or hint at self-glorification through speech, writing, or advertising, be it direct or subtle. This principle implies that all medical activity and education are but one fiber in the mesh of belief centered on God. Other kinds of medicine are woven into this fabric as well, and it is for this reason that other healers are sometimes consulted by the patient. Moreover, since faith and religious practice are essential elements of wellness, all medical prescriptions or interventions must take religious duties into account, and a basic knowledge of the Muslim perspective of wholeness and well-being is needed by every medical doctor trying to heal patients who are Muslim. A case in point is the tradition of fasting during Ramadan, when, as we have seen, it is common to take neither medicines nor injections during the day. Misdirected psychological pressure on the patient to break these rules will certainly not lead to the restoration of full health; medical doctors should measure the real impact of both religious duties and medical techniques on the patient and the healing process. Indeed, the human relationship between a well-informed, understanding medical doctor and such a patient—a patient thoroughly devoted to observance of religious duty—will bring about restoration of health more surely than technically sophisticated medical techniques are capable of doing. Often the psychological problems of the patient are willfully neglected and replaced with the conviction that medicines and apparatuses alone will heal the sick. It is genuinely hoped that the preceding examples will contribute to a better understanding between the medical doctor and the Muslim patient so that the sick may become healthy once more within the living tradition of Islam.

Notes

1. Rotraud Wielandt, *Das Bild der Europäer in der modernen arabischen Erzähl- und Theaterliteratur* (Beirut, 1980), Summary, p. 645. *Beiruter Texte und Studien* 23:645.
2. Āl-i Aḥmad Djalāl, *Gharb zadigī* (Tehran, 1962).
3. Sayid Mujtaba Rukni Musawi Lari, *Western Civilisation through Muslim Eyes*, trans. F. J. Goulding (Guilford, Surrey, 1977).
4. Khalifa Abdul Hakim, *Islamic Ideology: The Fundamental Beliefs and Principles of Islam and Their Application to Practical Life* (Lahore, 1953), p. 148.
5. ʿAbd al-Ḳādir ʿAudah (ʿŪdah), *al-Islām wa-auḍāʿunā as-sāyāsiyya* (Cairo, 1951), p. 57.
6. M. Bernand, "Idjmāʿ," *Encyclopaedia of Islam*, new ed., vol. 3 (London, 1971), pp. 1023–1026.
7. M. Bernand, "Ḳiyās," *Encyclopaedia of Islam* 5 (1968):238–242.
8. Cf. N. J. Coulson, *A History of Islamic Law* (Edinburgh, 1964), pp. 36ff.
9. J. R. Walsh, "Fatwā," *Encyclopaedia of Islam* 2 (1965):866ff.
10. Miḳdād Yāldjin, *at-Tarbiya al-akhlāḳiyya al-islāmiyya* (Cairo, 1977), p. 54.
11. Ibid., p. 239.
12. See Gerd Overbeck, *Krankheit als Anpassung: Der sozio-psychosomatische Zirkel* (Frankfurt/Main, 1984).
13. Karl Opitz, *Die Medizin im Koran* (Stuttgart, 1906). For more information on Islamic medicine see Munawar A. Anees, "Bibliography on Islamic Medicine," *Muslim World Book Review* 5, no. 1 (Autumn 1984): 59–68; also see J. Christoph Bürgel, "Secular and Religious Features of Medieval Arabic Medicine," in *Asian Medical Systems*, ed. Charles Leslie (Berkeley, 1976), pp. 44–62.
14. Lari, pp. 25ff.
15. Richard Gramlich, *Die schiitischen Derwischorder Persiens* (Wiesbaden, 1976), Part 2 of *Abhandlungen für die Kunde des Morgeniandes*, pp. 113–115.
16. Gramlich, pp. 330, 359–365.
17. First International Conference on Islamic Medicine, *Islamic Code of Medical Ethics*, Kuwait Document, Kuwait Rabi 1, 1401 (January 1981):16f.
18. Ibid., p. 21.
19. Ibid., pp. 22f.
20. Ibid., p. 23.
21. Ibid., p. 24.
22. Ibid., p. 29.
23. Ibid., p. 30.
24. Ibid., p. 32.
25. Ibid., p. 45.
26. Ibid., p. 44.
27. Ibid., p. 43.
28. Ibid., p. 30.
29. Ibid., p. 87.
30. Ursula Brucks, Erdmann von Salisch, and Wulf-Bodo Wahl, "'Wir sind seelisch krank, automatisch—und körperlich auch': Zum Krankheitsverständnis türkischer Arbeiter," in *Gesundheit für alle: Die medizinische Versorgung türkischer Familien in der Bundesrepublik*, eds. Jürgen Collatz, Elçin Kürşat-Ahlers, and Johannes Korporal (Hamburg, 1985), p. 346.
31. Irmgard Theilen, "Überwindung der Sprachlosigkeit türkischer Patienten in der Bundesrepublik: Versuch einer gansheitlichen Medizin mit türk-

ischen Patienten als Beitrag zur transkulturellen Therapie," in *Gesundheit für alle*, pp. 293f.

32. Ibid., p. 297.
33. Johannes Benzing, *Islamische Rechtsgutachten als volkskundliche Quelle* (Wiesbaden, 1977), p. 8.
34. *Islamic Code of Medical Ethics*, p. 79.
35. Ibid., pp. 80f.
36. A facsimile of the Arabic text of the Azhar *fatwā* and a German translation are found in Abubakr Gad Ali, "Rechtliche Fragen der Hornhautübertragung in islamischen Ländern" (Med. diss., Westfälische Technische Hochschule Aachen, 1974), pp. 42–45, 50f.
37. *Islamic Code of Medical Ethics*, p. 64.
38. Ibid., p. 67.
39. Ibid., p. 66.
40. For example, Arslan Terzioğlu, "Mittelalterliche islamische Krankenhäuser unter Berücksichtigung der Frage nach den ältesten psychiatrischen Anstalten" (Diss., Technische Universität Berlin, Fakultät für Architektur, 1968), pp. 252ff.
41. Bedi N. Şehsuvaroğlu: "Bīmāristān," in *Encyclopaedia of Islam* 1 (1960): 1222–1226.
42. Angela Zink, "Türkische Frauen als Patientinnen: Interaktionsprobleme aus der Sicht der behandelnden Ärzte," in *Gesundheit für alle*, pp. 351–369; Jürgen Collatz, "Die Betreuung türkischer Familien im Rahmen des Modellversuches 'Aktion Familien-Hebamme,'" in *Gesundheit für alle*, pp. 370–399.
43. Vincent Crapanzano, *The Hamadsha: A Study in Moroccan Ethnopsychiatry* (Berkeley, 1973).
44. Zakia Ghanjaoui, "Les représentations de la maladie mentale au Maroc" (Representations of mental illness in Morocco), *Cahiers d'Anthropologie et Biométrie Humaine* 2, no. 4 (1984):59.
45. Zakia Ghanjaoui, "Les représentations de la maladie mentale au Maroc" (Doctoral thesis, University 5 of Paris, 1985), pp. 181–183, Ghanjaoui, Journal article (1984), pp. 53f.
46. Ghanjaoui, Journal article (1984), pp. 60f.; doctoral thesis (1985), pp. 183ff.
47. Ghanjaoui, Doctoral thesis (1985), pp. 201f.
48. Ibid., pp. 210–212.
49. For a long list of terms describing psychic behaviors see Omar Samaoli, "Pratiques traditionnelles de prise en charge des troubles mentaux au Maroc" (Doctoral thesis, University 5 of Paris, 1985), pp. 183f.
50. Ghanjaoui, Doctoral thesis, pp. 213ff.
51. Samaoli, pp. 86ff.; for information on the Aïssaoua see J. L. Michon, "'Īsāwā," in *Encyclopaedia of Islam* 4 (1978):93–95.
52. Ghanjaoui, Doctoral thesis (1985), pp. 64ff.
53. Ibid., p. 69.
54. Horst Lison and Rüdiger Lorentzen, "Medizinische Versorgung türkischer Kinder und Jugendlicher," in *Gesundheit für alle*, p. 457.
55. *Islamic Code of Medical Ethics*, pp. 71f.
56. Ibid., p. 88.
57. See M. A. Draz, *La Morale du Koran: Etude comparée de la morale théorique du Koran, suivie d'une classification de versets choisis, formant le code complet de la morale pratique* (Le Caire, 1950); Peter Antes, *Ethik und Politik im Islam* (Stuttgart, 1982); Peter Antes, "Islamische Ethik," in *Ethik in*

nichtchristlichen Kulturen, eds. Peter Antes et al. (Stuttgart, 1984), pp. 48–81.

58. *Islamic Code of Medical Ethics,* p. 73.
59. Ibid., p. 88.
60. Ibid., pp. 58f.
61. Ibid., p. 68.
62. Ibid., p. 44.
63. Ibid., p. 52.
64. Ibid., p. 53.
65. Ibid., pp. 31f.
66. Lison and Lorentzen, pp. 456f.
67. Shams ad-dīn Muḥammad Ibn Ḳayyim al-Ghawziyya, *Tuḥfat al-mawdūd bi-aḥkām al-mawlūd,* ed. ʿAbdal-ḥakīm Sharaf ad-dīn (Bombay, 1961), pp. 174f.
68. Ibid., p. 183. For the terminology of classical Arabic see also G. Adamek, "Das Kleinkind in Glaube und Sitte der Araber im Mittelalter" (Doctoral dissertation, Faculty of Philosophy, University of Bonn, 1968), pp. 17f.
69. Cf. Harald Motzki, "Das Kind und seine Sozialisation in der islamischen Familie des Mittelalters," in *Zur Sozialgeschichte der Kindheit,* eds. Jochen Martin and August Nitschke (Freiburg, 1986), p. 423.
70. See J. G. Peristiany, ed., *Honour and Shame: The Values of Mediterranean Society* (London, 1965).
71. Cf. A. J. Wensinck, "Khitān" in *Encyclopaedia of Islam* 5 (1986):20–22.
72. For an article dealing with the difficulties of understanding the verse correctly, see Harald Motzki, "Wal-muḥṣanātu mina n-nisāʾi illā mā malakat aimānukum (Koran 4:24) und die koranische Sexualethik, *Der Islam Zeitschrift für Geschichte und Kultur des islamischen Orients* 63 (1986): 192–218.
73. Reyhan Pietruschka, "Erfahrungen einer türkischen Frauenärztin in Berlin," in *Gesundheit für alle,* p. 445.
74. Abdelwahab Bouhdiba, "Islam et sexualité" (Thesis, University 5 of Paris, Lille, 1973), p. 95.
75. Cf. Iradj Khalifeh-Soltani, "Das Bild des idealen Herrschers in der iranischen Fürstenspiegelliteratur, dargestellt am Beispiel des Qābūs-Nāmé"(Doctoral dissertation, Faculty of Philosophy, University of Tübingen, 1971), pp. 161ff.
76. Werner Ende, "Ehe auf Zeit (mutʿa) in der innerislamischen Diskussion der Gegenwart," *Die Welt des Islams* 20 (1980): 1.
77. Zink, p. 356.
78. *Islamic Code of Medical Ethics,* p. 67.

CHAPTER 9

Religion and Healing in an African Community: The Akan of Ghana

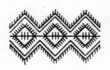

KOFI APPIAH-KUBI

My family has the gift of healing and has been a great source of inspiration and information regarding religious medicine. I learned from the practices of my grandmother, mother, and elder brother, and at times I practice the arts of healing as I acquired or inherited them from the family.

At national and international meetings I have shared and compared the material on the Akan of Ghana with other workers in the field from different parts of Ghana and the world. Research into Akan religious medicine is my lifetime occupation, and since 1970 these investigations have included a special focus on the healing activities of the Indigenous African Christian churches (often called Independent churches).

In this article I propose to deal with the following characteristic beliefs about health, disease, and healing practices among the Akan of Ghana: the holistic approach adopted by the Akan in restoring the otherwise strained harmony of relationship between individuals and their fellow human beings, their community, their environment—both natural and supernatural—and, above all, their God; the kinship link between humans and nature, together with the understanding that a relationship between these two can foster the good health of individuals and their society; the role of religion in healing and the need for the recognition or acknowledgment of the higher power in all facets of health care service; and the importance of the role of kin in times of crisis.

I intend to suggest answers to the following questions: What lessons can a Christian healing ministry and modern scientific medicine derive from this system? What are the possibilities for collaboration among the different dimensions of healing operative in Akanland? But before these questions can be answered, it is necessary to review the medical situation.

In Ghana, as in many African countries, there is uneven geographical distribution of health care services. Only about 15 percent of the approximately 12 million inhabitants enjoy 85 percent of the national health benefits, and the majority of those who are not served are the rural poor. In fact, modern medical services exist for those who can afford it and who happen to live in urban centers. Most adequately equipped medical facilities are located in the regional centers, with a few ill-equipped health posts scattered through the rural areas.

In the rural areas where the majority of the population live and where health hazards or problems are more acute, the national modern health facilities are often inadequate and in many instances nonexistent. In such areas maternal and child mortality and morbidity are very high. The life expectancy of the rural population is lower than that of the urban population. A quick review of the disturbing health situation is provided by the following Health Profile of Africa (*Development and Cooperation*, no. 3, 1984):

1. About 100 million people in Africa have no access to adequate drinking water.

2. Almost 70 percent of the African population do not get enough to eat.

3. About 72 million suffer from serious malnutrition.

4. Twenty-two of the thirty-six poorest nations in the world are in Africa.

5. The African population continues to be more exposed than other populations to endemic diseases such as malaria and to diseases caused by poor sanitation, malnutrition, and poverty.

6. Such waterborne and water-related diseases as intestinal parasites, gastrointestinal illnesses, and respiratory infections are the number one killers of African children.

7. About 90 percent of African children who die between the ages of one and four do so due to malnutrition, infectious diseases, and lack of hygiene.

8. In Africa one child in seven dies prior to completing its first year of life. In Asia it is one in ten, in Latin America one in fifteen, and in the industrialized countries one in forty.

9. Nearly all African countries have infant mortality rates well above 50 percent.

10. Life expectancy in Africa is less than that of other developing countries and about twenty-seven years shorter than that of Western countries.

In such perturbing health situations it is the traditional priest-healer who meets the challenge and thus becomes the main source of health services for the rural population.

The Priest-Healer of Akanland

There is a great deal of confusion in the literature over the use of such terms as "witch doctor," "fetish priest," "medicine man," "magician," and "sorcerer" to signify a priest or diviner. These terms are usually meant to be derogatory—to imply that the practitioner is ignorant, disreputable, or worse—and understandably there is no Akan equivalent for them. The Akan use terms such as Okomfo, Obosomfo, Odusini, and Sumankwafo to designate the various functions of the priest or diviner and the so-called medicine man. In order to avoid confusion I have decided to use the term "priest-healer," which adequately covers the work of the various types of healers in the Akan community. These individuals are both priest and healer because they combine religious activities as priests with healing ceremonials. Religion and healing are two sides of the same coin.

Priest-healers are often the first to be contacted whenever any trouble or crisis occurs in the community. They provide health needs, social comfort, and spiritual solace for the sick, confused, and lost individuals in the community. In this respect, they are often seen in the community as healers, priests, social workers, and legal advisers to individuals and their families. They live in the community and are fully informed of the socioeconomic, political, and religious realities of the people. They are readily available, and the good ones seldom charge for the services provided. Instead, the practice has been that clients and their families pledge a handsome reward to the priest-healer should the latter be able to satisfy their need. Often payment is in the form of gifts or services and rarely in cash.

In Akan society traditional priest-healers have stood the test of time and have achieved fame, respect, and success in providing for basic health needs. These priest-healers possess a variety of healing skills, and they make an immense contribution, particularly in meeting the health needs of the rural population. Their services have full cultural meaning and provide satisfaction for the questions and needs of the people who utilize them.

TYPES OF PRIEST-HEALERS

The following are recognized types of healers who handle various health needs in the traditional setting:

The doctor/physician, who is typically referred to as the *herbalist*, uses the traditional Akan herbal remedies.

The *diviner* or diagnostician, whose duty is to diagnose, operates both on psychological and on spiritual or religious levels. Through special techniques the diviner tries to elicit the details of the illness in terms of cause and effect. This work is so delicate that a diviner must be careful both socially and religiously to avoid exaggeration, gossip, and slander and must command respect in the community.

The *traditional birth attendant*, who is almost always a woman, specializes in maternity needs. She can prescribe medicines for childless couples after the necessary spiritual requirements have been met. She could, but normally would not, induce abortions. She helps women in menopause and young girls with painful menstruation. She also specializes in other types of women's and children's medical needs. She combines the work of a gynecologist and a pediatrician and is skilled in family medicine generally. It is estimated that about 80 percent of all rural deliveries are done by traditional birth attendants.

Bone-setters function as orthopedic doctors, specializing in repairing broken limbs. Most are also skilled in handling rheumatism and arthritis.

The *exorcist*, who has come to be known in the literature of the social sciences and comparative religion as the "witch doctor," has the main duties of exorcising the devil or evil spirit, warding off a curse or spell, and at times "catching the witch."

BECOMING A PRIEST-HEALER

People who become priest-healers are believed to have been set apart for divine service to the gods for the benefit of the community. Only the best is good enough for God and humanity; to become a priest-healer, a person must undergo several years of training involving seclusion from the world, observance of strict taboos and other disciplines, instruction in natural and religious law, and sometimes controlled "possession" by the deity. Some ordinary healers learn the art from their parents without any formal training, but for the profession of priest-healer formal training is needed, though the methods used and the time required may vary.

In undertaking the training some people give themselves voluntarily to the service of the gods, while others are "selected" by the gods through possession of some inexplicable illness. It is customary for novices to dedicate themselves to the deity for life, although they may also have secular occupations. During the period of training the novice is said to be married to the deity (there are both male and female deities). The training may last three or four years and takes place in the shrine house of a more experienced and powerful healer.

During this period the novice is expected to keep strict sexual and food prohibitions. The novice may not have a sexual relationship even if married. This prohibition is surrounded by strong taboos, and if it is broken, the novice is severely punished; sacrifices may be required to appease the offended deity, and the novice may have to begin training all over again.

The first year of training is often taken up with ceremonial ablutions. The novice washes with various mixtures of leaves sacred to the deity. Certain leaves strengthen the joints, especially the ankles, for dancing; others are for arousing possession. The novice washes his or her eyes and ears with herbs that make it possible to see the normally unseen and to hear the normally unheard. Special graveyard plants foster contact with the dead and other spirits. The novice's hair, which has sacred significance, is left uncut and unkempt. No secrets are given a novice at this stage; they are withheld until full trust can be assured.

During the second year of instruction the laws and taboos of the deity are revealed and explained. The novice must refrain from quarreling or any disgraceful acts and should avoid all forms of litigation. It is forbidden to use the name of the cult in cursing anyone, to go out alone at night, to touch a dead body or have contact with a menstruating woman, or to drink while in training and at any later time if consulting the cult. These rules are meant to emphasize the seclusion of the training period and to mark the absolute claim of the deity. The novice is often seen wearing charms of significance to this deity.

Learning to communicate with nature—plants, animals, mountains, and rivers—begins in the third year. The novice learns the art of divination and incantation. Some secrets about herbs, plants, and the spiritual world as well as the cult and ordinary community life are given to the novice by the chief priest-healer, and the novice is permitted to try some of the powers of his or her deity while the chief priest-healer looks on.

The final ceremony of induction as a full priest-healer comes in the third or fourth year. The novice is ceremonially accepted as a priest-healer with great celebration amidst music and drumming. Relatives, neighbors, and younger novices and devotees accompany the new priest-healer home to the village, where the cult will be established.

At this time the final payment is made to the trainer, and a male novice, if married before his training, may now "remarry" and bring home his wife (or wives) and children. The newly inducted priest-healer offers a sacrifice to his or her deity, saying, "Today you have finished marrying me." Thus, the completion of training frees the novice to marry if he or she desires. For a year or two the young, inexperienced priest-healer relies on the trainer for help in matters of great importance, often attending the annual festival of the trainer and sharing much with him.

The priest-healers are expert doctors, and they administer medicine by drawing on a wide knowledge of the properties of many roots, herbs, leaves, and barks. At the same time they seek to interpret the mysteries of life, convey the messages of the gods, give guidance in the daily lives of the people, settle disputes, uncover the past, explain the present, and foretell the future. With a profound belief in the spiritual world, the priest-healer and the patient look upon the treatment as not purely material, but also social and spiritual. Therefore, the priest-healer's power of thought and will and the patient's faith are the most essential ingredients in the cure. Above all, there is an absolute belief in the invisible efficacy of the medicine and treatment, provided that the right word is spoken over it or the true invocation is made. To the Akan, the importance of the spoken word and the human touch in healing cannot be overstated.

John Mbiti's description of the medicine man in Africa helps to complete the picture of the healer's work:

> First and foremost medicine-men are concerned with sickness, disease and misfortune. In African societies, these are generally believed to be caused by ill-will or ill-action of one person against another. Normally, through the agencies of witchcraft and magic. The medicine-man has, therefore, to discover the cause of the sickness, find out who the criminal is, diagnose the nature of the disease, apply right treatment and supply a means of preventing the misfortune from occurring again. This is the process that the medicine-

men follow in dealing with illness and misfortune: it is partly psychological and partly physical. Thus, the medicine-man applies both physical and spiritual treatment which assures the sufferer that all is and will be well. The medicine-man is in fact both doctor and pastor to the sick person. His medicines are made from plants, herbs, powders, bone, seeds, roots, juices, leaves, liquids, minerals, charcoal and the like; and in dealing with a patient, he may apply massages, needles or thorns to bleed the patient, he may jump over the patient, he may use incantations and ventriloquism, and he may ask the patient to perform various things like sacrificing a chicken or goat, observing some taboos or avoiding certain food and persons—all these are in addition to giving the patient physical medicine.

In African villages, disease and misfortune are religious experiences and it requires a religious approach to deal with them.[1]

The Akan Worldview

The Akan are the dominant ethnic group in Ghana, living predominantly in the Ashanti, Brong Ahafo, central and western regions, and part of the eastern region. They form about 40 percent of the Ghanaian population. Their main occupation is farming, although some of the coastal dwellers are fishermen. Akan farmers produce more than half the world's supply of cocoa. Some Akan are engaged in trading or employed in government service. Generally speaking, the language of the Akan can be said to be Akan. There are however various dialects such as Fanti, Twi, and Nzima. Most Akan speak and understand Twi and Fanti, but Nzima needs to be learned.

With few exceptions Akan are a matrilineal society. Ancestors are the custodians of the moral and ethical behavior of the people, punishing evil and rewarding good. To prosper, people should sacrifice to the ancestors, but they can do this only when they live in harmony with others. There is therefore pressure on all, especially the rich and the leaders of the community, to be generous in sharing. The ancestors are said to be the rightful owners of the land and the stool. (The stool enshrines the ancestral power and is a religious as well as politico-social emblem of the Akan.) The chief or the king, who is the embodiment of the ancestors, holds the land in trust for the kin group, who have an inalienable right to the use of the land.

The chief should be pure of heart and mind and must uphold the very high ethical and moral standards portrayed in the lives of the ancestors, who are revered by the Akan for complete moral and ethical inspiration and who are models of political, economic, and social success. In short, the ancestors are said to bring peace and harmony into society through the upright and spiritual rule of the monarch. Thus the successes and fertility of the chief affect the fertility of the people, the animals, and the land. As a consequence, infertility in any of these situations casts doubt and suspicion on the moral, religious, and ethical life of the chief.

Whenever problems such as ill health, epidemic, or natural disaster strike, the need to approach the ancestors becomes urgent. They are approached through divination, and the root of the problem is found and extirpated.

THE AKAN CONCEPT OF PERSON

The individual is viewed by the Akan as a composite of *mogya* (blood), which is inherited from the mother; *sumsum* (spirit), which is received from the father; and *okra* (soul), which is received from God the creator. Without *okra*, the life-giving force, the individual is merely *mogya* and *sumsum*. In fact, it is the *okra* that gives meaning to the life of the individual. An Akan proverb expresses this belief: "Nipa nyinaa ye Onyame mma obi nnye asaase ba" (All human beings are God's Children, none is the child of the earth). The child's lineage ties are gained through the mother's *mogya*. The *sumsum* from the father molds the child, giving it a personality.

Indeed, through *sumsum* a person is believed to receive the same temperament and spirit as his or her father. This spirit is the source of distinctive personal gifts and virtues, as expressed in the proverb, "Oba se ose nanso owo nkyi" (The child is like the father but he has his [maternal] kinship ties). The Akan sing the following song:

> The eggs of the crab
> Do not hatch into birds
> It is an abomination
> Should the eggs of a crab
> Hatch into birds
> For we all know that
> The crab always hatches crabs
> But never birds.[2]

So close is the tie of *sumsum* that the anger of the child's father can result in the illness of the child. In some cases a severe offense to the father can cause the death of the child. Supreme respect for the father and the paternal kin group is expected of every individual if health, peace, and tranquillity are to prevail.

The *okra* is believed to be the guiding spirit of the individual through his or her earthly life's journey. It is said to come from the day on which the individual is born. For example, if one is born on Friday (Kofi), one refers to one's *okra* as *okra* Kofi. When misfortune strikes, the individual is asked to cleanse the *okra* in case it has been offended in one way or another. The *okra* leaves the person at death to join the spirit world.

Destiny, according to the Akan, is concerned with the general quality and ultimate end of one's life. It is said that when God gives the *okra* he also gives *nkrabea* (destiny), but one's destiny is known only to God, and no one but God can change it. Thus, the Akan say, "When one was taking leave of one's God no one else was there."[3] This Akan saying emphasizes that an individual's destiny is between that person and God, who confers the *okra* that shapes or determines destiny. God-given destiny is said to be unavoidable. Some people are destined to be healthy, strong, hard-working, honest, and wealthy; others are destined to be sickly, weak, lazy, poor, and dishonest. It is believed that one's destiny can change only when one is born again after death. This belief is reflected in proverbs and in songs of daily life such as the following:

The destiny of a man in this world
Is known only to God.
Some came into this world to achieve greatness;
Others came to be rich and noble;
But the evil forces in the world often prevent them.[4]

Belief in reincarnation is strong. The Akan say that any ancestor who considered his or her work on this earth unfinished at death may decide to come and finish it. Some people are believed to be reincarnations of the ancestors. If a woman loses several babies in succession it is believed that the same child keeps coming and going, especially if the babies die at birth or are stillborn. To stop this occurrence, the child is given several cuts on the cheek and is also given a strange name; this procedure is believed to render the child ashamed to return from the spirit world.

In the Akan community the complete and perfect individual is the one who is successful in farming or business, who is not maimed in any way, who has no incurable diseases, and who is potent and able to produce many children. Barrenness is the greatest curse that can befall an individual. The worth of a person is therefore measured in terms of health and social relationships. Health is seen in terms of fulfilling one's social, moral, and biological obligations. Thus, to be healthy implies health of mind, body, and spirit, and it calls for living in harmony with one's neighbors, with the environment, and with oneself—a total harmony that encompasses physical, social, spiritual, natural, and supernatural realities.

Barrenness and some other permanent disabilities such as blindness, impotence, and so forth are considered dreadful misfortune. While a blind man may be seen as handicapped and therefore as deserving of sympathy from society, a barren woman or an impotent man is sometimes despised. In general terms, all these are said to be ill, for it is believed that one's inability to give optimum output may be due to the malfunctioning of a system or subsystem in the body (for example, the reproductive system in impotency). Thus an Akan prays: "Do not let me die in the day (Do not make me blind); Do not let me die at night (Do not make me impotent); Do not let me die at all (Make me fruitful and not barren or childless)."[5]

Consumption is mostly communal, while in some respects production is individualistic. Akan sayings reflect this fact: "It is only one man (hunter) who kills the elephant for the entire community"; "One has an uneasy feeling in the stomach if one eats a pot of honey all by oneself"; "We can only lick the sweetness of the world and not swallow it all up because of its taste."[6] Though the Akan support communal life, they encourage individual achievement with their strong belief that we shall each have to account to the Creator for our earthly life and destiny. They say, "Obra ne wo ara abo" (Life is what you make it). However, the communal life is so strong that the idea of the individual would be meaningless without the total idea of the community. The Akan maintain that the phrase "it is for me" is meaningless unless it is linked with the idea "it is for us." The individual *is* because his or her family, kinship ties, extended family, and clan *are*. The family is the basic unit and consists of the living, the dead, and the yet-unborn. The present, past, and future life of the community are very important. The "life together," or communal life, comes to the fore during ceremonies of birth, naming, marriage, and death. The communal life ensures physical security and comfort, economic cooperation, and social life for the individual and the community.

Thus, from birth through puberty and adulthood the kin group is constantly involved with the individual, whose world is a cosmic reality. Akan society is by definition communalistic. Descartes spoke for Westerners when he said, "Cogito ergo sum" (I think, therefore I exist), whereas Akan ontology is expressed by the words "Cognatus ergo sum" (I am related by blood, therefore I exist, or I exist because I belong to a family).

The individual Akan lives in a "weistic" community with a "weistic" philosophy, and "weism," not communism, is the key to this philosophy of "life together." It is "weism with God, nature, and man" that forms the cosmic reality.[7]

THE AKAN CONCEPT OF HEALTH AND DISEASE

Among the Akan good health is symptomatic of correct relationships between persons and their natural environment, the supernatural environment, and their fellow men and women. Health is associated with good, blessing, and beauty—all that is positively valued in life.

Illness on the other hand indicates that a person has fallen out of this delicate balance; this is normally attributed to the breaking of a taboo.

Illness may also be due to the malevolence of an evil spirit or evil eye. Health and disease are inextricably connected with socially approved behavior and moral conduct. To enjoy maximum health individuals must have good thoughts about their neighbors, try to avoid quarreling and aggressive acts, and conform to society's expectations. Sometimes disease is believed to be caused by a failure to perform the right religious act at the right time. It is also believed that the victim may not be the offender, but may be suffering from the offense of one of his or her kinsfolk. This explains society's concern for the illness of one of its members and the role of the kin group or family in the health of the individual.

Generally speaking, the Akan think of disease as a lack of equilibrium in the body as well as in society. Treatment is human-centered, unlike the Western medical system, which is disease-oriented. The theory of disease and methods of healing are, therefore, integral parts of the cultural world. Protecting spirits, evil spirits, supernatural powers, and magical spirits—all real to the Akan—form a coherent system that is the basis of the Akan concept of the universe.

Healing combines psychology, psychotherapy, religion, and herbal medication. The healing ceremonies involve confession, atonement, and forgiveness. The healing rituals elicit the confession of specific mistakes based on detailed reviews of the patient's history with special reference to the events surrounding the patient's illness.

The Akan view of the focus of disease is cosmic; the individual illness is thought to be derived from a sick or broken society. Society therefore becomes the point of departure for individual diagnosis. The damage in society must be repaired before the individual's health can be restored. The focus is on participation rather than achievement; this focus rejects the modern technological system that focuses on the individual in the quest for health.

The main point to be remembered here is that the Akan do not accept as the basis of health only that which can be felt, seen, and touched. This fact is quite understandable when one realizes that Akan do not make a distinction between disease and healing and religion; to the Akan they are one and the same thing. Though the Akan accepts physical illness empirically, it is believed that the whole person—body, mind, and spirit—is ill and not only part of the person; healing must therefore embrace the total person.

Among both healers and patients there is the firm belief that God, who is the giver or author of life and death, is the healer par excellence. Before embarking on any healing process the traditional healers often say: "God's will shall be done," and in fact, the prayer of libation mentions God as the final arbiter. As Akan proverbs have it, "It is God who grinds the maize for the chicken" and "When the chicken drinks it shows it to

God first"; and the most penetrating of all the Akan proverbs concerning God as a healer, "When God gives you a disease He gives the cure or medicine."[8]

THE ROLE OF KIN IN TIME OF CRISIS

As stated above, misfortune as well as good fortune is considered not only an individual problem or joy but a societal concern. An Akan proverb states: "If there is one wicked person in a community, that person enslaves the whole community."[9] This proverb demonstrates the Akan belief that an individual act has societal repercussions; this belief becomes highly manifest during times of individual illness or crisis.

When an Akan falls ill or is in a crisis situation, he or she turns to the immediate relatives living in the same household. Depending on the seriousness of the case, they may consult other relatives in the village or the wider kin group. The kinsfolk rally around the patient or the individual in need, take note of the sickness or the nature of the need, and pool all their human and material resources for care and comfort. The elders are summoned to a brief but serious meeting. They observe the symptoms, and if they realize that these will not respond to domestic remedies, as in the case of a laboring mother, they consult a specialist. It should be noted that in the Akan society some older people are gifted with certain healing techniques and have knowledge of techniques for delivering babies. Usually, the first consultation is with the old person in the family, the second with the traditional priest-healer.

Selected members of the kin group accompany the person in need to the treatment center and see to his or her welfare there. Plans are made to cater to the needs of the patient's dependents. In the case of a laboring mother, the younger children in the family are looked after and cared for. If the patient is privately or self-employed, care is taken that his or her work is continued until health is regained. The kin group also shares the expenses incurred during treatment, thus relieving the patient of a heavy psychological and/or financial burden.

If the problem is unusually complex, the specialist will recommend a more powerful specialist or a substitute. In this event the kin group, in accordance with Akan social ethics, express gratitude to the specialist, for, according to Akan belief, "The weak priest-healer who cared for the patient until a more powerful one came to his aid deserves some token of thanks."[10]

It is the matrilineal kin group that makes most of the decisions and takes the responsibility in consultation with the patient's father. In some cases the entire kin group will undergo certain ethical or dietary taboos, either temporarily or permanently, for the sake of the patient in their midst. The entire kin group can to some extent be considered the patient.

In some special cases the close relatives participate in the cure prescribed for the patient. This ensures that any evil that might be an agent of the misfortune or illness is warded off; in turn, the presence of the members of the kin group reassures the patient that the whole family is working to restore the patient's health.

When misfortune, including disease, strikes, the source must be found and uprooted. The traditional priest-healers help through divination to discover the cause and agent of the misfortune. At times it is suspected that the evildoers, operating through living or dead relatives or through evil spirits, may dwell in their midst.

Though the solidarity of the kin group is clearly manifest in times of illness, latent frictions and suspicions emerge, for "No one goes to another clan to bewitch people," and "When the house pebble cuts you it is sharper than the sharpest blade."[11] Parents are sometimes suspected of malevolence when their children fall ill, since curses on children by their parents are considered powerful and effective. Such a feeling is often summed up as follows: "When one is far away, one sees the forest as a body of trees; it is only when one gets nearer that one sees that they are separate trees."[12] Should the cause of the patient's illness be found to stem from parental anger, an appeal is made to the parent: "Akoko nan nkum ne ba" ("The hen's leg does not kill its chicks"). Yet, despite this fear and suspicion of close relatives as possible agents of evil, the role of the kin group in times of illness or crisis in the life of one of their members is a divine responsibility. Thus, the Akan sing: "To know whether your funeral will be grand when you die, look at how your relatives care for you in times of illness or crisis."[13]

The importance of the kin's role raises questions in relation to modern medical practices: how adequately are our modern medical centers and hospitals structured and organized to reap the benefits to the patient from the solicitude of the kin group? What are the Akan to make of visiting hours and isolation wards?

The Akan Belief in Holistic Healing

The Akan state that the whole person is ill, not only a part of the person. They further maintain that when one person is ill, the entire society is ill. Their comprehensive approach to medicine is a reflection of their worldview, their belief in a total concept of communal responsibility in matters of life, illness, birth, and death. Health is not an isolated phenomenon, not merely the absence of disease, but part of the magico-religious fabric of existence.

Consequently, healing must be comprehensive, involving the entirety of the individual, his or her family, and the society. Healing rituals include social, psychological, physical, religious, and herbal remedies—all the forces at one's disposal are called upon to combat illness. Any one-sided approach to healing, whether physical or spiritual, is considered by the Akan as incomplete and inadequate. The human being is seen not as divided into body-soul, spiritual-physical segments, but rather as a complete individual.

The Akan recognition of the multiple factors causing disease is an asset of traditional healing. Etiological factors identified in the somatic, psychic, constitutional, and genetic makeup, as well as in the social and cultural environment, argue very strongly for the comprehensive approach traditionally employed. The psychosomatic element in disease is recognized by Akan practitioners who, therefore, apply psychotherapy and multidimensional approaches to healing. In recent decades this approach has been given consideration by some groups in Western medicine, but efforts to develop it are still fragmentary at best. However, the fact that a person is an entity comprising body, mind, and spirit is being recognized in certain medical circles, even if they are unable at present to deal with the individual as a totality on a practical level.

The holistic approach is important because influential health policy-makers are beginning to understand the necessity of viewing human health as not only a physical and biochemical function but a grand total of all aspects of the human animal—how one lives, where one lives, with whom one lives, even what one believes. Today one can conceive of a social health policy that takes into consideration all of the social, political, economic, emotional, physical, and spiritual conditions that affect health.[14]

HEALING VERSUS CURING

Although the terms seem to be used interchangeably in modern medical discussions, according to the Akan there is a world of difference between curing and healing. A closer look at the terms reveals that curing is an event. For example, a doctor who cures a cut on a toe repairs a physically broken or afflicted part of the body. Curing is normally the work of humans, whether scientific physician, surgeon, or traditional healer. Healing, on the other hand, is a process entailing a long, complicated interaction of other human beings and of the community, and entailing, above all, the intervention of God. Thus, one can be cured of a disease but still remain unhealed. Healing implies the restoring of equilibrium in the otherwise strained relationship between a person, fellow human beings, the environment, and God. This process includes physical, emotional, social, and spiritual dimensions.

THE ROLE OF RELIGION IN HEALING

Much of Akan religion and medicine concentrates on achieving results for the individual in this life. Since illness is defined as religious dilemma, it must be solved by religious means. The attainment of total health in this world is, therefore, considered a proper duty of religion.

For every bit of good fortune as well as misfortune, the Akan ask two questions: How did it happen? Why? The "how" is often answered by common sense empirical knowledge, but the "why" is often very complicated and unclear. It is the "why me" question that is taken to the traditional priest-healer, who approaches the problem through religious means. The Akan do not consider evil or suffering as important in themselves; the vital question is the source of the evil or the cause of the suffering. They believe that natural phenomena are intimately linked with God and the spiritual world. Thus, Akan medicine has acknowledged the importance of both physical procedures of healing and a belief in a religious power involving forces beyond human comprehension. They attempt to maintain a balance between God, the spirits, the ancestors, and the living.

Hence, as previously stated, the Akan make little or no distinction between medicine and religion. In fact, it could be argued that everywhere and at all times religion has taken healing as one of its principal objectives. Religion is often described as the healing of alienation between humans and their creator, the world, and their fellow beings.

Rain is the most acknowledged token of God's providence. Rain is always a blessing and its supply is one of the most important activities of God. Rain is also believed to be the symbol of blessing so that, at ceremonies, especially after illness, the formal pronouncement of blessing is often accompanied by the sprinkling of water symbolizing peace, prosperity, health, happiness, and good welfare.

HARMONY WITH NATURE AS THE SOURCE OF HEALTH

The poem that follows sums up the philosophy of the Akan people of southern Ghana regarding our interaction with nature in our attempt to achieve wholeness and total health. The interdependence of human beings and their environment is stressed. The individual life is seen as a movement in the cyclical rhythm of nature. "The individual is born, grows, marries, bears children, becomes old, and dies. One returns to the spirit world of the ancestors, but is then reborn or reincarnated to begin another cycle in the world of the living. In like manner the trees blossom and flower; the fruits appear, ripen, and dry; and sometimes they fall on the ground and germinate again to produce trees, which will in turn produce more seeds."[15]

"Nature is a living thing; a river is not just a river; it is the repository of the divine spirit."[16] Akan tradition expresses the relationship that exists between the individual and nature in terms of kinship, identity, and mutual respect. As human beings, the Akan consider themselves part of creation and intimately bound to nature. Thus, our well-being in all spheres of life is dependent on how we treat nature, our fellow human beings, Mother Earth, and God our Creator. Health and disease are more complex than just the germ theory.

OH MOTHER EARTH

Oh Mother Earth,
We are fully dependent on you.
It is you who received us with your open arms at birth
When we were yet naked.

You supply our daily wants with your rich resources.
Indeed you nurture us throughout our earthly life.

And when the wicked death finally snatches us away,
You will still be there to open up your womb
And receive us all back.

Yet see what we have done to your loving-kindness in return.
We have in many ways raped, polluted, exploited
And wasted your rich gifts.

We have indeed treated you with greed and disrespect.
We have monopolized all your gifts at the expense of millions
Of our brothers and sisters.

We have grasped the mystery of the Atom Bomb
and ignored the Sermon on the Mount
And the Golden Rule.

We have indeed become Nuclear Giants
And Ethical Infants.
We reach out to the moon
While ignoring our Earthly duties.

We have constantly broken our covenant with you
To live with the ethics of learning to live with Nature
Rather than conquering Nature.

Thus our rivers smell, our environments stink,
Our fish and animals die,
We are plagued with diseases; the whole creation groans.

Mountains erupt and swallow our homes and farms
Like a roaring lion!
We are drowned by flooding rivers and oceans.

Your judgments elude our scientific knowledge.
We stand mouth-opened and repeatedly ask: How long, How long,
How long, Oh Mother Earth?

We least realize that the use of your gifts
Reflects our spiritual and social well-being,
Including our economic prosperity.

Our spiritual health is closely linked
To your health, Mother Earth,
And to that of the community too,
When we use your gifts justly.

Unjust use of these gifts brings about doom
Which is often accompanied by spiritual and social decay.

How do we expect to do violence to ourselves
And to you, Oh Mother Earth,
Without precipitating social, spiritual, and economic chaos?

Our constant plea therefore is:
Mother Earth
Forgive, Forgive, Forgive.
For the legs of the hen
Do not kill the chicks.
Shalom, Shalom, Shalom.[17]

Summary

Although present-day Akanland has undergone a tremendous, rapid social change due to the impact of colonialism, Westernism, and modernism through the spread of Christianity and Western education, the past of the Akan still prevails, especially in the areas of religious custom and healing. In many respects the ancestors are still considered the owners of the land and the custodians of law, ethics, and morality. The role of the chiefs and elders is still strong, especially in the regions and rural areas.

Although the mode of production has changed greatly, traditional communal life still persists, especially in the rural areas. The influence, concern, interest, and at times control of kin in social, economic, legal, political, and especially healing or medical matters remain very strong.

The services of the priest-healers continue to be used extensively by both rural and urban dwellers, in spite of the impact of modern scientific medicine. Many of the priest-healers have adapted themselves and their services to the modern demands and expectations of their clients. In contemporary Ghana many people use both the traditional and the modern medical systems.

Modern allopathic medicine was introduced into Ghana without serious consideration of the native people's concept of health and disease or of the general worldview of the Akan in particular. A typical consequence is the confused situation regarding health benefits among civil servants and other government workers in present-day Ghana. These workers use the traditional healing services for their health needs—yet, because the government demands an official written permission from a qualified medical officer before state employees are granted sick leave with pay, workers must go to the modern hospitals as well in order to get the official written permit that will enable them to obtain their insurance and other government benefits. The priest-healers, most of whom are semiliterate or illiterate, do not normally deal in written documents or keep records of the services rendered. The point is clearly made by the priest-healers and their clients that in these cases modern hospitals take credit for cures they have not accomplished, and both the clients and the priest-healers resent the hardship caused by this government regulation. Increasingly, the lack of record-keeping is seen as one of the weaknesses of the Akan traditional healing system in modern times.

In spite of the fact that Western-style surgery is not readily understood and accepted by the general Ghanaian public, it has had a tremendous effect. The efficacy of cesarean section as a measure of last resort is recognized and appreciated. On the whole, there is a genuine acceptance and craving for modern scientific medicine in Akanland. But people are quick to point out the shortcomings of modern medicine in meeting their needs and expectations. For example, the Akan do not consider childbirth a disease but a natural phenomenon, which requires the support of neighbors and close family members. To the Akan, childbirth is a biosocial event. Modern technological medicine, on the other hand, views childbirth as a potentially diseased condition that routinely requires the art of medicine to detect and treat deviations from the normal process.

The Western approach to medicine through high technology is a minority approach, contary to the communal concept of the Akan. Akan people complain of the high cost of maintaining a modern technological medical system. Such a system requires highy paid personnel and expensive equipment, making it difficult if not impossible for the rural poor to benefit from its services. This makes modern medicine the monopoly of those who can afford it—the rich.

In the course of giving treatment there is often some harm caused by the modern medical system itself, a phenomenon usually referred to as "doctor-caused disease" or "iatrogenic disease." In his *Medical Nemesis* Ivan Illich identifies the following aspects of iatrogenesis:

1. Postoperative complications of infection, or reaction to drugs

2. Cultural or social iatrogenesis—the system of making the population fully dependent on health personnel for all their health needs[18]

In its concentration on the management of disease, Western medicine has tended to ignore healing processes. Until quite recently, Western medicine was overwhelmingly self-assured, certain, and in many respects unaware of its limitations. Critics point out that the biomedical model of disease views the body as a machine with various parts and disease as a malfunctioning or broken part of that machine. This malfunctioning part needs to be detected and repaired by the mechanic—the doctor—through the use of drugs and other technological gadgets. The system thus deals primarily with curing disease rather than healing the individual.

In contrast, the Akan believe that when disease is present the whole person is ill and that therefore treatment must be comprehensive. This holistic approach to healing examines the individual's health by viewing his or her spiritual, emotional, psychological, social, economic, political, and intellectual realities and components as all interwoven into one. Thus René Dubos says:

> A holistic approach to healing, based on the concept of organismic and social adaptation, is certainly comparable with theoretical and practical scientific developments.
>
> This does not imply a rejection of the use of science in medicine. Rather, it points to the fact that there is more to medical science than the reductionist analysis of cellular structures and chemical mechanisms; more to medical care than procedures derived from the study of isolated body systems. In fact, the holistic attitude leads to the conclusion that the scientific medicine for our times is not scientific enough because it neglects, when it does not completely ignore, a multitude of environmental and emotional factors that affect the human organism in health and disease. Reducing the normal and pathological processes of life to the phenomena of molecular biology is simply not sufficient if we are to understand the human condition in health and disease.[19]

As Dubos emphasizes, health transcends biological fitness. Indeed, physical health is as much dependent on environmental and emotional factors as on measurements of blood pressure or temperature. Good health, therefore, is the individual's success in functioning within the given cultural, religious, and social set of values. To be healthy, according to the Akan, means to be fully integrated; that is, to be in correct relationship with oneself, one's neighbors, and the universe. The body is seen as the holy temple that harbors the essential elements of the human being—the mind and the spirit.

The key concept of Akan traditional healing is that of "balance." Healing emphasizes the restoration of harmony within nature, in human relationships, and in relationships with the spiritual world.

Disease is considered to have both natural and preternatural causes, and is usually attributed to an evil eye, an offense against the ancestral spirit, the breaking of a taboo, or the omitting of the correct religious rite at the appropriate time and place. Little or no distinction is drawn between religion and medicine. Furthermore, health and disease are inextricably linked with socially approved moral conduct; this view works as a stabilizing force and deterrent, pressing for social harmony and conformity. As a result, healing practices involve not only administration of medicine but also the process of confession, forgiveness, atonement, and sacrifice.

Plant medicine is the godfather or ancestor of modern synthetic medicine. Modern science can today count on many valuable drugs derived from ancient remedies such as digitalis, quinine, and atropine, to name but a few examples. The Akan believe that humans and plants are close biological kin. Plants act gently but surely to stimulate the body's own self-healing mechanisms. Medical substances carried in the plant can be safely assimilated by the body since plants are its natural food.

We can no longer afford to ignore the vital resources of natural, or plant, medicine. The usefulness of certain herbs and flora as healing agents has long been established in Akanland. Knowledge concerning their medicinal properties and instructions as to their correct usage have been handed down from one generation to another. These natural medicines are available and affordable and still command a great respect among the Akan. There is an urgent need for careful research into the use of plant medicine in order to provide it with the respect and recognition that it deserves in modern-day Akan. Such research will also avoid loss of the knowledge of this vast treasure of natural medicine, which is endangered as the modern, educated Akan turns to the use of synthetic medicine.

Much of Akan religion and medicine aims at achieving results for the individual in this life. Disease is largely considered to be a religious dilemma that must be solved by religious means. The attainment of total health in this world is, therefore, a proper duty of religion.

During the introduction of Christianity into Akanland, however, the all-embracing power of Christ and therefore of God was somewhat glossed over. Hence, the Akan converts to Christianity constantly complained of the conspicuous absence of God, the source and author of life, in all their life crises—childbirth, rites of passage, illness, and death. This may partly explain the popularity of the Indigenous African Christian churches (Independent churches) in Akanland. In all their activities they emphasize the unchallenged power of Jesus Christ in dealing with Akan religious, social, political, spiritual, and economic needs. Jesus is able to heal the sick, to protect the individual from the power of the devil and witches, to provide jobs for the unemployed, and to help people in all their undertakings. By so doing, these churches have fully met the Akan need for a unified worldview. Unfortunately, the modern medical system has no room for religion in the process of healing, and this lack causes their services to fall short of the Akan expectation of full healing activities.

It is quite clear that no one system of healing fully meets the needs of the Akan. There is therefore the need to blend the beneficial elements of the Akan traditional healing system and modern allopathic medicine. The words of Jelliffe and Jelliffe are relevant on this point:

> Recent considerations have clearly shown that rather than medicine being the monopoly of the western world with all the ideas flowing from industrialized countries to other parts of the world, the flow of ideas should be envisaged as occurring from many directions at the same time.
>
> Certainly, traditional societies have much to teach the western pediatrician and vice versa.
>
> The main end is for openmindedness and mental flexibility. It has been stated that western allopathy can be viewed as "linear" and bio-traditional practices as "curved." Recent considerations have clearly indicated that neither "linear" western nor "curved" bio-traditional methods have all the answers.[20]

The following account provides a good note on which to end:

> In a recent survey, the American Medical Association asked several thousand general practitioners across the country: "What percentage of the people that you see in a week have needs which you are qualified to treat with your medical skills?" Some replied 25 percent and some 1 percent but the average was 10 percent. In other words, by their estimate 90 percent of the people who see a general practitioner in an average week have no medically treatable problem. Certainly they are ill and suffering and in pain but their problem is not chemical or physical and defies normal medical procedure. The survey went on to ask what the doctor did for these people. Most of the respondents said they prescribed tranquilizers such as valium. When asked what they would like to do for these people most of the doctors said they would like to have had time to spend an hour a week talking to these patients about their lives, their families, and their jobs.[21]

Such dialogue is, in fact, recognized as the pivot of holistic healing and the strength of the Akan traditional priest-healer, who indeed makes the time for his or her clients in order to get to the root of their needs and fulfill them.

Notes

1. John Mbiti, *African Religion and Philosophy* (London, 1969), p. 196.
   This present article is based on my research in Ghana between January 1977 and August 1979. Some parts of the material have been updated through revisits to some of the shrines and priest-healers in the period from July 1984 to August 1985. Most of the informants were those interviewed in the 1977–1979 period.
2. This is a literal translation of the following: "Okoto nnwo anoma. / Onipa bone na owo oba bone / Onipa papa na owo oba pa. / Adofo momo

mmoden / Na monye papa. / Na papa ye yi mu ara / Na Onyame behyira mo / Okoto wo ho yi / Obiara nim se owo okoto / Okoto kowo anomaa a wokyiri."

3. "Obi rekra ne Nyame na obi nnyinaho."
4. "Wiase nkrabea mu nsem / Agya Onyame na onim. / Obi wo ho a obaa wiase / Se obegye din ansa na wawu / Obi wo ho a obaa wiase / Se orebepe sika / Ansa na wafi wiasse / Obiara nni ho a / Wamma wiase ammeye hwee / Nanso wiase mmonsafo / Wompe adepa."
5. "Mma mennwu awia; Mma mennwu anadwo; Mma mennwu koraa."
6. "Obaakofo na okum sone na amansan di"; "Obaakofo di ewe a etua ne yam"; "Ewiase yi ye taforo ho na yemmene."
7. John S. Pobee, *Towards African Theology* (Nashville, 1979), p. 49.
8. "Onyankipon na oyam akoko kyekyere"; "Akoko nom nsu a ode kyere Nyame"; "Onyame ma wo yare a na wama wo ano aduru."
9. "Se odeboneyefo baako to oman mu a ne nkoa ne amansan."
10. "Okomfe bone a wahwe oyarefo so ama Okomfopa abeto no aye bi na ose ayeyi."
11. "Obi nki obi abusua mu nkoyere"; "Ofie bosea twa wo a esen oyiwan."
12. "Wogyina akyirikyiri a wose kwae bom baako; woben ho na wohu se nnua so sisi maako maako."
13. "Se wowu na wayie beba a hwe wo yare bere mu."
14. R. Carlson, "Toward a New Understanding of Health within Limitations of Medicine," *Prepare* (Washington, DC), August 1980, pp. 15 ff.
15. Kofi Appiah-Kubi, "Oh Mother Earth," *Zygon* 19, no. 1 (March 1984): 61–63.
16. Ibid., p. 63.
17. I wrote this poem and first recited it at a conference on science and religion where I gave a paper on human health and environment. Later, it was published in *Zygon*. I conceived the idea for the poem at Spring Hill near Kansas City, Kansas, in 1983, when I heard and saw on television that volcanic action was taking human and animal life in Washington State, that somewhere in Indiana a whole township was moved because of the danger of toxicity, and that flooding in California had swallowed homes and farmlands. At the same time letters from my motherland of Ghana spoke of the serious drought situation there: bush fires were consuming livestock and wildlife, the rivers were drying up, and the entire nation faced starvation. In addition, governments around the world were spending tons of money building arms for eventual human destruction. I felt very strongly that, should humanity understand the Akan concept of human beings and nature and our ethics of living with nature rather than conquering it, the world would be a peaceful place in which to live. But is humanity ready for this understanding?
18. Ivan Illich, *Medical Nemesis: The Expropriation of Health* (Harmondsworth, Middlesex, England, 1977), pp. 22ff.
19. René Dubos, "Man, Medicine, and Environment" in *Ways of Health*, ed. David S. Sobel (London, 1979), pp. 12–13.
20. D. B. Jelliffe and E.F.P. Jelliffe, "The Cultural Cul-de-sac of Western Medicine towards a Curvi-Linear Compromise," *Journal of Tropical Pediatrics*, no. 26 (1980): 4.
21. Kofi Appiah-Kubi, "Traditional African Healing Practices and Modern Scientific Medicine: Integration or Articulation," p. 4.

CHAPTER 10

Health, Religion, and Medicine in Central and Southern African Traditions

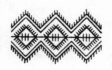

JOHN M. JANZEN

The societies of central and southern Africa that are grouped by linguists as speakers of Bantu languages offer a convenient focus for the examination of major African patterns of health, medicine, and religion. These societies, extending across the midcontinent at the equator and down to the Cape of Good Hope, display extensive linguistic and symbolic homo-geneity with somewhat greater variability at the institutional level.

The present essay examines the culture of health, medicine, and reli-gion of these sub-Saharan Bantu-speakers by examining the following: (1) verbs denoting well-being and affliction, from a stock of common cog-nates in the Bantu languages; (2) the worldview that interprets misfortune by differentiating "natural" afflictions or misfortunes "of God" from mis-fortunes caused by human intention; (3) divination and diagnosis, which are highly specialized features in African religion and health with a range of techniques and specialists; and (4) specific therapeutic practices, both those with a matter-of-fact empirical emphasis and those with a more elaborate ceremonial structure, including the collective therapeutic orders associated throughout the region with the term *ngoma* because of the type of drumming and singing that accompanies healing rites.

This core of assumptions and institutionalized behaviors may be stud-ied as it has persisted and changed over time and as it has guided the responses of individuals in their encounters with health, medicine, and religion introduced from outside their traditions. The Bantu-African cul-tural codes are also present in varying degrees in the Americas. A clearer picture of the classical roots of this tradition may help us to understand its more recent manifestations.

The Bantu-African Framework

Because of the ambiguity that surrounds extralinguistic uses of the con-cept "Bantu," we must clarify its recent uses in cultural history. The pres-ent project draws important material from the massive compendium of descriptive and historical linguistic work found in Malcolm Guthrie's *Comparative Bantu*, including recent historical writing, colloquia, and selected monographs on health, medicine, and religion done in the region.[1]

My own field research, begun in a western Bantu society, the BaKongo of coastal Zaire, has led to the study of African therapeutics in an increas-ingly more expansive cultural and historical framework on the subconti-nent. In a 1982–1983 field research project I explored the commonalities of therapeutics among selected Bantu-speakers in western Zaire, coastal Tanzania, Swaziland, and the western cape of South Africa. Preliminary findings of this survey are incorporated into the interpretations of the present writing.

The term *Bantu*, a plural form meaning "people," took on its wider classificatory meaning in the nineteenth century when linguists recog-nized it as one of the many common cognates found in languages of cen-tral and southern Africa. Their designation of these languages as a family carried with it the presumption of a common origin. Subsequent research has confirmed the view that the Bantu languages have a strong affinity with, and a presumed common origin from, the historic parent languages of the Cameroon grassfields and the Cross River region in Nigeria. It has also led to the inclusion of the Bantu languages within the more extensive Niger-Congo grouping that includes West African languages. Nineteenth-century racial and cultural doctrines led some writers to speak of "the Bantu" as a more clear-cut biological grouping than the original linguistic evidence warranted, a history that has given the term derogatory connotations in some settings, especially in South Africa, where it has labeled blacks. On the other hand, it is used as a term of pride for ancestral culture in Central and West Africa, as the formation of the International Center of Bantu Civilizations in Gabon suggests.

The recognition of far-reaching commonality in basic features of the Bantu languages within the Niger-Congo grouping of languages has continued to tantalize scholars over the prospect of other, nonlinguistic cultural features that may be part of the original or widespread derived system. The extent to which cultural systems are inferred or reconstructed from Bantu language features is thus debated, domain by domain. For example, specialized research has established underlying common vocabulary and techniques in livestock tending and the cultivation of food crops.[2] However, the practice of iron mining, smelting, and smithing, an important African cultural historical system in its own right, once thought to relate closely to the expansion of Bantu languages and culture, is much more problematic.[3] Further research is needed to establish which cultural domains do in fact reflect a common Bantu-related basis. The domains of health, medicine, and religion remain to be fully explored in this connection, although early work suggests that they fall somewhere between the affirmative and the null hypothesis of being couched in terms common to the wider Bantu-speaking cultural tradition.

In Africa, as elsewhere, the concept of health and the interpretation of affliction are embedded within robust cultural and religious realities that shape the focus and scope of attention, the modality of operation or function of such modes, and the emotions and values that relate to health and illness. These realities define therapeutic responses that are ultimately part of a vast set of assumptions and institutions, including science and medicine. A broad focus such as this is particularly important in the African setting, where doubt has too often been cast on the sophistication of its forms and where scholarship has tended to concentrate on localized rather than regional or more widely represented institutions.

To understand the integrative patterns, assumptions, and values in African cultures, which have over the centuries been confronted by, yet have often absorbed, external medical and religious influences, we do well to see them as African civilizational traditions. These historically deep, environmentally adapted traditions are agricultural, technological, social, political, religious, and therapeutic institutions bearing rich linguistic, ritual, and artistic expressiveness.[4] The main lines of the relevant African civilizational traditions and the stages of their florescence are given here for the general reader.

African Civilizational Traditions

Along the inland Niger River course in West Africa, cultigens of a distinctive horticultural system were domesticated between 4000 and 2000 BCE, giving rise to numerous regional cultural traditions often oriented toward city-state or empire capitals, surrounded by rural agrarian hinterlands and connected by trade routes. These are known to have been in contact with the Greco-Roman civilization of the Mediterranean coast as well as with the eastern Sudanic societies of Kush, Meroe, and Darfur, which had drawn some of their influence from ancient Egypt and the Near East. Later in the first millennium CE, Christianity and Islam would become important features of African civilization. Several recent influential authors have highlighted the ecumenical character of African civilization, not only in reflecting distinctive indigenous forms but also in sharing, over the long term, major world religious and cultural traditions.[5]

Prior to the adoption in West Africa of Near Eastern ironworking technology and the subsequent impulses gained by further food crops and of cultural techniques from India, Malaysia, and Indonesia, the agricultural-based Sudanic civilization spread southward across and around the rain forests onto the southern savanna. This movement was a cultural expansion into existing hunting and gathering societies as well as a part of the expansion of Bantu-speaking peoples. However, the later adoption of iron technology for warfare and agriculture and adoption of the outside tropical food crops considerably enhanced the cultural adaptiveness that was at hand, giving rise to the transformation of decentralized societies at particular times and places into centralized chiefdoms and states and, especially on the coasts, to large permanent mercantile settlements. As in the Sudan, so in the eastern and southern regions—and wherever the absence of the tsetse fly meant the absence of sleeping sickness—pastoralism, that is, a form of social organization based on raising livestock, provided a mode of livelihood complementing that of cultivation, even though hunting and gathering continued to play a role in most places.

For the past thousand years these civilizational forms have shaped African life, slowly and surely evolving sets of their own distinctive therapeutic ideas, practices, and institutions and adapting to local environmental dictates. It has often been these distinctive features that have determined how therapeutic and religious notions from the Islamic East, Western science, and Christianity would be received.

In Africa, as in most regions of the world, the forces of industrialization have been introduced. European colonialism brought industrialism and some of its attendant social forms: wage and migrant labor, the state, a new form of urbanization, mass production. As elsewhere, the manner in which the older classical civilizations interpenetrate industrial society and its values is complicated and varying. In therapeutics there has been found much mutual shaping and a forging of unique syntheses. Many themes and features of the classical civilizations continue, fused with or alongside themes of scientific-industrial civilization: wage labor alongside kinship and community cooperation, localized place spirits together with Christianity and Islam, laboratory tests side by side with divination, mass-produced pills and handmade herbal treatment.

Approaches to Health

Despite the unique mix of cultural features from historic and industrial civilizations, it is the historic that largely continues to determine the manner in which people cope with misfortune and interpret affliction, though they may utilize biomedicine and share its technical scientific ideas in some dimensions of life. Classic African cultural tenets are, however, adaptable in their own right, and they continue to provide compelling interpretive ideas and values. The examination of health, medicine, and religion in Africa must be seen from a framework of totality that encompasses the combined analytical and substantive scope of pertinent ideas, assumptions, and institutions represented in society. Such an exercise in the articulation of health concepts requires both a philosophical and a religious perspective, since there is no universal definition of health nor even an agreement of operating definitions in the scientific canons of the West or the literature of Christianity, Islam, and Africa.

The notion that "health is what the healers do" underlies a widespread stereotypic North American view of the basis of health and—for related reasons—a common perspective on the study of African health, but it is neither a very accurate nor an adequate notion. Just as some North Americans expect their physicians to keep them healthy or to patch up their bodies when they are ill, so many Western scholarly studies of health in Africa have concentrated on the customs of healers. The "medicine-is-health" view has often pervaded the budgetary decisions of African ministries of health, the major share going to pay for centralized hospitals, the training of physicians, and the maintenance of large institutions in lieu of preventive measures, nutritional surveys, Well Baby Clinics, or primary health care.

The concept of health as the absence of disease, a view traceable to classical antiquity in Western medicine,[6] flourished in the late nineteenth century with the discovery of the bacterial causes of the major contagious diseases and of related techniques for their elimination. This view is still salient in Africa today, for although some of the great scourges such as malaria, smallpox, cholera, sleeping sickness, tuberculosis, and typhus are less pervasive than formerly, most are still found. The exclusive focus on the elimination of the organismic pathology that this view entails may, however, obscure some of the socioeconomic factors that precipitate or exacerbate these contagious diseases. The elimination of organismic pathology may lend support to the misleading policy of "magic bullet" cures for diseases that respond best to improved work and living conditions. The epidemiology of tuberculosis in southern Africa related to mining work and to deplorable living conditions in reserves and slums illustrates this point.

Health may also be defined as "functional normality" and thus avoid some of the problems inherent in the above negative definitions of health.[7] In this view the core of health is a cohort peer group—for example, all children below two years, all adult males—and the normal functioning of the person or composite organisms. Normality, however, proves difficult to define in a way that is both measurable and manageable. Also, what is "normal" is not always healthful: a population may—as with yaws, malaria, or intestinal parasites in nineteenth–century Africa—be resigned to enduring a disease as a constant companion. "Normalcy" in this sense should not thus become a justification for inaction on the part of health authorities or scholars. The health norm, according to some, must be defined in a comparative or relative manner so that the reference group or cohort is wide enough to detect localized extreme cases of disease or pathology. If normalcy is defined in terms of organisms, normal functioning may entail a teleological goal and a typical developmental course. Health defined teleologically may raise other problems, although a health program or policy without end goals would hardly be possible.

"Health as adaptation" is another orientation based on the ecological perspective that has seen currency in studies of African health and health care.[8] This perspective has much to contribute, for it takes into account the environment as a factor in health and shows the human community interacting with the environment. However, the ecological definition of health has many of the same pitfalls as that of functional normalcy in that not all that is adaptive is healthful, as for example sickle-cell anemia, which is an adaptation to malaria.

The foregoing health concepts are mainly Western biomedical and social science constructs introduced in various ways into the African setting during colonial or postcolonial national development. Several other health concepts that follow, while Western in their formulation, may resonate more fully with African health views.

"Social reproduction as health" refers to the perpetuation of a particular social order in terms of the quantity and quality of health indicators. The work of demographers has provided a basis for examining the link between a society's ability to perpetuate itself and the health of its members. At least two schools of thought offer interpretations of this issue in the African context. Some Marxists use social reproduction to refer exclusively to the reproduction of labor in the interest of those who control the means of production. The continually high rate, or even increase, of fertility and the attendant rise in population and stress on resources are attributed to the increasing marginalization of those sectors of society who, in order to survive, must serve both their kin-oriented peasant productive base and the capitalist wage-giver.[9] This perspective leads to the pessimistic conclusion that until there is improvement in the distribution of limited resources and the risks of infant mortality are alleviated through good nutrition, housing, and other opportunities for all, Africa will experience increasing population expansion and the further erosion of its resource base. Another view, also based on demography, identifies the conditions of increasing fertility, population increase, and deteriorating health with societies that have abandoned traditional support structures that offered cushions of child spacing and more equitable access to society's resources.[10] Conversion to Christianity, these studies have shown, has frequently been accompanied by population increase due to the breakdown of preexisting religious sanctions. Other factors, such as urbanization, the collapse of the extended lineage kin unit, labor migration, and the like, have also contributed to the loss of social structures that might have formerly provided the social fabric and support systems inherent in "health." Clearly biological reproduction is not the only measure of health; measures of the quality of social and economic settings and the ability of people to perpetuate their social institutions and cultural patterns are required as well.[11] Social reproduction analyses have studied investments of time, creativity, and resources into the lineage community, the neighborhood, the ceremonial society, and other institutions. Although social reproduction comes out of a Western scholarly setting, it resonates with the association in African thought between well-being and social continuity, a topic taken up later at greater length.

"Positive health" and "health utopias" are proposed by some scholars as health definitions that openly recognize the central role of value-charged ideals and goals in culture at large and in health, development, and maintenance programs.[12] Certainly the World Health Organization's campaign of "health for all by the year 2000" is, in this perspective, incorporating the WHO's concept of health as not merely the absence of disease but the "well-being of body, mind and society." In the African context such a perspective may also account for the health programs and medical interventions brought in by Christian missions and taken over by Independent African churches. Moreover, many of the indigenous health concepts and practices would appear to fit under this general rubric. The "positive health" and "health utopian" views are explicitly value-related, goal-oriented, particularistic, and often associated with particular thera-peutic techniques and social arrangements. In the indigenous African tra-ditions, notions such as "balance," "purity," "harmony," "coolness," and "power," which address the quality of life in the community and the sta-tus of the individual in relation to others, may be examined in this connection.

Health, Healing, and Religion in the Bantu-Speaking Traditions

VERBS OF WELL-BEING AND AFFLICTION

Verbal categories alone cannot portray the sophistication of Central African ideas about well-being and affliction, but they do constitute the enabling constituent parts of such ideas. In order to illustrate this asser-tion more effectively and to avoid offering mere bits and pieces of a cul-tural perspective, a somewhat detailed analysis is necessary.

In Bantu-African thinking the interconnected fates of healthiness and of affliction or misfortune are traced to a central source of power (or life) in God and nature. This source of life is mediated by middle-range spirits, ancestors, and consecrated priests who maintain contact with or receive inspiration from that source. Evil and misfortune, including sickness, are present in any social, personal, physical, or psychic condition that falls short of the ordered and energized universe of full life. Some affliction is in the natural order of God-given life. Much of it, however, is attributed to the evil and chaos in human nature and society rather than to an anti-God or devil.

Although there are many terms that describe this condition of short-coming or chaos, thus permitting people to deal with it, one of the most widespread cognate verb stems in proto-Bantu and one that appears throughout the Bantu-speaking region is *duad, duadi, duade*[13] or *lwala* (in Kongo) and *kuhalwa* (in Ndembu of Zambia). It means to become ill or suffer misfortune and refers to the existential state of suffering due to affliction. Suffering is often borne stoically, relatively free of anesthetics or the hope of sudden relief.

The above existential level of suffering is distinguished from a wound or physical injury, which is everywhere identified by the Bantu cognate stem *puta* or *pute*.[14] Other particular types of afflictions receive specific names or labels.

The widespread presence of another cognate stem in Bantu languages reflects the fact that central attention is given not only to the existential nature of suffering and the physical wound, but to the invisible cause of misfortune and injury arising from the specifically human social dimension of evil-wishing, envy, gossiping, cursing, and mystical hurt projected within social relations. These notions are contained in the Bantu cognate stem *dog, doga, dogi,* or *dogo.*[15] In Kongo society the central reference of this cognate is to the use and misuse of powerful words *(loka). Lokila loka* is to utter a curse, spell, or oath; *kindoki* is the act or talent of using words and powers to rule effectively as chief or other instituted leader—or of using the same power, where it is illegitimate or errant, in a destructive and malicious manner. The individual who has such powers, an *ndoki,* is called a witch or a sorcerer in European languages, but these terms do not really encompass the emphasis on words and mystical power transmitted between people. At the extreme southern region of Bantu language expansion, among Nguni-speakers such as Zulu, this stem becomes *thak* or *ubuthakathi* for "sorcery" with much the same meaning as in Kongo.[16] Coextensive with this cognate in the Swahili east of the Bantu-speaking region is the term *cabi.*[17]

These terms, reflective of varying levels of affliction and their causes, are matched by a comparable range of concepts and corresponding verbal cognates that denote conditions of health and well-being. Although the Bantu languages have terms for health in a narrow sense—such as the Kongo term *mavimpi,* which is often heard as the greeting, "Mavimpi maku!" (Health to you)—there are other terminologically marked concepts dealing with the ceremonial or ritual states of "purity," "balance," and "coolness" that embody health consciousness in a far more embracing manner. They are also held to open the way to or serve as a precondition for access to power and efficacy in life. The absence of purity, balance, or coolness is a negative state reflecting a symptomatic or ritual condition of ill health.

Purity and pollution codes are known to be widespread in Bantu Africa, but only a few studies have elaborated them in any detail.[18] Guthrie's work does not identify a cognate stem of Bantu that might translate as "purity." However, the proto-Bantu term *pod* ("to cool down, to become well")[19] serves as the verbal core of the term that describes the action of the cupping horn in some Western Bantu traditions *(mpoka)* and of the medicine used in preparation for initiation *(mpolo).* The Kongo verb describes the action of the cupping horn doctor *(nganga mpodi)* as *hola mpoka,* to suck out with the cupping horn. Sucking is a generic healing act seen as removing an evil, pollution, or sickness. *Mpolo,* then, is this generic quality of health or vitality. It is also the term of character. To give someone *mpolo* in initiation is to recognize that person's character, a use with striking parallels in Yoruba culture.[20]

Purification is widely seen as a prerequisite condition for priestly or other mediatory roles. Among the Kongo, for example, purification *(veela* or *mvelela*) was required for those in charge of the powers of the spirit world and was an integral step in the initiation to ritual states in medicine cults such as Lemba and in curing rites.[21] Thus a crucial stage of many rituals was the opening purification medicine, which prepared the way for the composition of the central medicines. These "openers" were called *mpolo* or *mbonza* in Kongo, Teke, and related Western Bantu languages. The state of purity gave the initiator or priest enhanced powers of clair-voyance and invincibility in a range of affairs.

Among the Zulu, pollution *(umnyama)* is considered to be a mystical force that diminishes resistance to disease and creates conditions of poor luck, misfortune, disagreeableness, and repulsiveness; in its worst form it is a contagious force. Ngubane notes that the state of ritual pollution is most acute among women in menstruation and in the process of child-birth, although it also includes men and sexual intercourse.[22] A range of treatments exists to purify polluted individuals; frequently these entail some form of washing of the persons or their clothing or ritual parapher-nalia, as an "opener" to therapeutic initiation.

Broadly, then, purity may be seen as a religious concept and an attri-bute of health in the Bantu African tradition. Christian missionaries often adopted the purity and pollution vocabulary for their translations of the Bible and their theological work. Missionary linguists to the BaKongo used *mvelela* (purity) to translate Christian "grace" and *masumu* (pollut-edness) for "sin."

Pod, the cognate stem under discussion, also carries strong connota-tions of "coolness" and "cooling down" in association with being healed or being healthy. As in North America, where the African aesthetic of the cool has become pervasive in arts and style, so in its original setting it has to do with a certain way of carrying oneself, of movement and dance, and of getting along with others. Coolness is a quintessential quality of the ancestors, and their presence is usually invoked to end the "hotness" of strained relationships, witchcraft, and pollution.[23]

The concept of "balance" or "complementarity" is found in another verb in Bantu language and thought that may be regarded as a code of health and well-being. One widespread term that represents this in both Kongo and Zulu is *lunga*. Ngubane describes *lunga* as a Zulu concept that combines ecological systemlike links between individual persons and between humans and their natural environment. It is a concept of health maintenance that may be found in many actions designed to alleviate sickness and restore well-being.[24] In Kongo *lunga* is recognized as the name of a comprehensive healing practice employed by appropriately skilled and widely recognized healers called *nganga lunga*. The concept of complementarity is present in a wide range of allusions and practices, from recognizing the maleness in females and the femaleness in males, to emphasizing that medicines be composed of elements including both sides of dichotomies such as hot/cold, wild/domestic, ancestors/ humans, water/land, and the like.

The symbolic constructs suggested by purity/pollution, balance/ imbalance, and cool/hot dichotomies in Bantu-speaking languages and thought systems, each with their own classic vocabulary, raise the issue of whether these expressive codes or vocabularies are descriptive of coterminous or of separate realms. In the present discussion they certainly could be seen as glosses of the health/illness dichotomy. However, this is not to suggest that African health cosmologies may be represented by two simple columns of oppositions. The quite independent code of color expresses at least two of the above domains, that of purity and coolness with a common correlation of white:cool:pure::black:hot:impure, with red being a mediatory color. In the logic of central and southern African ritual color symbolism that has been so masterfully analyzed by Victor Turner among the Ndembu of Zambia,[25] we learn that "white" is not just the color but the quality of clarity, purity, and perfection represented in river clay *(pembe, pemba)*[26] and water; that black is not so much the color as the quality represented in charcoal and in the ashes of the spent fire; and similarly, redness is the quality of ambiguity, power, and blood represented in the kula tree's bark. When it comes to balance and complementarity, these colors may be used differentially and inversely to represent varying states or statuses; they are not permanently aligned with other levels of representation. They are all, in fact, subsumed to a further set of questions bearing on the source of events in experience, whether fortune or misfortune, health or disease.

AN AFRICAN WORLDVIEW

Throughout Central and South Africa, health experience and misfortune are subjected to higher-level questions on the predisposition of events and the relationships between persons. In Bantu Africa the question is often formulated in terms of whether afflictions are "caused by God" or are "human-caused."[27] According to one author, the afflictions and misfortunes caused by God "just happen" or are "in the order of things," such as the death of a very old person or an affliction with readily recognized symptoms and signs, which heals as expected.[28] The idea "caused by God"—translated, for example, by *kimbevo kia Nzambi* in Western Bantu (Guthrie's cognate stem *jambe, yambe,* or *nyambe*)[29] and by *umkhuhlane,* after Khuhlu, the Ancient One, in Zulu[30]—does not refer to retributive punishment, nor is there an Enlightenment type of understanding of the natural universe as a machine whose parts may need repair by some master creator. Rather, it is the regularity of the world as experienced that stands behind the concept. God, as creator, is also the ongoing source of life.[31]

As the conventional experience of affliction gives way to loss of control or of a sense of rising arbitrariness in one's life, the Bantu-African worldview suggests that misfortune or affliction is caused by chaos in the human world or in the relationship of humans to their environment: *kimbevo kia muntu* in Kongo, *ukufa kwa bantu* in Zulu.[32] Both express the cognate *ntu* (human), the very basis of the word *Bantu*, as pointed out earlier. A range of agents may be at play in this "human" causation: self, kin, strangers, ancestors, and spirits.

The widespread verbal concept of *dog*,[33] *lok*,[34] or *thak*,[35] commonly translated as sorcery or witchcraft, is but one of the many types of causes expressed here. Individuals may bring sickness upon themselves by disregarding social etiquette, ignoring good hygiene, or by turning their backs on kin, elders, ancestors, and spirits. Much human-caused affliction is, however, attributed to the evil intentions of others, through conscious machinations or unconscious urges. The notion also applies to situations of contradiction in a social relationship or institution in which persons are at odds with one another, as for example in the struggle to distribute land equitably in a bounded estate at a time when the population dependent on that land is increasing, or in the launching of an enterprise for profit in the face of a strong ethic of redistribution of goods. Such situations are believed to incur the ill will or envy of others, leading to the breakdown of health, to visible physical sickness, and even to death. These beliefs in the mystically channeled powers of individuals over one another operate to reinforce the ethics of social redistribution and loyalty to family, kin, and polity.

The ancestors and certain classes of spirits are the logical extensions of these beliefs and social values. Ancestral spirits, more closely linked to structures of family, lineage, and kin, are held to intervene in human affairs to perpetuate corporate kin interests and to reprimand those who betray familial trusts, secrets, and traditions. The term *kulu* or *nkulu* is widespread in this context as a word for elder, ancient, and even God. Perhaps the most widespread ancestor-shade term in the Bantu-speaking region is *dimu*,[36] which some readers will recognize from Shona rituals in the *bira zavadzimu* or the Venda *ngoma dzamidzimu* traditions.[37]

The "of God"/"of society" causal distinction is not so much a dichotomy as a continuum on which these two terms represent polar opposites. In Kongo society the complete range of etiological agents would need to include the nature spirits, in particular those of water and auspicious places; derived from these, the spirits of medicines; errant ghosts of the dead; and special types of ancestors in lineage and cult contexts. A portrayal of this Kongo worldview of causal agents of disease and affliction might appear as follows: (1) *nzambi*—God and the created order; (2) *bisimbi*—water, place, and nature spirits; (3) *bakisi*—medicine and disease spirits; (4) *bankuyu*—errant ghosts of the dead; (5) *bakulu*—ancestor shades of lineage and cult; and (6) *bandoki*—human witches.[38]

This worldview for the placement of agents in the causal sequence of fortune and misfortune has proven amazingly resilient in the face of Christianity and Islam and the introduction of science. The basic dichotomy remains, but in the face of new knowledge, new or outside-introduced diseases, and far-reaching change, the content of the two categories has shifted and changed. Conditions that were once placed under the human-caused category—such as the consequences of sickle-cell anemia and malaria, which brought seemingly arbitrary mortality into the human community—have shifted to the God-caused or "natural" category because they are now better understood and accepted in the biomedical mode.[39] On the other hand, new sources of so-called human-caused affliction and misfortune have arisen. With the decline of lineage and kin in urban industrial Africa, new and chaotic social settings—divorce, labor migration, joblessness, social disintegration, political instability, displaced persons—and the corresponding afflictions have frequently come to be explained in terms of human causes, where they apply, or in terms of alien spirits.[40]

A more open, synthesized worldview presents issues raised commonly in comparative religion and philosophy. The process of dealing existentially with unheaval, change, and renewal as well as the self-conscious grappling with the process of change and renewal are upon us in the central and southern African setting. The present paper can do little more than mention obliquely the approaches taken by scholars who consider this problem. A range of works on African religion seeks to show the impact of the dramatic changes of the past century. One area has been the emergence of middle-range cults and spirits that transcend the ancestors. In accordance with a strict Durkheimian perspective, these reflect the widening, expanding context of life and of domains in which thought must be focused on life and work. Many of these new cults or movements have reflected popular resistance to early colonial intrusion or to the involvement of a populace with new life conditions such as migrant labor and industrial work. Of the former sort, the Shona spirit-medium-led revolts of the 1890s were a remarkable example of coming to terms with a new dilemma—foreign occupation—through an old method.[41] More recently, one notes the widespread existence of alien spirits in mediumship in southern Africa, notably in Mozambique and Swaziland, societies that have experienced significant involvement in the industrial economy of South Africa alongside efforts to build up their own national societies and maintain certain traditions.

However, efforts by African and non-African authors to go beyond the study of these settings and to engage in the conscious, critical, or polemical construction of models of reality to deal with events and structures at hand have gone in at least two directions. There have been those who have asserted a unique African cultural reality around which projects must be built. A number of African Christian theologians have, for example, posited a Bantu worldview—not unlike that sketched here—in order to relate Christianity to the African cultural context.[42] The claim that an ethnographically or linguistically distinct system produces distinct thought and reality is rejected by a number of other African philosophers,[43] who argue that there is no more an African philosophy based on distinct cultural logics than there is a distinct European or Asian philosophy. Universal philosophy, for common human perceptions and approaches to reality, is in their view the only philosophy. They argue that in order to create an authentic and appropriate African thought it is necessary to master European science and philosophy, then transcend it to resolve Africa's unique problems.[44]

These matters are pertinent to the present focus insofar as they grapple with analysis of social, political, and scientific issues facing a vast continent. They are the same issues that ultimately face individuals dealing with misfortune, affliction, and other moral dilemmas. For many Africans in the late twentieth century, diviners and mediums are the main analysts. Thus we are interested in the reality they posit and how they use it to counsel their clients.

DIVINATION AND THE DIAGNOSIS OF MISFORTUNE

The African worldview that has been sketched here arises from basic assumptions and values in the cultures of Central and South Africa—for example, that human relations may cause affliction. Experience as lived is never neat and clean in this regard; it must be interpreted. This is particularly true in the realm of illness. Given the importance of the illness-causation dichotomy "of God"/"of society," an essential part of the healing process is to establish the nature of the agent, the type, and its relationship to sign or symptom. The highly developed art of African divination steps in to provide the methods and perspectives for this task.[45]

In most cases of affliction the basic questions about causation are answered by sufferers and their kin. Conventional afflictions—occasional malaria attacks, intestinal parasites in children—are tolerated and considered quite routine, that is, in the order of things. Family and kin usually provide the interpretive expertise in the selection of appropriate healers and doctors and support for longer-term treatment and care at the therapeutic retreat or the hospital. I have written of this process as "therapy management," a process that demonstrates the contextual nature of this knowledge and the social embeddedness of health care decisions in the "therapy management group."[46]

Diviners are consulted in especially difficult cases when the illness fails to respond to treatment or when dispute over the meaning of an affliction or other source of disagreement threatens to paralyze the community around a sufferer. With more seriousness, the proposition is entertained that the affliction might be "unusual," that "there is something else going on," and that it might be "caused by other people." Not only would diviners be able to sort out the issues involved in this type of consideration, they would be able to help the sufferer and his or her family select the most appropriate combination of treatments among the myriad therapies and specialties offered by African and non-African medicine. Some therapeutic specialties have their own specialized divination. However, almost everywhere diviners are specialists in generality, clearing house experts in divination and diagnosis for which there is no Western parallel.

As noteworthy as the pervasiveness of divination in Africa is the dizzying range of techniques that are used by the diviners. Perhaps the best known is the Ifa tray or cup among the Yoruba of Nigeria, used with a set of symbols that are thrown into the receptacle as sets of verses are spoken in keeping with the configuration of objects.[47] A comparable approach in the Bantu-speaking region known from the coastal Kongo along the southern savanna to the historic Lunda societies is the Ngombo divining basket. Its contents, representative of society's and life's articulation points, are shaken out before the client in response to queries about causes, relationships, and events.[48] In southern Africa among Nguni-speakers (Zulu, Xhosa, Swazi) and Sotho-Tswana groups, divination signs are usually animal vertebrate bones shaken out of a bag onto a mat, where the configuration is again studied for relationships and causes.

The details of divination techniques are, however, less significant than the invisible reality brought forth through an ostensibly objective, detached mechanism. The divinatory operator is put forward as a mediator of spiritual messages and insights. This premise also permits the diviner to deny personal involvement in disputes that may arise, claiming to be merely giving the will of ancestors or spirits. It is not surprising that new divination techniques should appear as improvements over old methods or that multiple techniques and specialties should exist in parallel or hierarchic relationship. Further, it is not surprising that classical divination methods are cast aside and replaced by appropriate techniques from Islam, Christianity, or science, adapted to the African setting. Thus in Kongo where the Ngombo basket was once common, today some Christian diviners or prophets use the Bible and its verses to divine and counsel.[49]

Throughout central and southern Africa mechanistic divining has been supplanted or complemented by "inspirational" divination, as new types of mediums make their appearance. Some claim inspiration from nature spirits, others from new alien and unknown spirits. Others draw directly from Christianity and Islam for their spiritual patronage. There has been a tendency for ancestral spirit mediums to be replaced by more "distant" and encompassing spirits as people have moved out of kin communities and as social dislocation has affected millions.

Divination, in the face of major social changes, has remained a constant offering of African religion and thought. The criterion of the skilled diviner continues to be the ability to steer judgment between broad cultural generalities and individualistic particulars—in other words, to recognize individual problems, family dynamics, and broader societal issues, but to put them into the more general rubric of the great question, "Is it of God or of society?"

THE TECHNIQUES OF A THERAPEUTIC TRADITION

Throughout the Bantu-speaking world healers are named by forms of the verbal noun *ganga*[50] (e.g., *nganga* in Kongo, *mganga* in Swahili, *inyanga* in Nguni languages). Other terms appear as regional role-definers for healers: *mbanda*[51] and *buki* or *mbuki*[52] in Western Bantu and *iggira* in Xhosa. The concept of the healer in central and southern Africa is that of a specialist, the bearer of knowledge and practitioner of skills, whether these have been acquired by apprenticeship, spiritual inspiration or possession, inheritance, or the purchase of techniques. If the concept of the healer is generic, language conventions and social structures recognize the specialized practice of the healer. Most healers carry a hyphenated second term attached to *ganga*. Thus in Western Bantu the *nganga ngombo* is the practitioner of the divining basket, the *nganga nkisi*, of consecrated medicines.

Generic terms for medicine or the practice of medicine suggest that these are merely the actions of the healers, that is, medicine is "what doctors do." Thus in some traditions *ganga* also refers to medicine.[53] Very widely, *buka*[54] refers to the action of treating or healing, and in Eastern Bantu *dagud*[55] (to practice medicine, to divine) is such a term.

The classic medicines of Bantu-speaking Africa, as if they flow from the same assumptions as divination and diagnosis, represent both matter-of-fact "natural" substances and highly charged ritual symbolic treatments. If we review medicinal terms in Guthrie's listing of cognates, this spectrum is clearly in evidence, suggesting that it is a very old feature of this medicine. *Ti*[56] (also *nti* or *miti*) refers to a plant or tree, often but not exclusively with reference to medicinal use. *Kag*[57] or *kaya*, widespread among Central Bantu, refers to leaves or the foliage of the plant. These terms reflect the presence of herbalists throughout the entire continent and the extensive knowledge of plants as foods and healing ingredients.

Plant-based medicines may or may not have a symbolic "overload" in a particular setting or use. However, because the African knowledge of plants and natural substances is profound, some of these plants may constitute poisons under certain uses. This fact, along with the perception that affliction may contain social tension, anger, and anxiety, leads to the incorporation of substances into compounds or "packages" that have ritualistic connotations. In one Kongo medicine for psychosis—"madness"— four plants with anesthetic qualities are labeled "calmers" and given a color code to suggest that they bring the individual from the "wild" into the "domestic" realm and combine opposing forces into one orderly, controlled focus.[58]

Thus it is not surprising that part of the classic proto-Bantu cognate vocabulary hypothesized by Guthrie also includes, in addition to common plants and ingredients, more highly charged medicines such as *pemba* or *pembe*,[59] the white clay, noted earlier, that represents purity and is widely used in connection with ancestral protection. It also includes the related techniques of bleeding by small incisions, sucking out blood or impurities with the cupping horn,[60] and related practices of rubbing plant substances into the incisions. This pragmatic or empirical practice of African medicine includes a host of common practices that deal with fractured bones and bonesetting, immunization against smallpox, lactogenic medicines for women with insufficient milk, midwifery and child care, treatments for intestinal parasites, and much more. The richness of this knowledge has been described by other authors.[61]

Although there is no single term in Bantu languages to describe the medicines that are explicitly charged with symbolic messages and intentions, this process is present everywhere. It is intended to deal with the arena of human-caused afflictions and misfortunes and with related emotions such as anger, conflict, evil-wishing, sorcery, and witchcraft. Western Bantu languages use the term *kisi* or *kiti*[62] to describe charms, spirits, and illness: in Kongo *nkisi*, the charm; *bakisi*, the spirits or shades associated with the charm and the infliction. In the northern and eastern Bantu regions, the terms *pingo*,[63] *cango*,[64] and *dawa* (from the Arabic) are widespread in this connection.

The fact that African disease etiology acknowledges the place of emotions, communications, interpersonal relations, and symbols in causing and alleviating affliction leads to the use of rather different measures in dealing with what Westerners might regard as "mere" physical affliction. Indeed, the distinction of physical and psychological or psychical and social diseases is not drawn. The concept behind the term *muntu* (person) is that of an individual linked integrally to lineage and thus to those who passed ahead and those who will follow, as well as to those in the immediate surroundings of life and work. Thus the attribution of an affliction to human or mystical causes requires both "empiric" and "symbolic" attention. This may mean, for example, that a man who has fallen from a palm tree and broken a leg requires routine bonesetting, splints and massaging, and rest, as well as ritual protection from the individuals who may have wished his accident and calming from hallucinations he may have had about his having offended the ancestors.

The Kongo understanding of these medicines is that they are explicitly magical, that is, they are put together as messages in power to achieve a given effect. They are not seen to be magical in the sense that they work mysteriously; they are *designed* to be magical. One characteristic of the *nkisi* is the use of words and spells to impute function to the combination of objects. Selections of plants or other objects are made on the basis of alliterative verbal or visual punning. Thus, in one account, *luyala*, a fruit, is included because its name contains the verb *yala* (to govern). The kola nut *(mukazu)* is included to indicate biting *(kazuwa)*. These ingredients are illustrations or visual-iconic representations of the verbalized intention. With an awareness of *lok*, the power of words, utterances are crafted to have a deliberative effect, which is then reiterated with plants. Other ingredients represent persons both as social role categories and as concrete individuals, whence the attractiveness of bodily hair, nails, or effluvia in the composition of charm medicines. The origin or charter of a medicine is important, especially those deriving from a vision or dream. Many magical medicines in Kongo are accompanied by a song composed by the inventor. The entire collection of named ingredients, combined into a statement and presented publicly with a chant that may voice its "origin myth" (that is, the charter of its inventor, source, and legitimation) offers a powerful rhetorical vehicle for either good or evil. *Minkisi* (pl. of *nkisi*) are, accordingly, regarded with considerable ambivalence by BaKongo. Frequently mentioned as the suspected cause of sickness, they are nevertheless also a final recourse of healing when the situation becomes desperate. For Christians who are taught the inefficacy of these magical substances they may still remain a hypothesis for the onset of sickness. The healing rites of Independent churches often ritualize their treatments in a manner that substitutes for the *nkisi* treatment.

Across the Bantu-speaking region a subset of magical medicines and related techniques fits into the rubric sometimes called "cults of affliction" or "drums of affliction" after the term *ngoma*, the drum-dance ritual involving a collectivity around the afflicted individual or individuals. The term *ngoma*[65] extends throughout the Bantu-speaking region and is presumably a part of that classical cultural and therapeutic complex. Because of its implications for the organization of African medicine, its relationship to religion and politics, and because of this author's research on the subject, a separate section is devoted to it.

NGOMA: THE RITUALS OF HEALTH MAINTENANCE

Western scholarship was first introduced to the "drum of affliction" or "cult of affliction" by Victor Turner's brilliant book, *The Drums of Affliction,*[66] based on his field research among the Lunda-Ndembu of Zambia. Since then it has become apparent that the institution exists very widely but with major variations. Across the midcontinent, where it appears that the common therapeutic culture derived from a "secondary" dispersion of the Bantu languages and cultures south of the rain forest, *ngoma* refers most specifically to the elongated wooden cylinder drum with a single leather membrane at one end affixed into the wood with small pegs. This type of drum is also the most frequently used drum in therapeutic rituals, along with shakers, other drums, song, and dance. In the eastern and southern regions of the Bantu-speaking societies, that is, from the Swahili coast down to South Africa, *ngoma* refers not only to therapeutic and divinatory rites and the cells and networks into which they are organized, but to secularized musical ensembles and dance groups as well. In southern Africa the drum type mentioned above is replaced by a cowhide on a frame or, in the twentieth century, by a metal barrel. In these southern regions, among Nguni-speakers, the practitioners become *isa-ngoma* (those who do *ngoma*), the notion referring mainly to a phenomenon that may be called "song-dance."

One of the common features of *ngoma* ritual therapy is its focus on chronic, spirit-caused, or human-caused affliction. It is thus often used as a "final recourse" therapy that enables the sufferer or the society at large to adjust to a lifelong relationship to the condition. Within this broad rubric a range of particular conditions have been addressed in *ngoma* therapeutic groups.

Among the Lunda-Ndembu, whom Turner studied in the fifties, hunting was an important economic and status activity. Chronic hunting failure was considered grounds for initiation to one of two hunting *ngoma* groups. In more industrialized societies at present, chronic inability to retain a job and the alienation experienced in urban life are regarded as syndromes appropriate for initiation to an *ngoma* order. In many societies of the region, impotence in men and infertility in women, various gynecological and obstetric problems, and the rearing of infants, particularly twins and triplets, are conditions directed into *ngoma.*[67] Epilepsy and other chronic and debilitating handicaps may be similarly dealt with in *ngoma.*

The collective social body may be as much a focus of the *ngoma* therapy and initiation as the individual. In Western Bantu–speaking societies of Zaire, Angola, and Congo, lineage segmentation and attendant conflicts are considered a process that often victimizes individuals in the community. Misfortunes in this connection, especially numerous sicknesses and deaths among children, are held to be symptoms of the collective affliction and recognized as reason for the lineage to perform the Nkita sequence of therapies and rituals.[68] In the Nkita diagnosis the sicknesses and misfortunes surrounding lineage crisis are deemed to be caused by a lack of proper authority in the community—in particular, a severing of the link between the living and the ancestors. Part of the Nkita rite is the reconsecration of lineage authority within the new segment.

Some *ngoma* cults have focused beyond the individual and kin group to emphasize the general public order and have even taken on aspects of government. The Lemba rite, which emerged on the Congo coast in the mid–seventeenth century and extended inland to the major markets and trade routes as far east as the Kinshasa-Brazzaville area, addressed the role of merchants in trade—and questions of wealth and wealth redistri-bution in a society that otherwise valued egalitarian relations. Individuals involved in trade and in the accumulation of wealth were vulnerable to the envy of their subordinates and often felt torn between the opposing values of accumulation and redistribution. Lemba worked out the psy-chological, economic, social, and political dilemma and literally became the governing public order of the region. Especially strict marriage vows were drawn between influential local lineages, reinforcing both the trade and market networks and the alliances that knit the society together regionally and channelled redistribution.[69] A rather similar *ngoma* order emerged somewhat later on the East African coast and along inland trade routes; it was known as the Beni-Ngoma.[70]

Despite the scope of *ngoma* therapeutic attention, which ranges from individual to kin group to public, and the specificity of afflictions dealt with—from snakebite to nonspecific totality of affliction and misfor-tune—there are a number of distinctive modalities of treatment, ritual, and support-group formation that merit attention.

In all *ngoma* orders the therapeutic course of the afflicted serves as an initiation process whereby the patient becomes the healer. Initial treat-ment, counseling, and acceptance of the affliction give way to instruction in the ways of being a novice. If the therapy is successful and the novice is persistent, the patient will graduate as a full-fledged healer of the afflic-tion he or she originally suffered. This therapeutic-initiatory course may vary from a few days to many years, depending on the nature of the afflic-tion, the intricacy of the stages of learning, the efficacy of the therapy, and the financial means of the sufferer.

Another central feature of *ngoma* is the use of song in the testing of dreams and visions and in the refashioning of the sufferer-novice's iden-tity. The pervasive use of music in the therapeutic rites heightens affect and provides a performance framework in which inchoate feelings and contradictory emotions are sorted out, given a new valence, and "moved" from a state of sickness to a state of health. All *ngoma* therapy thus has

what the West would call a psychotherapeutic dimension, although label-
ing of disease and therapy are not identified as explicitly psychic. The
physical-psychical dichotomy is not a typical central African distinction.
Rather, the whole person and the person's environment are involved. In
most *ngoma* therapeutic courses the subject literally creates a new song-
identity based on experience of suffering and healing. The song and the
rhythm are picked up by ritual partners, and the song-identity is mirrored
back and tested in the ritual setting, which combines patient-students and
therapist-teachers. The strong rhythm of drumming and dancing that
always accompanies the singing may affect brain patterns. It may also
facilitate dissociation and psychic and cognitive learning, as well as acceptance of a new role.

The therapeutic techniques and approaches taken to identification of
illness in *ngoma* are also anchored in a wider system of beliefs, values,
and cognitive realities held within the society at large. Ancestors are most
often considered to be behind the disease leading to *ngoma* entry, and it
is they who also show the way to healing or to stabilization of the
patient's relationship to the disease. In Turner's portrayal of Ndembu
ngoma groups, the shades who possess the living with sickness or misfortune are usually direct lineal ancestors who wish to have their place in
the *ngoma* order filled by a descendant. Acknowledgment of ancestral
"calling" and entry into the order represents the reestablishment of the
norm in the community of the living.

A variety of nature spirits and alien spirits may also be associated with
ngoma orders, particularly where violent psychopathologic manifestations
are dealt with or where disorders are seen to be due to rapid and hurtful
social dislocation in association with the breakup of a community or an
institution. Colonial rule, epidemics, the new influences of trade routes
and urban life as well as postindependence living have all been associated
with *ngoma* orders or ephemeral movements that may precede them.
Some authors have explained the shift from ancestral spirits to alien spirits in sickness and misfortune as being due to the opening up of the cultural categories to include the wider perspective of a pluralistic society in
the place of a more particularistic kin-based society.[71] Other authors have
interpreted the relationship of ancestors to nature spirits and alien spirits
in *ngoma*-type cults to be due to the distinction between norm-reinforcing
leadership recruitment in the former instance and recognition of psycho-
pathology, deviance, and sickness in the latter. Some *ngoma* settings relate
to a wide spectrum of spirits and ancestors, varying the individual ritual
on a case-by-case basis. This appears to be the perspective of a quite new
school of diviners operating in Swaziland, the so-called Takoza movement. Their divinatory evaluation of a case begins with an ancestral cause
for the affliction or misfortune but then moves to increasingly distant and
obscure (and more expensive) sources in the realm of nature spirits,

shades of enemies of the Swazi people, those who died a violent death, and unknown spirits beyond.

Whether the spirits in *ngoma* are ancestral, alien, or natural may be academic hairsplitting, since often spirits, like humans, are organized into whole communities or cultures associated with an entire cosmology, a religious or cultural tradition, or a political order (or the memory thereof). Thus the widespread Bucwezi cult complex of the lake region of Uganda, Burundi, Rwanda, and Tanzania is associated with a range of spirits held to be the dynasty and associated ancestors of the legendary Cwezi kingdom.[72] Spirit movement in relation to therapeutic communities is exceedingly dynamic, with much borrowing across political, language, ethnic, and even religious boundaries. In the Tanzanian capital of Dar es Salaam, spirits aligned with *ngoma* therapeutic groups are called *sheitani*, an Arabic term with negative connotations (although within the *ngoma* groups there are no such connotations).[73] Islamic communities, which may or may not harbor *ngoma* groups, describe the spirit world as *majini*, but these are organized into ancestral, water, and land groupings and are articulated the same way as African-derived *ngoma* spirit groups. The same spirits, controlled or approached by orthodox Muslims, relate not to *ngoma* communities but to Sufi brotherhoods. Equally intricate are the lines of articulation between *ngoma* and Christianity. In South Africa, possession attributed to ancestral shades may be channeled into Independent Christian churches and into the role of the prophet rather than into the role of the *ngoma* healer.[74] There are reports of Christian *ngoma*,[75] and many are the African churches that lump all spiritual power under the rubric of the Holy Spirit in order to deal with the transformation of the sickness experience into the career of a healer.

If, as has been seen, *ngoma* orders may be anchored in many types of spirits representing different values and concepts, both of affliction and health, then this may be because they are essentially congregations (in a Durkheimian sense) within a religious tradition. They appear to be infinitely flexible in representing the community of concern within which societal and individual problems are worked out. It is not surprising, therefore, that the basic *ngoma* institution can be Christianized and become an Independent church or Islamized and become a Sufi brotherhood, or that it can be rooted within ancestors or other types of spirits.

Lest we rest the case of *ngoma* flexibility with these religious examples, we must add yet another type of direction. In some settings the *ngoma* model is amenable to becoming the institutional framework for the perpetuation of technical knowledge. A good example of this is Mungano of western Tanzania. Nicknamed a "snake dance," Mungano addresses the problem of the prevalence of several types of deadly vipers in western Tanzania. Members of Mungano, recruited either through cures from snakebite or through other more formal means, learn to handle the snakes, dance with them, and use the venom to inoculate and immunize themselves and others. The dances serve the purpose of countering the public fear of vipers. The spirit-possession vocabulary of *ngoma,* in general, may seem incongruous in the face of knowledge of poisons and antidotes and immunization. However, the case of Mungano, by its very incongruity, demonstrates the importance of seeing the traditions of knowledge embedded in the *ngoma* communities as arising out of problem-solving in real life yet legitimated by a structure that continues to give credence, value, and authority to this type of institution.

The last major feature of the *ngoma* institution in central and southern Africa is its networklike character: the bringing together of patient-novice with healer-teacher, the manner in which patient-novice peers meet, and the multiplying and interrelating of these cells over time. A given *ngoma* order may literally constitute a social fabric across its reach, dotted by periodic temporary nodes as events occur and individuals come together. These node-events occasion communal singing and dancing and the sharing of concerns and joys, technical knowledge, and food and drink. It is literally the case that *ngoma* cells and networks create and reproduce society. Thus if we define health as "social reproduction," *ngoma* directly exercises this function.

There are, however, two variations on these general observations about *ngoma* and networks. In the first, *ngoma* networks come to be supported by government. In Tanzania, where this has been the case, healers' networks have turned into healers' organizations. The courtyards where periodic *ngoma* cell gatherings are held have become "*ngoma* dispensaries," where fee-for-service *ngoma*-healing is performed. Very few of the clients become novices of the order. The *ngoma* resource, namely access to and interpretation of spirit possession and affliction, is controlled as a commodity. Perhaps one may even speak of the bureaucratization of *ngoma.*

In the other instance, *ngoma* networks have developed into centrally controlled divination schools or services. Swaziland represents this direction. With the support of the king, a few reputable *ngoma* practitioners—the *isangoma*—have succeeded in establishing training colleges for novice diviners. Located near cities today, they have sizable clienteles, most of whom pay their fees and receive diagnostic expertise but few of whom become initiates. Here too the "resource"—the interpretation of misfortune—is controlled. It is apparent that the *ngoma* mode of dealing with affliction and misfortune, often of a chronic nature, lends itself well to either a decentralized or a centralized setting.

Conclusion

This essay has charted the health, medicine, and religion of central and southern Africa as a synthesis of classical Bantu-African civilization embedded in verbal concepts, lexica, patterned behaviors, and institutional arrangements. Fieldwork on this subject in western and southwestern Zaire, coastal Tanzania, Swaziland, and South Africa has permitted the comparison of local settings and the testing of a number of issues that link health, medicine, and religion to the societies, cultures, and environments of the region. These may be reiterated as they reflect issues of the present project with its emphasis on wellness and illness, caring and curing, ethics and justice, and life-course passages.

The oft-heard phrase in African discourse that an action must take into account "not only the living, but the dead and the yet unborn" provides an axiomatic point of entry into one of the central assumptions of African thinking about ethics and caring. The individual person, recognized as an ontological being in his or her own right, with an eternal identity, much as in Greco-Hebrew-Jewish thought, is also seen to be embedded in an enduring social body. This is the basis of ethical, epistemological, and etiological ideas in African health and medicine.

Further evidence that the social order is considered an important dimension in the maintenance of health is evident in the pervasiveness of the question of whether an illness or misfortune is "caused by God" or "human-caused." Implicit in the assumption that others can cause illness lies a keen appreciation for justice in the human community and for the affirmation of ancestral and spiritual norms to protect the rights of the living and the unfulfilled rights of the yet unborn. The fact that current health conditions and resource abuses in some settings may fall short of such a timeless ethic does not negate its presence in the value structure of the society.

The impact of health concepts and values upon behaviors and consequences has also been considered in this essay. Although positive health values such as purity, balance, and coolness are elusive and impossible to establish objectively, it is clear that in central and southern African society illness often calls forth a response from the social group around the individual, often the immediate family or lineage, in terms of an ethic of caring that is deeply rooted in society's norms.

Current scholarship and health care planning are increasingly concerned with the fate of individuals and cohort groups in settings where this customary procedure of looking for health in society and for therapeutic support in one's primary social group may be inoperative for either temporary or permanent reasons. What happens to this pattern of support when—as under conditions of a refugee camp, increasing labor migration, or urban professionalization—structures of the family, household, or wider lineage community have eroded or been subjected to severe strain? What are the consequences of this on objective health indicators? Demographers and public health scholars have debated shifts in household composition, fertility trends, and other social patterns and their impact on the health of the populace. Here the analytical concept of "social reproduction" as health finds resonance in the value system of African society.

The widespread presence in central and southern Africa of extrakin support communities, of which the *ngoma* cells, networks, communities, and derivatives of the classic *ngoma* form are an example, manifests the importance placed upon the social dimension of individuals' health and well-being. The core characteristics of *ngoma*, such as spirit-calling of the afflicted, transformation of the sufferer into the healer or of the novice into the leader, and the reconstitution of the society around its affliction provide powerful ritual techniques for the renewal of society. Recognition of the "power of the margins" reflected in these characteristics offers a unique model of caring and curing in the midst of adversity; every indication is that this principle operates as strongly in the new Africa as in the old.

The central and southern African approach to ritual is integral to the healing process, not merely in the extended *ngoma* rites, but also in more mundane therapies. There are a keen awareness and use made of such features as situational repurification, boundary-setting and role redefinition, name-changing, and other methods of transforming the individual for reentering society at another level, reflecting rites-of-passage patterns observed worldwide. Here is a unique model offering potential for social rehabilitation or readaptation in a changing society.

In the background of this emphasis on the unique relationship of the individual to society in the African perspective of health, medicine, and religion, there is a continuing presence of the natural world. This presence is evident in the pharmacopoeia at the basis of many of the symbols of healing rooted in a cosmology of plants, topographic features, and nature spirits. At the same time there has been considerable loss of common knowledge and understanding of the natural world reflected in the experience of many African elites of alienation from their lands, traditions, and peoples. This alienation is accompanied by overcultivation, soil erosion, deforestation, desertification, and by the crisis in agricultural production. These trends, although very serious, do not obviate the importance of the natural world in African thought. International attention directed to this issue has contributed to an awareness that corrective measures must be taken. The beginnings of an African "Green" movement are apparent in the writings of some African intelligentsia.[76]

The crisis mentality over conditions of health, nutrition, environmental degradation, and social and political collapse is not exaggerated. The analysis of reasons for the present state of affairs includes the centuries of foreign economic and human exploitation suffered by the continent, leading to a crisis of will because of the acceptance by today's elites and rulers of the colonial attack on everything African. It is imperative to rediscover the African cultural bedrock beneath the surface of African life and to allow it to shape policies in health care, agriculture, and the rehabilitation of the marginalized. We may celebrate the tremendous resilience of the fundamental metaphors of African culture that persist within or alongside Christianity, Islam, and modern science. This makes it worthwhile to identify the "classical" formulations of African culture. With these clearly in view, we may ask many questions of this tradition and emerge much enriched from the encounter.

Notes

1. The principal modern works to be used in sketching a Bantu-African framework include: Malcolm Guthrie, *Comparative Bantu* (Ridgewood, New Jersey, 1967); Larry M. Hyman and Jan Voorhoeve, eds., *L'Expansion bantoue*, 3 vols. (Paris, 1980); *Muntu: Revue scientifique et culturelle du CICBA* (Libreville, Gabon). This periodical, published by the Centre Internationale des Civilisations Bantoues, was begun in 1984.
2. Chris Ehret, "Cattle-Keeping and Milking in Eastern and Southern African History: The Linguistic Evidence," *Journal of African History* 9 (1967):213–221; same author, "Agricultural History in Central and Southern Africa, c. 1000 B.C. to A.C. 500," *Transafrican Journal of History* 4 (1974):1–25.
3. Pierre de Maret, "Bribes, debris et bricolage," in Hyman and Voorhoeve, pp. 715–730.
4. African civilization is thought of here both in the sense of Heinrich Baumann and Diedrich Westermann's *Les Peuples et les civilisations de l'Afrique* (Paris, 1962), as distinctive linguistic and cultural systems, and in the sense of Jacques Maquet's *Civilizations of Africa* (New York, 1972), as a food production–related way of life. Maquet's approach includes industrialization—his "civilization of industry"—as a civilization comparable to pastoralism, hunting and gathering, cultivation with surrounding cities, shifting cultivation in forest clearings, and grain farming of the southern savannas.
5. Jan Vansina, *Art History in Africa* (London, 1984), differentiates between Africa's "Oikoumenical traditions" along the Mediterranean coast and its "regional traditions," which are more closely correlated with vegetative zones; Ali Mazrui combines the Islamic, the Christian-Western, and the indigenous traditions as Africa's "triple heritage" in his study *The Africans: A Triple Heritage* (Boston, 1986).
6. Osewi Temkin, "Health and Disease," *Dictionary of the History of Ideas* (New York, 1973), pp. 395–407.
7. Christopher Boorse, "Health as a Theoretical Concept," *Philosophy of Science* 44 (1977):542–573.
8. Alexander Alland, *Adaptation in Cultural Evolution: An Approach to Medical Anthropology* (New York, 1970).
9. Joel Gregory and Victor Piché, "African Population: Reproduction for Whom?" *Daedalus* 111, 2 (Spring 1982): pp. 179–209.
10. Ron Lesthaege, "Demographic Regimes in Africa" (Unpublished, 1985).
11. Authors who have used a social reproduction perspective include Colin Murray, "The Work of Men, Women and the Ancestors: Social Reproduction in the Periphery of Southern Africa," in *The Social Anthropology of*

Work, ed. Sandra Wallman (London, 1979), pp. 337–363, and Murray, *Families Divided: The Impact of Migrant Labour in Lesotho* (Johannesburg, 1981); and Pierre Bordieu, *Outline of a Theory of Practice* (Cambridge, England, 1977), who offers a "social reproduction" analysis of Kabyle society of Algeria and a systematic theory of the notion.

12. I have attempted this in my paper entitled "The Need for a Taxonomy of Health in the Study of African Therapeutics," in *Social Science and Medicine* 15B (1981):185–194, which draws heavily from a historical survey by Oscar Koehler, "Die Utopie der absoluten Gesundheit," in *Krankheit, Heilkunst, Heilung*, eds. Heinrich Schipperges, Eduard Seidler, and Paul U. Unschuld (Munich, 1978), pp. 619–652.

13. Designated in Guthrie's *Comparative Bantu* with cognate stem numbers 677 and 678.

14. Guthrie, 1607–1608.

15. Guthrie, 644–647.

16. Harriet Ngubane, *Body and Mind in Zulu Medicine* (New York, 1977), pp. 30–48; Axel I. Berglund, *Zulu Thought Patterns and Symbolism* (London, 1976), pp. 266–277, 286–288.

17. Guthrie, 240. In the Benue region of Nigeria among the Tiv, a related term is *tsawi*.

18. Mary Douglas, *Purity and Danger: An Analysis of Concepts of Pollution and Taboo* (New York, 1966), offers a comparison of pollution and purity codes among the Old Testament Hebrews and the Lele of the Kasai in Zaire; Ngubane, pp. 77–99, analyzes the religion of the Zulu of Natal in South Africa; John M. Janzen, *Lemba 1650–1930: A Drum of Affliction in Africa and the New World* (New York, 1982), pp. 13–14, 110–115, reviews this dimension in a historic Kongo healing cult; Luc de Heusch, *Sacrifice in Africa* (Bloomington, IN, 1985), includes purity and pollution in a wide-ranging discussion of ritual across the continent.

19. Guthrie, 1565.

20. Robert F. Thompson, *Flash of the Spirit* (New York, 1983), pp. 9–16.

21. Janzen, *Lemba*, pp. 110–115.

22. Ngubane, p. 78.

23. See De Heusch, pp. 53–56, for an analysis of the central symbolism of thermodynamic codes in Central Bantu ritual and myth; for Ndembu of Zambia see Victor W. Turner, *The Ritual Process* (Chicago, 1969), pp. 27–31.

24. Ngubane, pp. 26–27, 131–132.

25. Victor W. Turner, "Colour Classification in Ndembu Ritual," in *Anthropological Approaches to the Study of Religion*, ASA Monograph no. 3, ed. Michael Banton (New York, 1966), pp. 47–84.

26. Guthrie, 1474, 1477.

27. Victor W. Turner, *The Drums of Affliction: Religious Processes among the Ndembu of Zambia* (Oxford, 1968), p. 52; John Orley, "African Medical Taxonomy: With Special Reference to Mental Illness," in *Journal of the Anthropological Society of Oxford* 1 (1970):137; Marja-Lisa Swantz, *Ritual and Symbol in Transitional Zaramo Society* (Uppsala, 1970); Ngubane, pp. 22–24; Eva Gilles, "Causal Criteria in African Classifications of Diseases," in *Social Anthropology and Medicine*, ASA Monograph no. 13, ed. Joe B. Loudon (London/New York, 1976), pp. 358–369; John M. Janzen, *The Quest for Therapy in Lower Zaire* (Berkeley, 1978), pp. 44–49, 67–74.

28. Ngubane, p. 23.

29. Guthrie, 925, 1917.

30. Ngubane, p. 23.
31. How to render this causal category in more universal analytical terms has been a subject of some debate in the relevant literature. Some analysts have misleadingly adopted the distinction made by George Foster and Barbara Anderson in their *Medical Anthropology* (New York, 1978), pp. 53–78, between personalistic and naturalistic causation that they say exists in most "traditional" ethnomedical settings. Not only does their survey omit African material from discussion, but it is not clear how their suggested distinction would apply. Both poles of the Bantu-African dichotomy are in a sense personalistic. Others, myself included, have used the word "natural" to gloss the etiology "caused by God." An extensive summary of conference proceedings on the subject is included in *Causality and Classification in African Medicine and Health,* eds. John M. Janzen and Gwyn Prins, special issue, *Social Science and Medicine* 15B, no. 3 (1981):429–431. Historical variations and alternative uses in the Western concept of "nature" make this issue too complex to develop here.
32. Ngubane, p. 23.
33. Guthrie, 644–647.
34. Luc de Heusch, in his article "Pour une approache structuraliste de la pensée magico-religieuse bantoue," in *Pourquoi l'epouser?* (Paris, 1971), pp. 170–188, has discussed this proto-Bantu verb and its various derivations among the Mongo (*lok*), Luba (*lo*), and Rundi (*rog*).
35. Ngubane, pp. 30–46.
36. Guthrie, 619.
37. Paul Berliner, *The Soul of Mbira: Music and Traditions of the Shona People of Zimbabwe* (Berkeley, 1981); John Blacking, *How Musical Is Man?* (Seattle, 1973), p. 77.
38. Janzen and Prins, p. 181.
39. See my discussion of such an etiological shift in a case study of affliction in Kongo society in Janzen, *The Quest for Therapy,* pp. 67–74 (chap. 3, "Disease of God, Disease of Man").
40. John M. Janzen, "The Meeting of Allopathic and Indigenous Medicine in the African Context," in *The Social History of the Biomedical Sciences,* ed. Massimo Piattelli-Palmarini (Milan, forthcoming).
41. Peter Fry, *Spirits of Protest: Spirit-Mediums and the Articulation of Consensus amongst the Zezuru of Southern Rhodesia (Zimbabwe)* (Cambridge, England, 1976).
42. For example, Alexis Kagame's *La Philosophie bantou-rwandaise de l'etre* (Brussels, 1956); or Father Placide Tempels's *Bantu Philosophy* (Brussels, 1945).
43. Paulin J. Hountondji, *African Philosophy* (Bloomington, IN, 1983); V. Y. Mudimbe, "Signes therapeutiques et prose de la vie en Afrique noire," in *Social Science and Medicine* 15B, no. 3 (1981):195–211; Kwasi Wiredu, *Philosophy and African Culture* (Cambridge, England, 1980).
44. For example, V. Y. Mudimbe, in his *L'Odeur du pere* (Paris, 1982), takes a middle position, suggesting that although Africans may long for an analytical thought system of their own origin, the reality is that much of the scientific and cultural agenda in Africa is determined elsewhere. He does not agree with the African romantics who see only good in the African past. Indeed, in his "Signes therapeutiques et prose de la vie en Afrique noire," he identifies many excesses and abuses in African therapeutics.
45. The classic studies on this subject include E. E. Evans-Pritchard, *Witchcraft, Oracles and Magic among the Azande* (Oxford, 1937); Victor W.

Turner, *Revelation and Divination in Ndembu Ritual* (Ithaca, NY, 1975); William Bascom, *Ifa Divination* (Bloomington, IN, 1969); and more recently, Eugene Mendonsa, *The Politics of Divination: A Processual View of Reactions to Illness and Deviance among the Sisala of Northern Ghana* (Berkeley, 1982).

46. The "therapy managing group," considered regarding its composition and character, is presented in Janzen, *The Quest for Therapy*, pp. 3–11, 139–150, and in J. M. Janzen, "Therapy Management: Concept, Reality, Process," *Medical Anthropology Quarterly* 1 (1987):1.

47. Bascom, *Ifa Divination*.

48. Turner, *Revelation and Divination*.

49. Janzen, *The Quest for Therapy*, pp. 107–111.

50. Guthrie, 786.

51. Guthrie, 42.

52. Guthrie, 195–196.

53. Guthrie, 787.

54. Guthrie, 196.

55. Guthrie, 250.

56. Guthrie, 1730.

57. Guthrie, 990.

58. Janzen, *The Quest for Therapy*, p. 199.

59. Guthrie, 1474, 1477.

60. In addition to its association with the cognate *pod* discussed earlier, the cupping horn is called *cuku, cumo;* to bleed, and cup, *dumik* or *cumik.* These are found in Guthrie, 412, 440, 700, 439.

61. J. Kerharo, "La Pharmacopée africaine traditionelle et recherche scientifique," in *Presence africaine* (1972):475–499; I. van Puyvelde, *La Pharmacopée et la médecine africaine traditionnelles* (Butare [Rwanda], 1974); A. F. Banghawe, E. N. Mingola, and G. Maina, *The Use and Abuse of Drugs and Chemicals in Tropical Africa* (Nairobi, 1972); J. M. Watt and M. B. Breyer-Brandwijk, *The Medicinal and Poisonous Plants of Southern and Eastern Africa* (Edinburgh and London, 1962); J. O. Kokowaro, *Medicinal Plants of East Africa* (Kampala, Nairobi, and Dar es Salaam, 1976); and Oku Ampofo, "Plants That Heal," *World Health* (November 1977): 26–30.

62. Guthrie, 1072–1073.

63. Guthrie, 1534.

64. Guthrie, 293.

65. Guthrie, 844, 1401.

66. Turner, *The Drums of Affliction* (Oxford, 1968).

67. Ibid.

68. Renat Devisch, *Se recreer femme: Manipulation semantique d'une situation d'infecondite chez les Yaka du Zaire* (Berlin, 1984); Janzen, *The Quest for Therapy*, pp. 112–113.

69. Janzen, *Lemba*.

70. Terence O. Ranger, *Dance and Society in Eastern Africa: The Beni Ngoma* (London, 1975).

71. Richard P. Werbner, ed., *Regional Cults*, ASA Monograph no. 16 (London, 1975).

72. Hans Cory, "The Buswezi," in *American Anthropologist* 57 (1955):923–952; Iris Berger, *Religion and Resistance: East African Kingdoms in the Precolonial Period*, Musée Royale de l'Afrique Centrale, Annales, no. 105 (Tervuren, Belgium 1981).

73. Swantz; Hans Cory, "Ngoma ya Sheitani," *Journal of the Royal Anthropological Institute* 66 (1936):209–217.
74. Martin West, *Bishops and Prophets in a Black City: African Independent Churches in Soweto* (Johannesburg, 1975).
75. Terence O. Ranger, "Healing and Society in Colonial Southern Africa" (Unpublished).
76. One local work I am aware of in Lower Zaire is Dianzungu dia Biniakunu's KiKongo book, *Nei yankatu ngongo eto: tuzolele nsi zalubutu, zantoko ze zicilumukanga maza* (Desolate land, we protest: We want a fruitful and beautiful land flowing with water) (Kinshasa, Zaire, 1987). On an international scale, writings by Kenyan novelist Ngugi address this issue.

CHAPTER 11

Afro-Caribbean

Spirituality:

A Haitian

Case Study

KAREN McCARTHY BROWN

Haitian views of healing and wholeness as revealed in the religious system called Vodou provide the focus for this study. While the specifics of the discussion would differ if it were centered in other Caribbean locales, there are certain basic attitudes and understandings about the nature of the human condition and the causes and cures of human suffering that are broadly shared among descendants of African slaves throughout the Caribbean—areas that may be collectively named the Afro-Caribbean. Before turning to Haiti, I will first consider briefly the factors that create

the differences among Afro-Caribbean cultures and then attempt to outline the common foundation on which their various healing systems rest.

Traditional attitudes and practices surrounding health and spirituality
vary from one area of the Caribbean to another for several reasons. Of
first-level importance is the place (or places) in Africa from which the
slave populations were drawn and the resulting ideas about health and
spirituality that the slaves brought with them. For example, in Haiti there
are three clear lines of African influence: those of the Fon peoples, most
of whom live in the area we now call Benin; the Yoruba peoples (Nigeria);
and the Kongo peoples (Angola and Bas-Zaire). By contrast Cuban traditional religion is dominated by Yoruba influence, while that of Jamaica
has its deepest roots among the Akan of Ghana. Other factors that
account for the differences are the nature of the slave systems under
which the first generations labored, including the brand of Christianity
practiced by the slaveholders; the geography, plant and animal life of the
New World setting and the differences and similarities that the slaves
found between these and the ecologies of their homelands; and the social,
political and economic history subsequent to slavery.

In relation to Haiti, the last point warrants special comment. Haiti was
the second independent republic in the Western Hemisphere and the first
Black one. After its successful slave revolution (1791–1804) and mainly
as the result of trade boycotts, Haiti was effectively cut off from contact
with the United States and Europe for nearly a century. Furthermore,
even though the French colonists had established Catholicism as the official religion of the people of the island, including its slave population,
Haiti was denied priests by the church for more than fifty years following
the revolution. At the opening of the nineteenth century, when the long
struggle for independence ended, it is possible that as many as three-
quarters of the slave population of Haiti had been born in Africa. Therefore, for a substantial period of time following the expulsion of the
French, several strong African cultural traditions interacted in Haiti in an
atmosphere relatively free of outside influence. This phenomenon sharply
distinguishes Haiti from the rest of the Caribbean and particularly from
places such as Jamaica. Jamaica experienced a continuing colonial presence well into the twentieth century. As a result, the influences of Africa
in Jamaican traditional spirituality are subtler and more diffuse than those
in Haiti. However, the ubiquitous "balm yards" or healing centers in contemporary Jamaica are significant African survivals. It is likely that their
existence is a testament to the durability of a level of religious practice
that does not require elaborate temples or rituals, or the participation of
large numbers of persons. More importantly, their survival is also evidence of the centrality of healing for African-based spirituality.

In spite of diverse input from Africa and divergent experiences during
and after the period of slavery, the various Afro-Caribbean communities
share a broad range of traditional assumptions, attitudes, and practices

relating to health and healing. I have identified six such factors, which I believe to be common to the healing traditions of the Afro-Caribbean.

First, healing is the *primary* business of these religious systems. In fact, it is not an overstatement to say that spirituality and healing are synonymous in the Afro-Caribbean. Client-practitioner interactions occasioned by problems in the lives of individual persons occupy much of the time of spiritual leaders. Furthermore, even large ritual events that occur on a regular basis can be understood as healing ceremonies when placed in their proper context.

Second, the understanding of personhood operative within these Afro-Caribbean healing traditions is a fundamentally relational one. The individual person is defined by a web of relationships that includes not only the extended family but also the ancestors and the spirits or saints. Furthermore, the individual *qua* individual is also understood in relational terms. Personhood is seen as constituted by a dynamic balance of diverse spiritual energies or tendencies.

Third, healing within Afro-Caribbean traditions takes place through ritual adjustments in these relational webs. To be more specific, healing involves adjusting or reactivating the reciprocal gift-giving that characterizes all relationships in the Afro-Caribbean, whether they are relationships with the living, the dead, or the divine.

Fourth, these African-based religious traditions address a wide variety of maladies. The expertise of the healer extends beyond physical problems to include social problems arising from such areas as love, work, and family life. While a person with physical symptoms could well be given herbal treatment appropriate to those symptoms, herbs would not represent the main part of the cure. In fact, the distinction between physical and social maladies is finally an insignificant one. Basic diagnostic categories are concerned with the *origins* of problems, and problems are virtually always seen as due to disruptions in relationships. The major curative action is therefore, as we have seen, directed at healing relationships. Further, the connection between a specific cause (the root problem) and a particular set of symptoms (the presenting problem) is by no means a necessary one. In other words, failure to honor the spirits could equally well result in the loss of a job or in digestive difficulties.

Fifth, these healing systems have a penchant for working through what Lévi-Strauss called "the science of the concrete."[1] The harmful emotional states that cause disruptions in relationships—such as jealousy, despair, fear, anger—are addressed in ways that appeal to the nonrational and even nonverbal dimensions of human interaction. Emotional or relational states are concretized in sounds, gestures, or objects that are laden with the highly condensed metaphoric referents of such things as taste, smell, and color. Adjustments are then made in the externalized or concretized relational situation. For example, in Haiti, a marriage threatened by the destructive anger of the husband could be treated by placing ice and a little sugar syrup in a jar that also contains a slip of paper with his name written on it several times. The jar is then inverted, the basic signal within the Vodou science of the concrete that a situation is to be changed. The wife, who desires to "cool down" and "sweeten" her husband, "works the point" several times a day. She lights a candle by the jar, prays over it, and concentrates her energy on the desired end. Scientific and social-scientific thinkers alike have tended to label this sort of healing practice "magic" or "superstition," thus dismissing it from the larger psychotherapeutic discussion, where it could well suggest middle-range alternatives to drug therapy and the talking cure.

Finally, all of these traditions are involved in one stage or another of negotiation with Great Atlantic culture, that is, with the Western world. Scientific medicine, capitalism, individualism, and modern technology all present challenges to customary attitudes and practices in the area of health. In some parts of the Caribbean, exposure to these forces has been substantial and long-term (Puerto Rico, for example), and as a result, traditional healers have circumscribed their activity, focusing on problems that would be considered insignificant by the church and by Western medical institutions, such as broken love affairs, predictive dreams, and chains of bad luck. By contrast, in rural Haiti the majority of problems of all sorts are still treated by traditional healers. Yet no area in the Caribbean has been without some contact with the trappings of modern life. African-based systems of spiritual healing characteristically accommodate elements of modernity in their worldview rather than react to them competitively or with hostility. For example, a traditional healer may advise a patient to go to a hospital or get a shot of penicillin from the local clinic. Unfortunately, there has not been the same openness in the other direction.

This summary view of the Caribbean context serves as background to a more detailed discussion of traditional healing in Haiti, which will begin with sections on the centrality of family and the view of person. The focus on exchange relationships emerging from these two topics will provide the organizing motif for discussions of Vodou rituals and of the Vodou spirits. A more specific treatment of the Haitian Vodou understandings of the causes and cures of human suffering will follow. This will touch on a variety of topics, including the etiology of problems, the sources of authority used in treatment, and the questions of morality that arise in the quest for healing.

Serving the Spirits in Haiti

Haitians do not often call their religion "Vodou," a term that in the rural areas at least is still reserved for a particular subtype of dance and ritualizing. (*Vodou* comes from the Fon language and means "spirit.") When Haitians refer to the religious dimension of their lives they refer to a form of activity rather than an institutional entity. They say they "serve the spirits." I have come to believe that human suffering is the major impetus for serving the spirits and, furthermore, that an understanding of Vodou ritualizing in terms of the ways in which it both comprehends suffering and ameliorates suffering yields greater insight than any other.

"Moun fèt pou mouri" (People are born to die), Haitians are fond of saying with a shrug of the shoulders. This proverb comments on the suffering and death that are commonplace occurrences in poverty-stricken Haiti and shows the stoic acceptance that, on one level at least, characterizes the Haitian attitude toward such a life. Haitians have no vision of heaven in their religion,[2] no ideology of progress shaping their understanding of history, and virtually no experience of upward mobility in their lives or the lives of their children. Suffering is an expected, recurrent condition. It is not an exaggeration to say that problem-free periods in life are pervaded with an anxiety that anticipates crisis just around the corner. Life as a whole is thus characterized by cycles of luck and the absence of luck. The clever, faithful, and/or powerful person is one who manages by a juggling of scarce resources to give generously to the living, the dead, and the spirits. The resulting network of dependents who are obliged to serve and elders or social superiors who are obliged to give sustenance and protection—even though subject to the inherent unpredictability of personal relationships—provides the only means any Haitian has of controlling his or her "luck." At the very least, the obligations created by these gifts construct the safety net that is essential for survival, given the uncertainties of life in Haiti.

Haiti occupies the western third of Hispaniola, an island it shares with the Dominican Republic. It is a small country—about the size of the state of Maryland—that is home to 5.5 to 6 million people. Haiti is still largely an agricultural country, although much of its land has been rendered nearly useless by short-range farming techniques and soil erosion caused by cutting trees to produce the charcoal most people still use to cook their food. Diseases such as tuberculosis, malaria, yaws, syphilis, and elephantiasis, which have been virtually eliminated in most of the Western Hemisphere, afflict the population in Haiti still. In parts of Haiti the infant mortality rate is above 50 percent, and anyone reaching the age of fifty-five or sixty is considered among the fortunate. The majority of children show some signs of malnutrition: spindly arms and legs, swollen bellies, reddish brittle hair. Social disease is also rampant in Haiti, a country that has survived a succession of brutal dictators who have increased their personal wealth at the expense of the people and maintained their power through random violence and intimidation. It is estimated that 80 percent of the population is illiterate and that the average annual income for a

Haitian is somewhere between $200 and $300. When the considerable wealth of the 8 to 9 percent of the population known as "the elite" is taken into account, it appears most persons in Haiti get by on little more than $100 a year—and yet a chicken purchased in Port-au-Prince can cost as much as $5.

"Mizè mennen parespè," the Haitians say, meaning, if you show you are suffering people lose respect for you. Mizè (literally, "misery") is an interesting word choice here, for while it can be used to refer to suffering in general, it is used most often to refer to poverty with all its attendant pains and indignities. There are many beggars in Haiti. One sees them everywhere, but most often in markets, cemeteries, and churchyards. In spite of their numbers, there is a special shame associated with begging. This becomes apparent in the way begging is used within the Vodou system. When the spirits want to teach a lesson in humility to a devotee, they command that person to don the ritual version of rags and go to the market and beg. The ignominy of begging comes largely from the fact that beggars are seen as isolated individuals whose activity announces to the world that they have been abandoned by the extended kin group and now must forage on their own. Even if the family were lost through death rather than discord, the person who must beg can easily be seen as someone who was not clever enough or respectful enough or sufficiently hardworking to find a place as adopted kin in another family.

The Centrality of Family

For the slaves taken from Africa, the loss of extended family was so great that they apparently made efforts to recreate that family before they had even set foot on the shores of the New World. It is reported that some slaves recognized an incest prohibition as existing between males and females who had undergone the Middle Passage on the same ship. We know almost nothing about the interactions among slaves in the early part of the eighteenth century, when large numbers of them arrived in Haiti to work the plantations. However, knowledge of the crucial role of the extended family throughout West Africa easily leads to the conclusion that whatever blending among Fon, Yoruba, and Kongo cultures took place during that period must have been compelled in large part by the need for family. In the early stages this need would have been met through fictive kinship structures in which putative "mothers" and "fathers," "aunts" and "uncles," and "cousins" provided the individual with both identity (a place in society) and protection. Since the contributing African cultures defined family as including the ancestors and the spirits, the need for family was both a social and a spiritual need.

The slaves' loss of access to family land in Africa was as great as their loss of the African family itself. Indeed, from one perspective family and land were inseparable. Prevented from visiting family graves and from leaving food offerings and pouring libations at ancestral shrines, the enslaved African had also been denied the means of ensuring the spiritual blessing and protection of the ancestors. Thus when slaves could bring no other possessions with them, some nevertheless managed to carry away small sacks of the soil of their motherland. This connection of family, land, and religion persists in rural Haiti today.

Unlike most of the other Caribbean nations Haiti is predominantly a country of peasant farmers, many of whom own their own land. Where the social structures have not been decimated by the combined pressures of overpopulation, depleted soil, and corrupt politics, rural people in Haiti tend to live in large, patriarchal, extended families. Even moderately successful men in the countryside may enter into multiple *plasaj* or common-law unions with women. Each of these women is set up in a house of her own in which she raises the children born of their union. Thus a multi-generational extended family can swell to considerable size even when counting only the blood kin. Such families, however, are not defined solely by blood ties. Large rural families invariably include adopted "god-mothers," "godfathers," and "cousins," as well as a number of "maids" and other workers who exchange their labor for a place to sleep and for meager rations. Included in this latter group are the *restavèk* (literally, the "stay-withs"), children whose parents could not afford to feed them and so either sold them or gave them away to slightly more prosperous families. Social hierarchy is relentless in Haiti. There is always someone poorer than oneself. Even the most minimal rural household with only one or two able-bodied adults to work an unproductive square of earth manages to have a servant.

The patriarch of the extended family functions as the *oungan* or priest when that family serves the spirits. He is often the one who treats family members when they become ill, although an outsider may be called in for such treatments if there is someone in the vicinity who has a reputation as one who "knows leaves." However, it is necessarily the patriarch who presides at the *gwo sèvis*, the big dancing and drumming events that include animal sacrifice. These ceremonies are held annually if family resources permit. More commonly they are held at longer intervals and then only in response to crises within the group. The purpose of the elaborate ritualizing is to honor, entertain, and feed the ancestors and the Vodou spirits which those ancestors served.

The family dead are buried on the family land and the cemetery is a major center for religious activity. In addition, a cult house for the ritual objects of the family is often built on a small, separate plot of land. Thus, to inherit land is also to inherit the bones of the ancestors and the duty to honor those ancestors as well as to serve the spirits represented in the cult house. Conversely, to be separated from the land is also to risk one's access to the power and protection that these spirit entities provide.

Separation from land and family is, however, an increasingly frequent experience for the younger generations of Haiti's rural poor. Inheritance laws in Haiti work to divide the land into smaller and smaller plots. This pressure, combined with that of the multiple problems cited earlier, has pushed large numbers of young people off the land and toward the elusive promise of a better life in the cities.

For young men urban life is often cruel. In the countryside they are reared to the expectations of male privilege and power. (Even the female-headed households that are prevalent in the cities perpetuate this ideology to a degree.) Yet some experts estimate unemployment among young urban males at 60 percent and others argue that the figure should be much higher. Women fare somewhat better in the urban environment. Most of the factory jobs available are of the piecework variety, and European and American employers seem to favor women for these repetitive tasks. Urban women also have a market tradition bequeathed to them by their rural sisters. In the country it is the women who take the excess produce to market, along with bread, candy, herbal teas, baskets, and other things they make with their own hands. The urban woman spun away from the rural extended family frequently ends up not only in charge of her house and her children—as she might well have been in the country—but also solely responsible for their financial support. In the countryside her market money would have been the "rainy-day savings" for times of drought and hunger or the means to fulfill a private dream for herself or her children. In the cities she must rely on the old market skills more centrally. The poor urban woman is constantly engaged in small-scale commerce, often in several such enterprises simultaneously. For example, even if she has a regular job, she may sell peanut candy at the door of her home or work as a seamstress or beautician in the evenings and on weekends.

Both men and women who no longer live with their extended families feel the loss acutely. In fact, this sense of loss can persist for generations. In the cities, it is the Vodou temple and the fictive kinship network it provides that compensates for the missing large rural family. The head of the temple is called "mother" or "father," and the initiates are known as "children of the house." The Vodou initiate owes service and loyalty to his or her Vodou parent after the pattern of filial piety owed all parents by their children in Haiti. In turn, Vodou parents, like actual ones, owe their children protection, care, and help in times of trouble. In certain circumstances this help is of a very tangible sort: food, a place to sleep, assistance in finding work. The urban Vodou temples are currently the closest thing to a social welfare system that exists in Haiti.

The differences between men's and women's lives in the cities have also left their mark on the practice of urban Vodou. While in some parts of rural Haiti women can gain recognition and prestige as *manbo* (priest-esses), herbalists, or *fanm saj* (midwives), nowhere in the countryside do they effectively challenge the spiritual hegemony of the male. This is not the case in the cities, where there are probably as many women as men in positions of religious leadership.

The urban Vodou temples run by men tend to mimic the patriarchal structure of the rural extended families. The urban *oungan* is notorious for fathering many children and recruiting desirable young women to be among his *ounsi*, brides of the gods, the ritual chorus and general work-force of a Vodou temple.[3] He thus creates a highly visible father role which he then operates out of in relation to all those who serve the spirits under his tutelage. While the female *manbo* who heads a temple is not necessarily more democratic in all of her relationships with those that serve the spirits in her house, she does tend to be so in the ways that a mother's role is normally less authoritarian than that of a father. For example, many temples headed by women function as day-care centers for the working mothers associated with them. In sum, the woman-headed temple tends to reiterate the tone and atmosphere inside the home, a place where women have usually been in charge. This is an atmosphere that allows for more flexibility in human relationships than is found in the male-headed temple, which recalls the more public and therefore more rigid social rules of the entire extended family. This shift toward greater authority for women in urban Vodou has undoubtedly had an effect on the nature of the care given to individuals who turn to tra-ditional religion to solve the many problems that urban life in Haiti can bring.

Whether the temple is headed by a man or a woman, it is clear that its appeal to the urban population is rooted in its ability to recreate family. A song sung at the beginning of Vodou ceremonies in Port-au-Prince illustrates this:

> *Lafanmi semble,*
> *Semble nan.*
> *Se Kreyòl nou yè,*
> *Pa genyen Gine enkò.*

> The family is assembled,
> Gathered in.
> We are Creoles,
> Who have Africa no longer.

The Vodou View of Person

In Vodou, persons are said to possess several "souls." In fact, there is no generic term in the Haitian Creole language that includes all of these spir-

itual entities or energies, even though each possesses some of the characteristics of what Westerners call soul. Furthermore, the word *nam*,
derivative of the French word for soul, is only one of the complex of forces
that constitute a person. A person's *nam* is usually understood as the animating force of the body. The most immediate effect of death is the departure of the *nam*, which is sometimes said to linger for a short period of
time around the corpse or grave. The *nam* is an evanescent thing that disappears soon after death.

By contrast the *gwo bonanj*, the big guardian angel, is capable of sus-
tained existence apart from the body it inhabits. One of the situations in
which the person is separated from his or her *gwo bonanj* occurs during
the possession trance, which is central to Vodou ritualizing. The struggle
that marks the onset of possession is understood as a struggle between a
person's *gwo bonanj* and the Vodou *lwa* (spirit), who desires to "ride" that
person and to use his or her body and voice to communicate with the
faithful. One who is thus ridden by the spirit is known as a *chwal* (horse)
of the spirit. Those who are possessed report that they lose consciousness
after this initial struggle. The loss of consciousness and the resulting
amnesia about what the spirit said and did while riding the *chwal* is
explained as due to the departure of the *gwo bonanj*.

Similarly, it is the *gwo bonanj* that wanders from the body during
sleep, even into the land of the dead, thus allowing deceased persons or
those living at a great distance to appear in dreams. The wanderings of
the big guardian angel during sleep are sometimes useful for information-
gathering. For example, a mother in Haiti said she learned from a dream
that her daughter in New York had met with an accident and broken her
arm. In like fashion, when a person is uneasy, she may say that her *gwo
bonanj* is agitated. This is an undesirable state mainly because it robs the
person of sound sleep and therefore of dreams, which are an important
vehicle for communication with the dispersed family, the ancestors, and
the spirits.

Finally, it is the *gwo bonanj* that must be ritually removed "from the
head" of a person shortly after death. The big guardian angel is then sent
"under the water" to dwell for a period of time until it (now referred to
as a *mò*, one of the dead) is "called up from the water," installed in a clay
pot known as a *govi*, and placed on the family altar. The Vodou ceremony
known as *rele mò nan dlo*, calling the dead from the water, calls them from
Gine, Africa, a watery land said to exist below the earth. The ceremony
ideally takes place a year and a day following the death. Because it is an
elaborate and expensive ceremony, however, in practice families wait
until there are several of their dead whom they may retrieve at once. As
a result the dead frequently emerge complaining of cold, dampness, and
neglect. In this ceremony, the dead speak through a kind of ventriloquism
possession and genuinely sound as if they come from both far away and

underwater. Their identity is confirmed by the intimate knowledge of family life which they display. The spirits called up from the waters of Africa inquire about family members and comment on problems within the group. Given these various understandings of the nature and activity of the *gwo bonanj*, it seems fair to conclude that this dimension of soul is both the consciousness and essential personality of the individual.

The *ti bonanj* (little guardian angel), which each person also possesses, is much more difficult to define. One urban *manbo*, or priestess, gave me two interesting responses to questions about the nature of the *ti bonanj*. "When you look at your shadow," she said, "you will see that sometimes it has a dark center. That is the *gwo bonanj*, but the paler shadow around the dark center is the *ti bonanj*." When asked what the little guardian angel does, she gave another concrete illustration: "When you are walking a long way or carrying something very heavy and feel so tired that you know you are not going to make it, it is the *ti bonanj* that takes over so you can do what you have to do." The *ti bonanj* is thus perhaps best described as a spiritual reserve tank. It is an energy or presence within the person that is dimmer or deeper than consciousness, but it is nevertheless there to be called upon in situations of stress and depletion.

Much less routinely, Vodou *oungan* and *manbo* speak of another dimension of the person called the *zetwal* or star. This is not an inner presence so much as it is a kind of celestial parallel self. The concept of the *zetwal* is rooted in the belief that each person is born with his or her fate already foreknown and unchangeable. The regular movements of the stars and their recurring patterns mimic, perhaps even direct, the larger contours of life in the human community. Whatever control an individual has over his or her life thus comes in specific moments and short-run situations. *Mizè* (suffering) may be held at bay only for a short time and *chans* (luck) only marginally enhanced. The overall shape and direction of a life are determined by fate.

The *nam*, the *gwo bonanj*, the *ti bonanj*, and the *zetwal* are the constitutive parts of a Haitian view of personhood that is clearly derivative of what ethnographers call the "multiple soul complex" in West Africa. The fact that Vodou contains European elements as well as African is also hinted at in this formulation. In addition to their Catholicism, the French planter class of Haiti was known for its participation in a variety of forms of marginal spirituality including Freemasonry and spiritualism. It seems likely that the astrological flavor of the *zetwal* concept also owes its parentage to this line of influence, even though the notion that individual persons are born with their fate already cast by the gods was a belief held by the Fon and to some extent also by the Yoruba.[4]

While Vodou devotees understand the dead body (*kòr kadav*) of a person to be a material substance separable from these various animating spiritual entities and therefore subject to decay and ultimate dissolution,

the body/soul or material/spiritual split is not central to their understanding of personhood. As an indication of this it is worth noting that
there is no division within the Vodou view of person between drives or
appetites that come from the body—for example, hunger and sexuality—
and those that come from the spirit or mind. In fact, sexuality is perhaps
the central aminating force in all of life. Much of Vodou ritualizing suggests that sexual and spiritual energy come from the same source.

What complicates the understanding of personhood is the realization
that individuals are not comprehensible apart from the Vodou spirits
associated with them. It is easiest to discuss this in the urban setting,
which I know best. Here, each person is said to have a *mèt tet*, master of
the head. This is the main spirit served by that person, and if the person
is one who serves as a "horse" of the spirits, it will be the *mèt tet* who
most often possesses that person. To a certain extent the personality of
the individual human being mirrors that of his or her *mèt tet*. For example,
a man who has Ogou as his *mèt tet* will be expected to exhibit some of
the warrior spirit's anger, strictness, and perseverence in his everyday
behavior. Yet he will also have been told that Ogou is "too hot" to be
served alone. The spirit of war and anger must be balanced by others, for
example, by a strong "sweet" spirit such as the ancient and venerable
snake spirit, Dambala.

In addition to a *mèt tet* each individual has a smaller number of other
spirits, usually two or three, from whom he or she receives special protection. This complex of spirits, which may consist of some that are
known only in that family and others that are recognized throughout
Haiti, differs from individual to individual. It is partly because of this that
Vodou, though centrally concerned with morality, could never produce a
codified moral law that would apply equally to all persons. In Vodou, an
individual lives a moral life by faithfully serving the particular configuration of spirits that "love" or "protect" that person. This includes following their advice, advice that will be consistent with the personalities of
the spirits. Thus it might be said that the Vodou ethic is an intensely contextual one.

It is the urban devotee's particular grouping of protective spirits that
determines the nature of ritual as well as moral obligations. Furthermore,
it is important to note that the choice of this penumbra of protective spirits
is not for "the living" to make; Vodou devotees insist that it is the spirits
who choose the persons they love or protect. Yet, priests and priestesses
do determine the choices the spirits have made, often through divination.

A question may well be raised as to whether the Vodou spirits are
truly distinct and separate from the persons who serve them. This question is answered in paradoxical ways within Vodou ritualizing. Beliefs
surrounding possession trance and the struggle of the *gwo bonanj* with the
possessing spirit, as well as the insistence that the person is chosen by the

spirit and not vice versa, point to a clear distinction between spirit and person. However, from the perspective of certain rituals such as those that occur during initiation and after death, the individual person cannot be separated from the spirits that reside "in the head" or "on" the person, these being equally common expressions among Vodou devotees. Initiation rituals simultaneously "feed the spirits in the head" and establish a repository for them outside the person. This repository is called a *pò tet* (head pot). After initiation it is placed on the Vodou family altar and becomes the focus of rituals designed to cool, soothe, and strengthen the person. Furthermore, when the spirit is removed from a person's head at death, this spirit is sometimes treated as if it were the *gwo bonanj* and sometimes as if it were the *lwa*, the Vodou spirit, who was the *mèt tet* of the dead person. Similarly, when the ancestor is called up from the waters and established on the family altar, the spirit is called both by the name of the ancestor and by the name of the *lwa*. For example, reference may be made to "Marie's Ogou" or to "Pierre's Dambala." Thus there is also a sense in which at least the head spirit is identified with the *gwo bonanj*, if not with the individual in a larger sense.

In fifteen years of work on Haitian traditional religion, I have learned that paradoxes of this sort are to be cherished rather than resolved, for it is invariably such paradoxical statements that provide the greatest insight into the religious system we call Vodou. If it is understood that within the Vodou worldview the individual is both a separate self and an inseparable part of a family, then it can be grasped how the spirits who are part of that extended family can be *both* other than and merged with those who serve them.

Rituals of Haitian Vodou

For some individuals, coexistence with their spirits presents no problems; life flows more or less smoothly. It may be the case that someone within their family serves the spirits and this is sufficient to fill the hungry bellies, slake the dry throats, and stroke the wounded pride of the ancestors and the *lwa*. However, if one is not so fortunate and life is not going well—and it often is not in a country such as Haiti—then more is required. Vodou offers a series of ritual steps that escalate the intensity of the individual's involvement with the spirits. Each of these ritual steps is based on an exchange. The person commits to service of one sort or another; in return the spirits proffer relief and protection.

Some problems can be handled with a onetime or at least a short-term commitment to the spirits. This type of commitment could be something as simple as lighting a candle before the image of a spirit, or it could be an elaborate and expensive feast for several spirits, which would include dancing, drumming, and animal sacrifice. Other problems require a more routinized and long-term relationship with one or more spirits. Such life-time commitments vary from "marriage" to a spirit to the decision to become a priest or priestess.[5]

In the process of escalating their commitments to the Vodou spirits, devotees accomplish two related things. First, they gradually increase the strength and stability of their own *gwo bonanj*. For those who move to the upper levels of initiation this means mastering the art of possession trance, which is the art of both letting go of the *gwo bonanj* and bringing it back. Second, devotees gradually increase their control over the Vodou spirits as well. Men and women who advance to the grade of *oungan* and *manbo* do so through a ceremony in which they "take the *asson*."[6] The *asson* is a small, hollow gourd covered with a mesh of glass beads and snake vertebrae. This rattle, which is the emblem of the Vodou priest-hood, is not used to make music but to signal key changes in the drum rhythms in a Vodou service, as well as to summon and send away the *lwa*. When a *lwa* tries to seat itself on an inexperienced horse, the struggle between the *gwo bonanj* and the spirit can become violent and even harm-ful to the horse. It is in situations such as these that the spirit must be sent away. Thus, within limits, Vodou priests and priestesses have power over the spirits. As one Vodou priest put it: "The spirits don't like the *asson*, but they give it to us anyway so we can work with them."

Although it is clear that overall the spirits have far greater powers than do the living, the relationship between devotees and spirits is neverthe-less characterized by reciprocity and mutual dependence. The *lwa*, like the ancestors, depend on the living to feed them. Hungry spirits are trou-blesome and destructive. The living, in turn, depend on the protection and luck that only the spirits can guarantee. This relationship is not unlike the one that exists between parents and children. While the greater power and authority of the parents is unquestioned, parental care in Haiti is not purely altruistic. In the rural areas children work from a young age and their work soon becomes essential to the ongoing family enterprise. Play for children four or five years old often consists of small fetching and car-rying tasks; and all over Haiti, the childless person is pitied mainly because there will be no one to take care of that individual in old age. For those reared in monotheistic religious traditions, the notion that the spirits are dependent on their devotees is an especially difficult one to grasp. Yet comprehending this principle is essential, for without understanding that the spirits need the living, it is all too easy to attribute the problems, ill-nesses, and general harassment that the spirits at times dole out to the living as due to their temperamental, or worse, evil nature.

Vodou is a blend of various African traditions with Catholicism. Although it can be argued that Catholicism has been Africanized in Vodou, and that this is a far truer statement than its reverse, this does not mean that the Catholic Church has no role in the life of the 85 to 90 percent of Haitians who serve the spirits. Pilgrimages to various churches and attendance at Mass are integrated into many complicated Vodou rituals. In addition, the church has taken over the major ceremonies of the life cycle. Birth, where it is ritualized at all, is celebrated through baptism. Also, ideally everyone should go through a First Communion. Pictures from this event are among a family's most treasured possessions. For economic reasons, most Haitians enter *plasaj* (common-law) partnerships rather than have legal marriages. However, where there is a wedding, it is understood that it should be a church wedding. The church also buries the dead, although Vodou rituals are woven in and out of the wake, the entombment (burial is aboveground in Haiti), and the memorial Mass that comes nine days following the death.

Vodou ritual pervades the life of the great majority of Haitian people. For example, candles are lighted and libations poured at countless family altars every day. There are also large ceremonies that have a more social and celebratory air. Among these are the sumptuous feasts for the spirits that occur with some frequency throughout the calendar year at large urban temples. These are a source of entertainment and celebration for curious onlookers and invited guests as well as for the members of that particular Vodou family. Even though all guests may not be offered drinks and plates of food, it is a tradition that the doors of the Vodou temple are closed to no one. Furthermore, the more people present at one of these events, the more chance it has of being a success. The spirits will not come until the crowd is *byen eshofe*, well heated up. When sweat is streaming down the bodies of the drummers and they have found that vast reserve of energy on the other side of fatigue, when their intricate polyrhythms drive the dancers to new heights of grace and spirit, when the voices of the leader of songs and the *ounsi* chorus challenge one another in an ascending spiral of statement and response, that is when the ceremony is *byen eshofe* and that is when the *lwa* will mount their horses and ride.

Spirit Possession

Once the spirit is in charge of the horse, the crescendo of energy stops and people settle in to watch the possession performance. The term "possession performance" is not used here to indicate that there is anything false or contrived about these visits from the spirits. Vodou priest and priestess alike condemn the occasional person in their midst who may *pran poz*, act disingenuously as if possessed. The term is used rather to indicate what has often been noticed about possession in the Vodou temple: it has a theatrical quality. The characters of the major Vodou spirits are well known. Even an outsider such as myself can identify the possessing spirit within moments of its arrival because of certain stereotypical behavior as well as the ritual garb and implements that the spirit requests. However, the Vodou priests and priestesses, the ones usually possessed at these large feasts, improvise freely within the character range of the spirit. Thus a *lwa* not only goes through standard ritual salutations and exhibits certain forms of behavior that are seen virtually every time this spirit possesses someone, but the spirit also addresses particular persons and gives advice about specific problems. The spirits hug, hold, and dance with the devotees. They give ritual blessings and sometimes ritual chastisement, both appropriate to the situation. They sing. They eat. They cry. At these large public events, the Vodou spirits process the problems of the community, fine-tuning human relationships. Sometimes an intimate problem can be whispered into the ear of a sympathetic *lwa*, and the spirit will take the devotee aside for a discreet and private audience. More frequently, these interactions with the spirits become the occasion for an individual's problems to be aired (and healed) in the larger community context.

One specific example of this process will serve to make several points. There was a *oungan* in Carrefour (a town on the coast road south and west of Port-au-Prince) who had a reputation for being a strict and dour disciplinarian in his Vodou family. Because she had angered him, he sent away a woman named Simone, the song leader in his temple, and told her never to return. At a ceremony not long after, this *oungan*, whose name was Cesaire, was possessed by the warrior spirit, Ogou. Ogou arrived in a rage and immediately began to berate Cesaire (the very horse he was riding). Who did Cesaire think he was, Ogou asked, that he could send Simone out of the temple? Simone was one of Ogou's favorites, and besides, it was he, Ogou, who was in charge of the temple, not Cesaire. The gathered faithful were instructed to convey this message to the ill-mannered *oungan* without fail, and then the spirit departed, leaving the body of Cesaire in a crumpled heap on the temple floor. When he had barely regained his senses, the reluctant Cesaire was carried along in a procession of all the temple dignitaries, complete with the brightly colored, sequined banners of the temple, right to the home of Simone. They stood outside and sang Vodou songs of invitation and reconciliation. After much coaxing, Simone agreed to come back to the temple, and, accompanied by the full parade, she was ritually reintegrated into the Vodou family.

This example shows something of the complexity of the possession process in which a *lwa* can chastise, even humiliate, his own horse. Yet, perhaps more significantly, it also shows the key role of the community in the interpretation and application of the wisdom of the spirits. Thus, the public airing of community problems and issues within the Vodou temple is a means of enforcing social sanctions, mobilizing the assistance of the community, and mending broken relationships. It is, in short, a way of healing.

Yet there are vast areas of Vodou ritual that are concerned with healing in a more direct way. These vary from the individual client-practitioner interactions (practices that will be discussed below in a section on the types of caring used in Vodou healing) to the expensive and elaborate cycles of initiation rituals.

Initiation

Vodou initiation ceremonies are never undertaken lightly or routinely. Almost always it is trouble with the spirits, manifesting in problems in the individual's life, that lead a person to undergo initiation. In the temples of the Port-au-Prince area there are four levels of initiation possible. Each level involves a period of seclusion that may vary from three to twenty-one days, and most temples have a small interior room set aside for such purposes. Persons tend to be initiated in small groups. The men and women in these groups become "brothers" and "sisters" in a special way. Above all, they are committed to helping each other with ritual duties. This is the case even when the groups contain individuals who are seeking different grades of initiation. All grades of initiation have public rituals that occur intermittently in the exterior temple dancing area as well as rituals reserved for the already-initiated members of the house that occur within the inner chamber.

The first level of initiation is called the *lave tet* (head-washing) and involves cooling and soothing as well as feeding the spirits in a person's head. The second level is *kanzo,* a word that refers to a rite in which initiates are briefly removed from the initiation chamber in order to undergo a ritual trial. In the semipublic part of the *kanzo* ritual, small, hard dumplings are snatched from boiling pots and pressed into the palm of the left hand and the sole of the left foot of the initiate. When this ceremony is completed, the initiates are told: "Now you are *kwit* [cooked]; no one can eat you," that is to say, no one can do harm to you. They are also admonished: "Never say hot again, say strong!"

The third level is called *sou pwen,* on the point. *Pwen* is a complex, multivocal concept in Haitian Vodou, as it is in Haitian culture in general. Within the general culture, "singing the point" or "sending the point" refers to a socially appropriate means of indirect communication that is especially useful for conveying difficult messages. For example, one young man in Haiti told me this story: he was courting a young woman who came from a family as impoverished as his own. The girl's mother decided that the match offered neither one any chance of advancement, and yet she was loathe to insult her daughter's suitor. So when he visited, she went about her household tasks singing a popular song, the refrain of which was "Dè mèg pa fri," (Two lean [pieces of meat] do not fry). The young man got "the point" and broke off his relationship. In and out of the temples, it is often Vodou songs that are used for the purpose of singing the point. These songs have a sparse, even cryptic quality to them that lends itself to communicating several different, sometimes contradictory, meanings at once. The person who "sends a song" in the Vodou temple, that is, the one who suggests the next song to be sung by the group, is not only following a closely prescribed ritual order in which each important *lwa* is saluted in the proper order with his or her own songs and rhythms, but quite frequently is also sending the point, *pwen*, to a person or group of persons present at the ceremony. Such an observation both reveals the extent to which Vodou ritual intertwines with and comments on the life of the community and suggests a preliminary definition for the troublesome word *pwen*. At a level of abstraction uncharacteristic of the way people who serve the spirits speak, *pwen* may be said to mean the condensation or pith of something. At a concrete, ritual level *pwen* are charms or medicines composed of words, objects, gestures, or some combination of the three. They may be drawn on the earth, spoken, sung over a person, placed under the skin, or ingested; they may be buried at the crossroads, in a cemetery, or in the courtyard of a house. When one is initiated "on the point," the reference is to the condensation of the power of a particular spirit who has been diagnosed as the *mèt tet.*

The fourth and final level of initiation is the one that gives a person license to begin practicing as a healer. It is called *assògwe*, literally, "with the *asson*," the beaded rattle that gives priests and priestesses some measure of leverage in the spirit realm.

In Haitian Creole, the verb *kouche* (to lie down, to sleep, to make love, to give birth—less commonly, to die) is the general word used to describe initiation. Entering the initiation chamber is like dying. Friends and family members cry as they line up to kiss the initiates goodbye. Shortly after this genuinely emotional leave-taking, the initiates are blindfolded and led through a dizzying dance of spirals and turns before being taken into the small room where they will *kouche*. As in many other sorts of initiation around the world, to *kouche* is to be forced by ritual means to regress, to become a child again, to be fed and cared for as a child would be, only to be brought rapidly back to adulthood, a new kind of adulthood, again by ritual means. When the initiates leave the inner chamber after days of seclusion and ritualizing, they have their heads covered. Initiates must keep their heads covered for forty days. Like newborn babies with vulnerable soft spots, new initiates must protect the tops of their heads. The spirits within have been fed and are still changing and strengthening day by day. On an altar inside, the initiates have left their *pò tet* (head pots), residues of the internal externalized, the self objectified, the spirits concretized. These *pò tet* generally remain on the altar of the priest or priest-ess who performed the initiation and who will be ever after the initiates' spiritual mother or father. Thus, through initiation rites, bonds among the living—as well as between the living and the spirits—are reinforced.

The Vodou Spirits

In the preceding discussion, I have been using the term "spirit" in a generic sense, as the Haitians often do, to refer to what are in fact three distinguishable groups: the *mò*, the dead; the *màwasa*, the divine twins; and the *mistè*, the mysteries, more often referred to as the *lwa*, or, using the term in a more specific sense, the *espri*, the spirits. Generally speaking, the dead and the divine twins are more central to rural than to urban Vodou. As the structure of the large extended families unravels, the sources from which people seek wisdom and assistance change. In the cities, possessions by specific powerful ancestors decline, while more energy is focused on possessions by the major Vodou *lwa*, most of whom are known and venerated throughout Haiti. In similar fashion, as children lose some importance for the work of the family, the divine children, the *màwasa*, also lose some ritual significance. However, neither the dead nor the *màwasa* disappear completely in the urban context.

The dead are still venerated in the cities. As was mentioned above, the *lwa* are inherited in urban families, where they will be remembered for some time as the *lwa* of a particular ancestor, for example, Marie's Ogou. Also, in the urban context family graves continue to be important, as do the annual celebrations for the dead that occur on and near All Souls' Day.

The *màwasa* also continue to have a role in urban Vodou. In addition to being routinely saluted in most large dancing and drumming ceremo-nies, the divine twins are given special attention in two contexts, both of which have to do with enhancing the luck of a particular group or a par-ticular enterprise. The first instance has to do with making a *promès* (promise). This is done when resources do not permit the immediate ful-fillment of an obligation to the spirits. In such a case a small *manje màwasa*, a meal for the divine twins, can be prepared. The dishes, favor-ites of children, will be fed to the actual children in the group. When they take obvious pleasure in the food this is taken as a sign that the spirits have agreed to accept the promise.

The second ritual in which the *màwasa* play a central role is the *manje pov* (feeding of the poor). This ritual is performed by families, both bio-logical ones and those created around the urban Vodou temples. Ideally it is performed annually to ensure the good fortune of the group. Large quantities of all sorts of food are prepared. A small portion of this—a pot

of soup, perhaps—along with coffee, soap, tobacco, and small change, is
then sent to a gathering place for the poor. The steps of a church or the
cemetery are likely places. These things are passed out to the poor along
with an invitation to come to the temple or the home later in the day for
a feast. Before any of those later assembled can eat from the overflowing
pots prepared for the ceremonial meal, the children of the poor (a group
doubly identified as the socially vulnerable) must first consume a separate
manje màwasa.

Within the realm of the spirits, the *màwasa* play a role parallel to that
of children in the social realm. They require more in terms of care and
material goods than they can give back in the same media of exchange.
However, because children are closely associated with the good fortune
of a family as well as with its vulnerability (youngsters are said to be the
most likely to "catch" destructive spirits sent against a family by its enemies), the exchange can be kept more or less balanced by the luck or
blessing that children can uniquely bestow.

The *manje pov* reveals the connection that is made within Haitian
Vodou between children and the poor. Both are socially vulnerable
groups in need of care. Furthermore, the poor, like children, are understood to be sources of blessing. Almsgiving, particularly when on pilgrimage, is highly recommended in Vodou circles. The identical rituals that
end both the *promès* and the *manje pov* reinforce the reading that helping
children and the destitute brings good fortune. When the respective meals
are finished, the guests—in one case the family children, in the other the
poor, both children and adults—wash their hands in a basin containing
water and basil leaves. The donor of the meal then stands in the center,
and all guests wipe their hands on his or her clothing, face, arms, and
legs.

By far the largest proportion of resources, time, and energy in the
urban Vodou context is expended on service to the *lwa*. These *lwa* are
both related to and different from their West African progenitors. The religious systems of the Fon and the Yoruba, both of which made central
contributions to Haitian Vodou, have complex pantheons of spirits. These
spirits have hegemony over a wide variety of life domains, including natural phenomena such as thunder, wind, rain, and smallpox, as well as
cultural activities such as farming and hunting. When these rich spiritual
systems were transported to the Caribbean, their considerable power to
make sense of the world came to focus almost exclusively on the most
problematic arena of life there, the social arena. For example, Shopona,
the powerful Yoruba figure associated with smallpox, was completely forgotten. Others similarly associated with the powers of nature were lost
unless their skills and proclivities translated readily into the social realm.
In related fashion, many spirits were redefined in the New World setting.
The Yoruba Ogun (the Fon Gu), a patron of metalsmithing, hunting, and

warfare, came to be understood exclusively as a warrior in Haiti. This pervasive socialization of the divine occurred when West Africans were brought to the New World, and it happened again in new ways when their descendants were forced from rural homelands into the cities. Among the Gède (generalized spirits of the dead) recognized in Port-au-Prince are an automobile mechanic, a dentist, and a Protestant missionary. And Azaka, a *lwa* who is a peasant farmer, functions in his urban incarnations mainly as a voice reminding the dispersed of the importance of maintaining contacts with the extended family.

In the Haitian countryside (probably to a greater extent in former times than now) the various *lwa* are organized into several *nanchò* (nations). The names of these—for example, Kongo, Ibo, Wangol, Nago, Rada, Petro—almost all point to specific areas or groups in the African homeland. In the cities this complex of spirit nations has been synthesized into two major groupings, the Rada and the Petro. Within Vodou lore and practice these two groups are understood as fundamentally different, even oppositional. For example, mixing of the altars of the two pantheons is prohibited. Furthermore, even though both may be saluted in the course of a single evening, clearly articulated ritual transitions create buffer zones between the two groups.

The opposition between Rada and Petro can be best understood as a contrast between the quite different modes of relationship that each group represents. The Rada *lwa* are the "sweet" spirits. They are served with sweet foods and drink. The ambiance of their possession performances is intimate and warm. Even those Rada *lwa* who are awesome in their wisdom and power are treated with a respect that is transparent to the affection that underlies it. Rada spirits are *rasin* ("root") *lwa*. They are also said to be *frangine* (African). They are, in short, family, and the mode in which one serves them reflects this. While fidelity and caution are required in the service of the Rada *lwa*, these spirits are not overly strict in their dealings with the living. If a promised feast cannot be offered to them one year, they can be persuaded to wait until the next. The Petro *lwa* by contrast are characterized as "hot" spirits. Their possession performances often play at the border of violence and destructiveness. In like fashion, the unfaithful or careless devotee does not escape punishment. Why then would anyone serve the Petro *lwa*? Because they have access to realms of life that the Rada spirits do not. The power of the Rada *lwa* derives from their wisdom, including herbal knowledge. The power of the Petro *lwa* by contrast extends over, but is not limited to, the arenas of money and commerce. The Petro *lwa*, whose iconographic repertoire includes intricate and intense drum rhythms as well as police whistles, whips, and knives, are the spiritual incarnation of the plantation owners and their neocolonial equivalents—the mulatto elite who control the wealth of the country and the American and European businesspeople who profit from the labor of the poor. The opposition between Rada and Petro is thus aptly described as that between family members and foreigners, or insiders and outsiders. Not incidentally, the Petro *lwa* also chart a course for the person who would assert his or her individual needs over and against the demands of family. The two pantheons, Rada and Petro, thus offer different rewards and are in turn characterized by different modes of sociality. Relationships with spirits in both realms require reciprocity. However, exchanges with the Rada spirits take place in a warm familial atmosphere characterized by compassion, while those with the Petro *lwa* operate according to impersonal and inflexible rules and are thus pervaded with caution and anxiety.

The difficulty ethnographers have experienced in attempting to create a definitive list of the Vodou *lwa* is well known. The reason for this difficulty is rather simple: no such list is possible because the *lwa* are inherently mercurial. They are more accurately described as ways of being in the world, subject to endless transmutation through experience, than as beings per se. For example, the Haitians will say that there is one Ogou; they will also say that there are seven or twenty-one. In fact, there are probably many more than twenty-one that could be identified in the Port-au-Prince region alone. Each is an extension and elaboration of the central character of the warrior spirit Ogou. In his various manifestations Ogou plays across the full range of the constructive and destructive uses of power and aggression. For example, there is the politician Ogou Panama. There is the drunkard Ogou Yamson. There is Ogou Fèray the general, and Ogou Badagri the heroic soldier. Moreover, the individual personalities of the *lwa* are not exactly mercurial but similarly multifaceted. A particular *lwa* can exhibit power, dispense wisdom, and give solace and practical advice. But the same spirit can also—the particulars of his or her personality permitting—whine, pout, needle, harass, and become wantonly destructive. It is impossible, therefore, to group the Vodou spirits according to the moral categories of good and evil. Each spirit, Petro as well as Rada, has both constructive and destructive dimensions, and these change as the character of a *lwa* is applied to a particular life situation through the medium of possession performance. The *lwa* thus do not so much set examples for the living as they hold up mirrors that clarify certain aspects of the lives of those who serve them.

Treatment in the Vodou System

Vodou priests and priestesses treat a wide variety of *pwoblèm*, "problems." Clients come to them for help with love, work, and family problems as well as with sickness. The first determination that a Vodou healer must make is whether the problem "comes from God." If a problem is determined to have been sent by God, it is then seen as "natural" in the sense of that which is meant to be, that which is unavoidable.

When Catholicism blended with African religious traditions to create Vodou, the great West African sky gods, progenitors of human and divine beings alike, were absorbed into Bondyè (God). Bondyè (literally, the "good god") is the one and only god and is clearly distinguishable from the *lwa*, who are sometimes said to be his "angels." A popular Haitian proverb emphasizes the message that is contained in the name of god itself: "Bondyè bon" (God is good). As a result, if a problem, usually a physical illness in this case, is understood as coming from Bondyè, then it works to the greater good, even though this fact is unlikely to be apparent to the sufferer. No priest or priestess will interfere in such a case.

However, if a problem is determined to come from what some Haitians call "supernatural" causes, it is then thought to be appropriate for treatment within the Vodou system. It is important to remember that Haitians do not live in a two-story universe. God and the spirits are an intersecting dimension of life; they are not denizens of a separate realm. When they call a problem "supernatural," it means two things: the problem is not part of the natural order, meaning part of what is fated to be, and it is likely to have been caused by the spirits. Health problems that have a history of being resistant to scientific medical treatment often end up in the Vodou temple, where that very resistance is taken as a sign of the spirit-connected nature of the ailment. In fact, most problems are diagnosed as supernatural in origin or, if not specifically caused by the spirits, then at least falling within the province of their curative powers.

Once the preliminary determination is made that a particular problem is suitable for treatment, the *manbo* or *oungan* sets out to discover more about its nature and origins. Clients do not present themselves to Vodou healers with a detailed list of their symptoms. According to tradition, nothing more is required than a statement such as: "M'pa bon. M'pa genyen chans" ("I'm not well. I don't have any luck"). From this point, it is up to the priest or priestess to determine the nature of the problem, as well as its cause and cure. This is usually accomplished through divination.

The most popular form of divination used in Port-au-Prince is card-reading. However, gazing into a candle flame may be used or other more exotic techniques, such as pouring a small amount of alcohol into the top of a human skull and then reading the patterns made by the liquid moving along the cranial grooves—a very graphic appeal to the wisdom of the ancestors! For card divination, an ordinary deck is used with all cards below the seven removed. After lighting a candle and praying, the *manbo* or *oungan* offers the cards to the client for cutting. These are then laid out in four rows of eight in front of the healer. The whole process is repeated twice, once to determine the best description of the problem and once to track down its supernatural connections. After the first spread, the healer begins tapping the cards in patterns dictated by his or her own inner perceptions. Occasionally a question will be raised or a statement made. For example: "There is trouble in your house. I see fighting." The client is free to say yes or no without prejudice. Gradually, through a series of such statements and responses, the contours of the problem reveal themselves. It should be emphasized that while this is clearly not a miraculous procedure or even one requiring extrasensory perception, it nevertheless calls on the intuitive skills of the practitioner and represents an important step in the curing. When the problem is articulated through this gradual dialectical process, its definition may well surprise even the client. I once witnessed a session in which a mother brought her young daughter for help because the child would not eat, was losing her hair, and had run away from home. In the course of settling on the appropriate description of the problem, the *manbo* uncovered something that was unknown to the mother and unspoken before by the daughter: the girl's stepfather was sexually abusing her.

Once a full picture of the problem emerges, the healer then lays out the cards once more to determine its cause or origin: "I see the spirits love you a lot. Ezili especially. Did you promise you were going to do something for her and then not do it?" By this means a complete diagnosis is made.

Diagnoses point to disruptions in relationships. Often the relation in question is with the spirits themselves. Broken promises, lax or insufficient offerings, or refusal of the spiritual vocation the *lwa* have chosen for a person can all be reasons for trouble. Many *manbo* and *oungan* have dramatic stories to tell about their own efforts to resist the desire of the *lwa* that they take the *asson*, that is, undergo initiation to the priesthood. One woman was hospitalized three times and given last rites on two occasions for an intestinal disorder, the cause of which medical doctors could never determine. (Eventually she obeyed the *lwa*, and thereafter she reported that she experienced no further health problems.) Obligations incurred or promises broken by family members generations back can emerge as the cause of the contemporary individual's troubles.

However, as was seen in the case of the sexually abused child, it is not always the spirits who cause a problem. For example, the cards often reveal that someone is suffering because of the "jealousy" of other persons. Jealousy is understood to be such a strong emotion that the lives of its targets can be seriously disrupted. Within the Vodou system the object of jealousy rarely escapes at least part of the burden of blame. Such an attitude reflects a society in which it is expected that anyone who has much should give much. Thus, a wealthy person is almost by definition thought to be stingy, and a very lucky person is suspected of having done "work with the left hand." A less serious but related diagnosis is that someone is suffering from "eyes." This mildly unsettling condition comes from the fact that too many people are paying attention to that individual. It may be that there is gossip circulating. With both jealousy and eyes, as with several other diagnostic categories, the troubled relationships are among the living. In such situations the spirits are called on for help, but there is no sense in which they are seen as causing the problem.

Sorcery and Ethics

Disruptions in relations with the spirits cause serious problems, yet in many ways it is an even more serious situation if, in the course of a "treatment," it is discovered that a person's problems arise from the fact that another human being has done "work" against them. The range of magical actions that fall under the category of "work" is considerable. It may only be that a rejected lover has gone to the *manbo* or *oungan* for a love charm, or it may be something more serious, such as an act of sorcery performed by a vengeful neighbor.

For example, sorcery is frequently implicated when a diagnosis is made that a woman has "fallen into perdition." "Perdition" is a condition that befalls a pregnant woman in which the child in her womb is "held" or "tied" to prevent it from growing. When a woman who has missed one or more menstrual periods and assumes herself to be pregnant experiences a discharge of blood, she suspects that she may have "fallen into perdition." In all pregnancies it is believed that the menstrual blood that would ordinarily exit from the body each month is held in the womb where it serves as nourishment for the child. In a state of perdition the nourishing blood bypasses the fetus. The fetus, however, is not expelled but held inside the mother. Fetuses are believed to be able to stay in a state of arrested growth for years until something is done to "cut off" the perdition or "untie" the child. When that is accomplished the monthly blood flow stops, and the child begins to do its "work" within the womb. The infant born nine months later is the one who was conceived before the state of perdition began. Falling into perdition can be caused by several things. It can be caused if "cold" is allowed to enter the womb. It can be caused by restive *lwa* or ancestral spirits. However, work of the left hand, specifically sorcery, is the most frequent diagnosis. All children, but especially the unborn, are said to be susceptible to being "caught" by a work of sorcery directed against a family.[7]

There is an underlying belief in what might be called an economy of energy in Haitian attitudes toward sorcery or the work of the left hand. A rather flat-footed way of articulating the content of this belief would be to say: nothing comes for free. For example, there is a significant distinction made in the types of powers that a person can call on for help in this life. There are first of all *espri fami* (family spirits), and then there are *pwe achte* (literally, "points that have been purchased"). Most often residing in some tangible object such as a stone or bottle (the "point"), these spirits are either the souls of persons who died without family, ceremony, or burial, or they are the free-floating spirits of another, often malevolent, sort.

Serving family spirits entails obligations that may strain resources and energy; however, the demands of family spirits theoretically never escalate beyond reason. Within a given family the living and the spirits are interdependent in a way that makes both parties exercise restraint. Powers that have been purchased are another matter. While it is understood that they may be extremely effective, they have neither history nor loyalty to curb their rapacious appetites. Consequently, working with the left hand leads all too easily to an ascending spiral of obligations. Stories are frequently told of *manbo* and *oungan* who turned to sorcery in a desperate moment and then found it impossible to extricate themselves. First they lost members of their family; finally they lost their own lives. This belief that a person ultimately pays for what is gained through illegitimate means is one moral force within Vodou that curbs the wanton practice of sorcery.

Another moral force is the belief that only in extreme circumstances may one use sorcery to harm another, and only if one is absolutely just in doing so. For example, there was a *manbo* who lost her home through the deception of a woman friend who stole the title papers. The former friend actually went to court in an effort to claim the house for herself. The *manbo* performed a very simple act of magic (there is a widespread belief that the simplest ritual acts are the most powerful)[8] that involved dropping a "point" or charm into a latrine. As a result of this, three people either fell sick or died: the judge, the lawyer, and the erstwhile friend. When this incident was discussed within the family, someone invariably noted that the *manbo* could do this with no fear of reprisal from humans or spirits because she was so clearly in the right. The house was hers.

Yet another belief that acts to curb destructive uses of spiritual power centers on that part of Vodou associated with cemeteries. Although a version of this system operates within the cities, the pattern is clearest in the rural areas where cemeteries are still family property. The first male to be buried in a cemetery is known as the Baron Simityè, Baron of the Cemetery. When a wrong has been done to an individual or family by someone from outside that group, a simple ritual performed in the cemetery calls on Baron to send a *mò*, one of the souls of the dead, to avenge that wrong. The Baron's power can never be used, by definition, by one family member against another.

What complicates this discussion of morality and the uses of power within Vodou is the fact that it is not always possible to keep the categories clear and distinct. What is sorcery from one person's perspective is no more than what was required for an effective treatment from another's point of view. For example, love magic may heal a broken heart or soothe wounded pride, but it also necessarily involves the manipulation of the will of another. Cemeteries in Haiti are littered with the evidence of this common sort of "work." Small male and female rag dolls bound face to face and stood on their heads (inversion creates change) in a jar or drinking glass are evidence of a work designed to bring about a reunion. The same dolls bound back to back indicate that the dissolution of a troublesome relationship was the desired result. One bound with its face to the back of the other is said to be in a position to "eat" the other, that is, to take revenge. Such routine magic is within the repertoire of most Vodou healers and does not involve trafficking with suspect or "purchased" spirits.

Understandably, most priests and priestesses claim to eschew the work of the left hand. Equally understandably, rumors circulate that this one or that one "serves with both hands." It is not unlikely that most sorcery rumors can be attributed to individuals or groups in conflict wherein each party, knowing their own spirituality to be rooted in family and tradition, can only assume that the practices of their enemies are not so rooted.

Knowledge and Power

In the course of treating a troubled person, Vodou priests and priestesses call on a variety of different types of knowledge and power. The word *konesans* (knowledge) is used to refer to learned skills such as herbalism and divination as well as to what might be called intuitive powers. The different degrees of initiation are seen as increasing *konesans*. At least part of what is meant by this is sensitivity to a sense of foreboding. The attuned person, the one with *konesans*, knows when to cancel a trip or a business appointment. At a higher level of development it may be the gift of "seeing" what is wrong with people just by looking at them. (Although called seeing, one *manbo* described its physical manifestation as a prickling in the scalp.) Many of the most sought-after Vodou healers are said to have this gift.

In addition to their own developed talents, priests and priestesses also call on a range of higher authorities in the healing process. Possession allows the healer access to the awesome wisdom and power of the *lwa*, and in fact it is often one of the *lwa* who prescribes the specifics of a cure. Quite detailed information about what should be done to treat a particular case can also come in dreams. One *manbo* said that it is usually her dead mother (a powerful *manbo* herself) appearing to her in dreams who provides the solutions to her most difficult cases.

Dreams can also function in healing ways in the lives of ordinary devotees. Dreams can give warnings about bad things to come, thus providing the means of possibly avoiding sickness or anger, robbery or accident. Both the dead and the *lwa* routinely appear in dreams to give warnings and advice. The spirits sometimes appear in dreams in the same form as they are depicted on Vodou altars. Individual *lwa* have been conflated with particular Catholic saints, and the inexpensive and popular chromolithographs of the saints have thus become the most common images of the spirits. However, it seems that even more frequently the *lwa* appear in dreams in disguise. Each dreamer has his or her own code which must be applied to interpret the dream. Often it is a friend who has a name or personal qualities reminiscent of the *lwa's* who comes to stand for that spirit in the dream world. Thus one *manbo* said: "Last night I dreamed about Gerard. [Saint Gerard is the Catholic saint conflated with Gède, the spirit of death.] Gerard asked me how my daughter was doing, if she was out of the hospital yet. That is when I got scared for my daughter. I was afraid she might really get sick because I know everytime I dream about Gerard, that's Papa Gède."

The care given by Vodou healers ranges from truly awesome displays of power to tender solace. I know of one *manbo* who brought her severely depressed female client into her home as part of the curing process. The woman had not spoken for nearly a year following the loss of a child. This mute condition, well known in Haiti and generally seen in young women, is considered especially difficult to treat. In the early stages of the treatment the *manbo* actually took the woman into her bed and held her until she slept. Yet treatments can also involve humiliation (e.g., being sent to the market to beg) and angry lectures from the spirits. In my experience, women healers routinely use the full range of care, from the solacing to the jarring, that is possible within the Vodou system. Male healers, by contrast, tend to remain authority figures throughout the healing process.

From a more general perspective, the jarring or confrontational aspects of Vodou healing are never separated from the overall context of familial care in which healing takes place. In fact, to make the distinction is to miss the coherence of the system. An image drawn from Haitian culture may make it easier to articulate this subtle point about the tone or ambience of caring within Vodou. Haiti is a child-centered culture. There are no events from which children are excluded. Yet the crying of infants and the misbehavior of older children are not tolerated. Crying babies are grabbed and rather roughly jostled into silence with unspoken messages that communicate at once the full attention of the caretaker and that person's unwillingness to tolerate the behavior. Older children can be given a harsh reproof at one moment and then a quick hug and kiss soon after. In a similar way traditional healers in Haiti can be possessed by an angry *lwa* without having that anger shape their personal relationship to the person seeking the cure.

The Creole verb *balanse* (to balance) has a special significance in Vodou and in healing within Vodou. When devotees take ritual objects off the altar they are instructed to *balanse*, to swing the objects from side to side. This is thought to awaken or enliven the objects and the spirits associated with them. The word can, however, be used in less constructive contexts. For example, when death touches a family it is said to "balance their house." The sense that balance is a dynamic condition is revealing, as is the notion that it comes out of opposition, whether that be the back-and-forth motion of the ritual *balanse* or the harsher clash of death against life. Within the Vodou view of things life is stirred up through opposition. This stirring and jarring, which can wound, is nevertheless healing when the clash of opposites is wisely orchestrated by the Vodou healer.

One example of a specific problem and cure will illustrate the confrontational dimension of Vodou healing. A young woman came to a *manbo* distraught, in fact nearly hysterical, because her husband had left her. In one moment the woman said she wanted her husband back; in the next she recounted a long history of his abuse. Finally, with a shrug of impatience, the *manbo* said harshly: "Pran tèt ou!" ("Get ahold of your head!") Three ritual baths were prescribed to be administered, one each week for the next three weeks. The first bath was made from warm milk in which cinnamon sticks had been steeped. About four cups of the liquid were placed in a small enamel basin and the woman was instructed to remove her clothes. Because this was a good luck bath, the liquid was applied to the body from bottom to top, starting at the feet and stroking upward. (The reverse would operate in a bath designed to remove bad luck, a more serious condition.) The second bath was composed of various liquors and perfumes. It was applied in a similar fashion, as was the third and final glorious combination of champagne, roses, and perfume.[9] After each treatment the woman was instructed to leave the infusion on her skin without washing for three days. The first bath, she reported, made her smell of sour milk "like a baby." After it she took to her bed and cried for most of a week. She said that the second bath, in which alcohol was the dominant ingredient, burned her eyes and genitals. The second ended the tears, but she was flooded with anger. She sought out her former husband and screamed and yelled at him until the neighbors intervened. She reported nothing remarkable from the third bath beyond the fact that she no longer felt so unhappy. This sequence of baths took a woman's ambivalence about the man in her life and concretized it. The first and second baths shook loose contradictory emotions; they jarred her into powerful and direct experiences of sadness and anger. From the resulting dynamic "balance" came the possibility of the third bath, which moved her beyond the extreme moods of the first two to a less precarious emotional state, one in which she gradually was able to let go of the destructive relationship. These baths, like so many of the Vodou treatments, can also

be seen as a ritual regression, a regression to infancy and then a movement back, or even as a ritual rebirth not entirely unlike that which is
accomplished through the initiation ceremonies.

Conclusion

"Moun fèt pou mouri," people are born to die—the saying reveals the
Haitian's sense that life is both short and painful. This verdict cannot
change; it can only be accepted. Yet in the midst of the struggle that is life
it is possible to enhance one's *chans* (luck) and minimize the *mizè* (suffering). This is accomplished in two ways: first, by respectful attention to the
web of sustaining human relationships that defines family, and second,
through conscientious service to the spirits who are after all members of
one's own extended family, even—from one perspective, at least—parts
of oneself. The spirits are served by the parent (fictive or actual) in the
name of the family. In order to serve the family well in this role, the priest
or priestess must have *konesans:* knowledge, intuition, insight into human
and spiritual affairs. Such knowledge is most often rooted in the *oungan*'s
or *manbo*'s own experience of suffering. To *kouche* (lie down, sleep, give
birth, die, and, specifically, to be initiated) is to take the risk necessary to
be healed oneself and through that process to enhance and focus one's
power and knowledge in order to heal others. Once gained, *konesans* carries with it a moral obligation that it be used justly and respectfully. Thus,
the *manbo* or *oungan* is one who knows how to *eshofe*, to raise the life
energy in individuals and groups, human and divine. Power thus mobi-
lized can then be concentrated in *pwe* (points) which are the concrete
embodiments of relationships human and divine. Problems properly
articulated in the concrete can be healed. One can pick up the *pwe* and
balanse—turn the point upside down and bring about change that heals.

Notes

1. Claude Lévi-Strauss, *The Savage Mind* (Chicago, 1966), pp. 1–33 (chap. 1,
   "The Science of the Concrete").
2. As will be seen below, there is a sense in which the dead continue to exist;
   however, none of the living would consider this existence superior to his
   or her own. Thus immortality does not function as a reward for sacrifices
   made in the present life.
3. A partial qualification to this characterization exists in the large numbers of
   homosexual priests who have genuine power and prestige within Vodou.
   This is somewhat surprising given the extreme homophobia in Haitian culture. However, it is only a partial qualification because many of these
   priests are more accurately described as bisexuals. They often have traditional families.

4. See William Bascom, *The Yoruba of Southwestern Nigeria* (New York, 1969); also Melville Herskovits, *Dahomey: An Ancient West African Kingdom*, 2 vols. (Evanston, IL, 1967).

5. Marriage to a Vodou spirit—a ritual complete with marriage license, an exchange of rings (wherein the spirit is represented by his or her *chwal*), a wedding cake, and, on occasion, champagne—is a ritual that does not demand that a person experience possession. It nevertheless involves a life-long commitment to the spirit. One day a week is dedicated to the spirit spouse. Special colors sacred to the *lwa* must be worn on that day, and the devotee must sleep alone so that the spirit may appear in dreams.

6. "Taking the *asson*" as a path to gaining status as a priest or priestess is a ritual performed mainly in the south of Haiti and in Port-au-Prince. In the northern part of the country such status is conferred by virtue of family position or reputation as a healer. The initiation rituals are costly for those who take the *asson*. It may be partly as a result of economic factors that individuals sometimes claim to have received priestly training in dreams, visions, or periods of time spent "under the water."

7. Gerald F. Murray, "Women in Perdition: Ritual Fertility Control in Haiti," in *Culture, Natality and Family Planning*, eds. John F. Marshall and Steven Polgar (Chapel Hill, NC: 1976), pp. 59–78.

    Murray points out that the socially useful part of this explanatory scheme is that, in providing the possibility of a pregnancy much longer than nine months, a woman can claim the father of her child to be almost anyone with whom she has ever had sexual relations. This in turn allows her to choose among fathers the one who is most likely to be able to give meaningful support. Given the current social instability all over Haiti, finding men with the means and temperament to be responsible fathers is one of the major problems faced by women.

8. See Serge Larose, "The Meaning of Africa in Haitian Vodu," in *Symbols and Sentiments: Cross-Cultural Studies in Symbolism*, ed. Ioan Lewis (New York, 1977), pp. 85–116.

9. The ingredients for Vodou treatments are paid for by the client. Fees for the healer beyond the cost of materials are understood to be gifts, and theoretically it is up to the client to decide how much he or she will offer. In practice, however, the range of what is appropriate is usually well known to clients without their asking. It is worth noting that many of the most sought-after healers are not prosperous persons. They adhere strictly to the tradition that healing powers are not to be used for inordinate profit.

CHAPTER 12

Polynesian Religious Foundations of Hawaiian Concepts Regarding Wellness and Illness

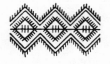

KATHARINE LUOMALA

Before the arrival of Westerners, the priesthood of eastern Polynesia had developed a highly refined religious philosophy of the universe. Every aspect of culture in this area, which includes the Hawaiian Islands,[1] expressed an elaborate and holistic worldview that shaped concepts of wellness and illness, life and death, for human beings and for the natural world. Within this perspective, medicine was inseparable from religion. David Malo (c. 1793–1853), a Hawaiian historian, wrote, "The medical treatment of the sick was a matter that belonged to the worship of the gods."[2] Despite some two hundred years of Western influence, the traditional philosophy, attenuated and modified, lives on in folk belief and medical practice.[3]

Hawaiians believed, as did other Polynesians, that human beings, natural and man-made objects, and nature itself (which was inhabited by innumerable beings) constituted a generically related, sentient totality.[4] Each object that possessed psychic, utilitarian, or aesthetic significance in daily life—each plant, animal, and feature of the earth, sea, sky, or underworld—was a person, not a thing. According to this philosophy, every existent being had a name, personality, soul, vital principle, power, feelings, and needs, just as did human beings. These phenomena embodied (kino lau) gods, nature spirits, and souls of the dead. If properly approached, they would respond, voluntarily or involuntarily, to human rituals, prayers, spells, and offerings. In addition, other natural phenomena, such as rocks, possessed no spirit but were animated by mana (extraordinary power) that could, through appropriate rites and sacrifices, contribute to human health and fertility. Some contemporary Hawaiians believe that such rocks give birth to pebbles. Many Hawaiians who were questioned in 1971 in a Hawaiian community near Honolulu drew no clear-cut or inflexible line between the natural and the supernatural; they "did not distinguish between man and nature, between one's own body and the rest of the environment, or between things living and nonliving."[5] For them, all these constituted an interconnected totality.

The traditional pantheon was large and ever increasing because priests knew how to create new spirits and gods, or new spirits chose them as their caretakers. The Hawaiian national gods, particularly Kāne, Kū, Lono, and Kanaloa (also worshiped throughout eastern Polynesia), took multiple forms, had many overlapping functions in daily and national life, and bore epithets descriptive of specific forms and functions. But, according to Samuel Kamakau (1815–1876), another Hawaiian historian, "the god for the day when a god was needed" was the ancestral aumakua who had the dual role of protecting or punishing his or her descendants in each extended family ('ohana).[6] It was to their aumakua (and the souls of their immediate ancestors) that individuals prayed that they might cure illness, resolve family troubles, increase the supply of plants and fish, give protection from black magic, and forgive every wrong. At a meal supplicants offered the aumakua the essence of their food and a beverage made from kava to strengthen its spirit, which then returned to possess a medium who named its embodiments and announced taboos to be observed; through this medium the aumakua promised to bring the family health, blessings, and freedom from danger and fear. An aumakua might be a primordial elemental force, as was Pele, who was embodied in the volcano but could take human form. She was the aumakua of her living, human descendants, and at death they joined her in the volcano. Shark aumakuas were numerous in this island environment, and a family could create a new shark guardian by having a priest transfigure the corpse of a family member, a stillborn child, or a miscarriage into a shark. Besides family aumakuas there were individual, occupational, and professional aumakuas. A medical practitioner recited the names of his aumakuas—deified healers—to add power and confidence to a treatment.

Because each element in the universe that was significant in daily life was in intimate, psychic rapport with every other, persons might deliberately or involuntarily strengthen or weaken that relationship to harm or benefit themselves, others, and nature. Numerous orders of priestly specialists called kahunas had been trained in an occupation, craft, or profession. They applied their practical skills and, more importantly, their relevant religious knowledge in order to adjust the equilibrium of relationships in the cosmos and thereby achieve the results desired by those who employed them.[7] Learned kahunas existed in each division of culture. The priests of the two highest orders, who were said to know all specialties, served paramount chiefs and gained political power through their superior knowledge and communion with the national gods. They officiated at all ceremonies related to a high-ranking chief or chiefess. The lower orders included the priestly medical doctors (*kāhuna lapa'au*), among whom were many suborders, organized according to specialty. Some kahunas acted as sorcerers and caused much illness; the healers had to discover their identity and overcome their evil work. Bodily health, the greatest blessing conferred by the gods, could be lost on account of one or more overlapping categories of illness or injury. The following summary of major categories shows that no matter what the category or the specific disorder it encompassed, both the cause and the cure were the work of gods. A priestly medical healer, dedicated to their service, had therefore to treat both the physical body and the psyche with the gods' powers.

Categories of Illness

BODY SICKNESS AND AUMAKUA SICKNESS

One category, "ordinary sickness" or "body sickness" (*ma'i kia'i kino*), consisted of ailments whose physical symptoms were generally responsive to the ministrations and prayers of a man or a woman *(kahuna lā'au lapa'au)* who specialized in herbs, massage, steambaths, and related treatments.[8] Whether or not the *ma'i kino* category was first conceptualized in post-European times is unimportant, because a priestly medical practitioner always believed that his ritually prepared potions and ointments were only the physical vehicles for the mana, or supernatural power, that his incantations and offerings to his god of medicine had activated. If a patient failed to improve, the kahuna suspected that he had a serious case of "aumakua sickness" and must be treated by a kahuna aumakua.

"Aumakua sickness" *(ma'i 'aumakua)* afflicted everyone at some time, was not amenable to medicine (in fact its mana might be fatal), and was most resistant to treatment.[9] It was a form of "sickness from inside" *(ma'i na loko)*, one that was usually caused by family troubles. To treat this illness the kahuna aumakua or the male head of the extended family used supernatural guidance and a religious ceremony of "mental cleansing" *(ho'oponopono)*. Each participant, including the patient, confessed any transgressions and sought human and divine forgiveness. A transgression *(hala)* within the family had, it was believed, angered the aumakua, who then punished the sufferer—who was not necessarily the guilty person. The sin might have been a broken promise to the god or a family member, a curse or other evil act, an entanglement of many bitter and hostile feelings, neglect of the aumakua, disrespect for consecrated and tabooed things, or defilement *(haumia)* from psychically polluting people or things.

The kahuna aumakua, who from the beginning (as in the case of any illness) had been in communication with his own gods through dreams, visions, omens, trances, male or female spirit mediums, or divination through pebbles or other mechanical means, announced (if he thought there was hope of a cure) what offerings, sacrifices, and prayers the aumakua required for atonement *(kalahala, "forgive fault")* before it restored health and harmony to the family. For the ceremonial closure *(pani)* of a successful treatment the kahuna might have the patient eat a seaweed called *kala*—a symbolic choice, since the word also means "free" and "untied." He also ceremonially cleansed *(ma'ema'e)* and purified *(hui-kala)* the patient in order to restore the former state of holiness by sprinkling the patient with consecrated salt water mixed with turmeric on which he had breathed or by having the patient immerse himself five times (the ritual number) in the sea.[10] A similar pattern was frequently part of the treatment of many other spirit-caused illnesses not only in Hawaii but throughout Polynesia.

An important category of conditions treated by priestly specialists related to pregnancy and childbirth, conditions that were always fraught with polluting psychic and physical dangers to a woman and to her male and female associates. Certain specialists also diagnosed by examining blotches and veins on a newborn infant, what they considered inherited or latent diseases that would afflict the child in adulthood unless treated immediately; treating the parents, however, was the same as treating the child.[11]

EVILS CAUSED BY SORCERY

A large and complex category was "sickness from outside" *(ma'i na waho mai)* caused by sorcery, which, in fact, was suspected in any illness or injury. Hawaiians shared the general Polynesian belief that malignant influences and malicious spirits, usually sent by sorcerers but sometimes by mischievous imps, could invade a person's body to cause havoc and bring on "visiting sickness" *(ma'i kipa)*. Medicines and offerings to the gods were of no avail until the healing kahuna had returned the evil to the originator and exorcised the unwelcome visiting demons. He would first, however, have his patient confess any transgressions in the matter and then purify the patient. The countersorcerer next pitted the mana of his gods and incantations against those of the sorcerer until one was victorious. All medical practice was really a battle of mana between healer and whoever or whatever had sent the disease. Each type of "outside sickness" was named, identified, defined in terms of its cause and cure, and connected with specialists. Among a variety of outside sicknesses, only a few types will be mentioned here.

The principal elements of sorcery techniques, according to Peter H. Buck, were similar throughout Polynesia except in the west.[12] In the west, in Tonga for instance, a sorcerer used imitative magic rather than spirits. He concealed in a man's house some leaves, which had previously been inserted into a bamboo tube or wrapped in tapa. While the leaves rotted the man would sicken and die. Elsewhere contagious magic was used, with the dominant element being some material thing that had been in contact with the proposed victim and therefore contained his or her vital essence. By means of this bait the sorcerer sent malicious spirits into the victim while he chanted repetitively his death-dealing and literally descriptive spells of what the victim was to suffer. This was *pule 'anā'anā*, "praying to death," the most feared type of sorcery among Hawaiians. Their aristocrats had the highest development in Polynesia of protective measures against assassination by sorcery. Hawaiian chiefs and chiefesses depended less than even the Tahitians on their inherited mana and personal taboos of sanctity to protect themselves. Like Tahitians, they had hereditary attendants of chiefly rank who carefully disposed of their refuse, although only Hawaiians had special utensils in which to deposit their food scraps and bodily wastes. In New Zealand, on the other hand, the chiefs, at least those of the highest rank, had sufficient mana to be automatically protected. Further, the system of village latrines, unique in

Polynesia, and the sanctions connected with them prevented the use of body wastes for sorcery.

Counteracting 'anā'anā was considered difficult, and Hawaiians, like Tahitians, combined a ceremony of confession by the patient with prayers to the gods for their forgiveness of sins and for the black magician's death. As usual, a sorcerer was not selective, in that any member of the family he hated should suffer. "Prayer," Kamakau wrote, "was the one great 'poultice,'" and it accompanied all remedies for curing and revenge.[13] Cases of individuals being prayed to death are frequently reported in the literature, and cases continue to be reported into the twentieth century. Western-trained physicians have described the effects on victims they have tried to treat.[14] Although there are still healing kahunas, the popular connotation of the term "kahuna" today is that of an evil sorcerer.

Sorcery, according to Kamakau, began in the eighteenth century on Molokai Island and spread throughout the rest of the Hawaiian group.[15] More than likely he meant certain types of sorcery, not sorcery as such. Origin myths tell of a female medium Ka-'alae-nui-a-Hina (Great Mudhen of Hina) and her two brothers Kāne-ka-huila-o-ka-lani (Kāne in the Lightning) and Kāne-i-kaulana-'ula (Kāne in the Red Sunset), who were sorcerers from mythical Kahiki across the sea and who scattered the first diseases over the islands. Many people were cured by the first priestly healers, who were Ka-maka-nui-'aha-'ilono (The Great Eye Messenger), Lono-pūhā (pūhā, "abscess"), and (Kāne)-kōlea-moku (muku), whose embodiment is the plover (kōlea).

Sorcery, it seems, increased in the eighteenth century, a period of warfare and of the rise of Kamehameha, the great Hawaiian king (1795–1819), who adopted the Molokai gods as well as other captured gods to gain their support. The most dangerous Molokai gods, the Kālaipāhoa (Cut with a Dagger), included the three Kahiki sorcerers, the goddesses Pua and Kapo of the Pele family, and others. These gods were embodied in three supernaturally poisonous trees, a mere scrap from which would sicken and kill a person. A victim could be restored to life with a bit of another supernatural but healing Molokai tree named for its god, Ma'iola (Cure Sickness). The sorcery gods' caretakers were said to send them like shooting stars over great distances to murder people. However, anyone with a Kālaipāhoa chip or image felt protected from sorcery-caused illness and paralysis. It is said that Kamehameha's own images when laid beside him helped in his illness; his righteousness and religious faith enabled the mana of his gods to overwhelm that of the hostile gods.[16]

In ho'ounauna ("sending" sorcery), Molokai kahunas created new sending gods (metaphorically, "biting sharks of the land") by transfiguring parts of a relative's corpse. A specialist could send these evil gods back to the originator by a ritual (kuehu) that included shaking a tapa or shredded ti leaves in a certain way over the victim. Frequently a kahuna created a familiar spirit ('unihipili) from the vital essence of a dead relative's hair, bones, or other parts either to steal a person's soul or to aid the person in some way; this dangerous spirit would turn on its caretaker if neglected. In *ho'opi'opi'o* sorcery, by touching a part of his own body in sight of his victim, a kahuna was said to be able to afflict his victim with pain in that part unless the gesture was noted and returned. In *ho'omanamana* a sorcerer imbued an object with destructive mana; the term also refers to imbuing a newly carved image with mana and sanctity. Suggestion and perhaps hypnotism were used by both the healing and killing kahunas. When fear alone failed to kill, genuinely poisonous concoctions were secretly administered.

A prominent chief's death was considered unnatural and the result of his having been prayed to death. A unique Hawaiian institution was the "burning" *(kuni)* ceremony held to identify the murderer. A specialist burned sacrifices as well as part of the corpse, chanted spells, and fought insanely with the sorcerer's spirits until supernatural signs revealed either the murderer's fate or his apparition, which a fearless kahuna announced regardless of the murderer's rank. *Kuni* was expensive. If forty dogs and eighty fowls were sacrificed, according to Malo, for "an ordinary person" (a wealthy commoner?), four hundred dogs and a very large number of fowls were required for a chief. A kahuna was very highly paid for such services.[17]

MADNESS

Like other Polynesians, Hawaiians distinguished between real insanity and temporary derangement such as evidenced by countersorcerers; by mediums possessed by a god; by inspired but eccentric prophets; by persons inspired to predict the future while in a delirium, trance, or ecstacy; and by mourners overcome with grief for a deceased chief. A countersorcerer in battling a rival kahuna's spirits often acted as if insane by eating filth and poisonous things to which his training had made him immune, by exposing his private parts, and by engaging in other peculiar behavior in order to distract his rival's gods from hearing his destructive incantations. By contrast, a truly insane person *(pupule)* and a raving maniac *(hehena)* continually ate filth, exposed and mutilated himself, and acted peculiarly.[18] This condition was a type of "outside sickness" because the craziness, raving, palsy, or imbecility was caused, it was believed, by Maka-kū-koa'e (Eye Set on Tropic Bird), a male sorcery god whose victims jumped over cliffs where tropic birds fly. Many people still fear to be out after dark because night-prowling, malevolent, homeless ghosts *(lapu)* are able to cause madness and disease.

Although the only function of the god Kāne-'ula'ula (Red Kāne) was to care for the insane, kahunas regarded insanity as very difficult to treat. They might try plant medicines such as kava, a relaxant; or try to exorcise the possessing spirit by chanting while rubbing the patient with excrement, so offensive to any spirit that it would flee.[19] For an afflicted chief they might try appeasing the gods with a human sacrifice; for a commoner the sacrifice was a speckled fowl called 'ōpulepule (a synonym for "crazy," pupule), which through the inherent mana of words and breath supposedly counteracted the insanity.[20] An unmanageable patient was tied up and sometimes left to die of hunger.[21] Some were beaten to death. That a heiau, that is, a temple area, at Waolani, Oahu, was a place of refuge for the insane, lame, bald, crippled, humpbacked, and sick may have added to its reputation as the home of 'e'epa, those peculiar supernatural beings gifted with incomprehensible and miraculous powers. Even into the twentieth century disabled persons might be insultingly told to go to Waolani where they belonged. Tahitians, believing that the insane were inspired or possessed by a god, respected but avoided them, and exercised no control over them since their actions were those of gods, not humans. They were abandoned, unmourned, and left to die of their own actions.[22]

SUICIDE

Until recent years reports of suicide among Hawaiians were extremely rare except among the insane and in the case of those individuals who, as was the custom, took their lives to be companions in death with a beloved chief or chiefess. Otherwise suicide was not socially sanctioned. Although suicide by defeated warriors occurred in some parts of Polynesia (in Pukapuka they asked relatives to bury them alive), Hawaiian warriors who escaped capture expected to fight another day.

Domestic life and sexual love occasionally led to suicide. A folktale about a woman leaping over a precipice to her death because of her lazy and improvident husband is unusual because in other domestic tales about a lazy or jealous husband the woman's family, particularly her brother, on hearing of domestic strife takes the woman back to her childhood home. Blighted love as a cause of suicide—sometimes by hanging—appears in romantic fictions, but the dead lover is usually restored to life. Love led Ka'ahumanu, Kamehameha's favorite wife, to attempt suicide when the king temporarily deserted her for her sister. One dark night the grief-stricken woman swam out to sea to drown and be eaten by sharks. Her attempt failed because of an exhausted male attendant who had insisted on accompanying her; twice she had to rescue him from drowning and get him safely ashore. Her response differed from that of a jealous co-wife who, according to a folktale, killed her rival; but her angry husband then beat her to death. Violence, including murder and destruction of property, was in the past often a jealous and angry man's reaction against a rival. Male violence is still a common reaction to frustration, but recently suicide has been added as another male response to such troubles.

Injured pride, often the cause of suicide in some parts of traditional Polynesia, led around 1809 to the most famous example of suicide in Hawaii. Kalaniakua was a sacred chiefess of the highest possible rank and was likened to a goddess because she had inherited the mana of both of her highborn parents, who were brother and sister. (Such marriages were permitted only—and in fact preferred—for royalty, in order to keep blood lines pure.) Kalaniakua died of "Kālaipāhoa poison," prepared by a chief at her request, because of "shame at the frequent jibes" from her elder half-sister on points of prestige and privilege and because of accusations that she had destroyed her unborn child fathered by Kamehameha the Great.[23]

A traditional institutionalized form of suicide was that by Hawaiians who demonstrated their love for a deceased chief or chiefess by starving themselves to death or having themselves strangled in order to become "companions in death" *(moepu'u)*. There were also forms of involuntary *moepu'u*, as when a man slew his junior companion at a chief's secret burial place to prevent him from revealing its location to those who might steal the mana-rich bones for fishhooks and other artifacts.[24] Also from one to forty war captives, taboo-violators, and members of a segregated, hereditary group of inferiors called *kauwā* might be sacrificed to honor the deceased and his gods. After Kamehameha the Great began to regard all people as taboo, that is, sacred to Liholiho (his firstborn son by his sacred wife Ke'ōpūolani and his chosen successor), he discouraged all forms of *moepu'u*. In 1815, when Keku'iapoiwa Liliha (Ke'ōpūolani's mother and Kalaniakua's elder sister) died and chiefs and chiefesses wanted her husband Pueo to be her death companion because they felt his taboo violations had killed her, Kamehameha said that anyone who tried to kill Pueo would become the death companion. Although people sought to be Kamehameha's *moepu'u* when he died in 1819, they were restrained. In 1823, when Ke'ōpūolani died, the *moepu'u* custom was prevented because of Kamehameha's earlier proclamation and because the queen had died a Christian.[25] Variations of the custom occurred elsewhere in Polynesia. Slaves were killed in New Zealand to serve a dead chief in the afterworld, and widows might strangle themselves. In Tonga, a great chief's widows were strangled, and one or two men were buried alive in the vault of the Tui Tonga, the most sacred personage in the kingdom.

EXOTIC DISEASE AND EPIDEMIC

A post-Western category of illness, "foreign disease" *(ma'i malihini)*, included all new diseases introduced after 1778, when Captain James Cook visited the islands. In Hawaii, as in other islands visited by his ships, his crew introduced venereal diseases. Ships that arrived later brought other infectious and contagious diseases (some more than once) such as Asiatic cholera(?), whooping cough, measles, mumps, smallpox, bubonic plague, scarlet fever, typhoid fever, yellow fever, influenza, and leprosy. Contagious and infectious diseases were called "jumping sickness" *(ma'i lele)* because of the rapidity with which they spread; each disease had a descriptive name. Because Hawaiians, like other Polynesians, had no immunity, the death toll was heavy among young and old, chiefs and commoners, and it further decimated a population whose fertility was already reduced by venereal diseases established previously. Two well-known deaths were those of King Kamehameha II (Liholiho) and Queen Kamehamalu, both of whom died of measles while visiting London in 1824.

The first of the three greatest epidemics in Hawaiian history was *'ōku'u* (perhaps Asiatic cholera) in the early 1800s, when according to various estimates probably fewer than 15,000 and perhaps under 5,000 died (although one estimate was 175,000). It weakened the people, the government, and the army. Kamehameha the Great lost enough soldiers to lead him to abandon his plan to conquer Kauai, the only militarily unconquered island. He himself was very ill. The second worst epidemic was during four months of 1848 when a combination of measles, whooping cough, diarrhea, and influenza killed an estimated 10,000. Then in 1853 the first of three smallpox epidemics killed between 5,000 and 6,000. Every year, however, outbreaks of one or more of the new diseases resulted in numerous deaths among Hawaiians and foreigners.[26]

Kahunas found their traditional treatments—herbal cathartics, enemas, and infusions; copious draughts of seawater; and immersion in the ocean (the universal remedy for physical and psychic cleansing and purification)—of little avail. Patients sought to cool their fevers and wash off cutaneous eruptions in cold streams and winds. One desperate kahuna had his smallpox patients bathe in a muddy pond from which a cow later drank—and died of smallpox. American Protestant missionaries, who had begun to arrive in 1820, fought against the medical kahunas' treatments and idolatry. Converts, including even the native pastors, the missionaries said, served Jehovah in health and their pagan gods in sickness. Although some converts included Jehovah and biblical phrases in prayers to aumakuas, they felt that Jehovah cared only for the soul and not for the body's ills. When a kahuna's patient recovered he attributed recovery to the aumakuas, whereas the missionary attributed it to the "True Physician," Jehovah.[27]

Social and Historical Conditions

Not only foreign diseases decimated the population. The commoners' hunger and poverty weakened their physical resistance, and yet the paramount chiefs, in order to buy foreign goods, demanded more and more tribute of food and other supplies for the ships and ordered the people away from their fishing and farming to cut sandalwood for export. This was a major departure from earlier custom; formerly a paramount chief redistributed the tribute to the gods and also to the chiefs who supervised his lands, passing on some of their share to commoners' households. War fatalities increased with foreign weapons until 1795, when Kamehameha had at last consolidated the chiefdoms he had conquered into a central- ized kingdom. His reallocation of lands dislocated both chiefs and com- moners, and a chief's traditional responsibility for his retainers' welfare deteriorated. After Kamehameha's death this responsibility further dete- riorated when Kamehameha II (Liholiho), abetted by two of his father's widows (his mother Ke'ōpūolani and foster mother and regent Ka'ahu- manu), the high priest, and the prime minister, abrogated the religious law (the taboo system) because of three decades of Western influence and social, economic, and political factors.[28] E. S. Craighill Handy has called the taboo system the keystone of the arch supporting Hawaiian culture.[29] Sanctioned by the gods, the taboo system had been a means of personal and social control and of responsibility at every level of authority in a society that was composed of hereditary, stratified, and endogamous social classes (some scholars call them castes). On top was a small group of chiefs *(ali'i)* ranked among themselves, then came numerous com- moners *(maka'āinana,* "people of the land") and a small group of segre- gated inferiors *(kauwā)* considered polluting to the other two classes.

In 1778 there was a homogeneous population estimated at between 250,000 and 300,000. Within forty-five years it had declined by over half. The 70,000 Hawaiians in 1853 represented for the last time the largest ethnic group in the islands; intermarriage with foreign residents was steadily increasing, and young men continued to leave the islands. By 1967 "probably not more than a thousand could accurately claim unmixed ancestry, in the strictest sense of the term."[30] The census began to eliminate its former distinction between "pure Hawaiian" and "part Hawaiian." Now Filipinos, Japanese, and Caucasians outnumbered them.

During the first half of the nineteenth century, Western medicine, available to a very few Hawaiians from mission and ship doctors, was scarcely developed enough to ameliorate health conditions.[31] Further, Hawaiians and other Polynesians believed that Western medicine might cure foreign diseases, but not if they were combined with indigenous dis- eases; the Western physician, they felt, treated only the body and not the spiritual cause. Even today a Hawaiian not medically ill, but still suffer- ing, will seek out a kahuna who is a healer, or he will be advised by an understanding Western-trained doctor to consult one. Although much acculturated, Hawaiians still emphasize the role of the supernatural as an adjustive mechanism in illness and other crises. They turn to it particularly when empirical knowledge and techniques have not solved the problem, and those who know little about either Western health or Hawaiian therapeutic knowledge depend on the supernatural more than do those who have either only much Western knowledge or only much Hawaiian knowledge. Hawaiians still distinguish between foreign disease (ma'i malihini) and indigenous disease (ma'i kama'āina). There is still the distinction between "body sickness" and "aumakua sickness."

In 1978, residents in a Hawaiian community near Honolulu believed that negative words and actions as well as negative and insincere thoughts and emotions can make the responsible individual or an innocent person in the household suffer from "retributive comeback" in the form of illness, misfortune, or death; or a third party may suffer from it if two individuals or groups dispute over a person or a possession. The spiritual activators are Hawaiian gods, the Christian God, or unnamed, unknown forces; the human activators use sorcery, a curse, or the return of evil to the originator. If self-examination to determine the cause of an illness or other trouble fails, an individual consults, perhaps, a kahuna or a Christian minister. The treatment is to ask the wronged person's forgiveness directly or through prayer (traditionally forgiveness must be granted), to change one's ways, and to seek outside spiritual support and allies.[32]

ALOCHOL AND TOBACCO

Alcohol abuse has been a major problem since Westerners introduced alcohol and knowledge of distilling spirits from sugar and ti roots (Cordyline terminalis). Hawaiians also learned to make beer from ti roots, sweet potatoes, mountain apples, and other plants. No evidence exists that islanders made fermented beverages in precontact times despite their fondness for fermented poi, a staple food made from taro root.[33] Rum was first introduced, it is said, around 1791 by a Captain Maxwell (no given name reported), who invited Kamehameha and his party aboard ship, where they became drunk. When Kamehameha returned ashore, people, terrified, thought he had gone mad. He and other chiefs as well as foreign residents built stills; rum drinking and drunkenness became common among chiefs and commoners of both sexes. Foreigners introduced other liquors besides rum. Kamehameha, at first "strongly addicted," later became a strictly temperate drinker, and is said to have passed a "stringent prohibitory law" in 1818. His queens, however, drank to excess when his religious duties required him to sleep two nights, four times a month, at a heiau, that is, a temple area.[34]

Port cities—Lahaina on Maui and Honolulu on Oahu—had the most drunkenness, but it became rare on Maui and its three neighboring islands after Hoapili, the stern governor, took charge. Legislation between 1826 and 1849 to eliminate stills and regulate grog shops in Honolulu was spearheaded by Christianized elder chiefs and chiefesses despite opposition from foreign residents, certain chiefs, and intermittently King Kamehameha III. In 1838 two liquor laws were passed, partly through the influence of the temperance movement in the United States and through the concern of some whaling captains. The laws sought to eliminate stills in the kingdom and to limit the number of grog shops in Honolulu; hours were regulated and liquor retailed by the glass only. That same year the kingdom's first import duty was on liquor. Yet alcohol abuse continued, especially among royalty and its court.[35]

Besides alcohol, Westerners introduced tobacco; pipe smoking became widespread, and the wealthy also smoked cigars. Tobacco grew readily, and smokers preferred it green. Tobacco, and by 1809 liquor, began to replace kava as an offering to the gods. In 1838, Dr. Alonzo Chapin described the phenomenon he had observed between 1832 and 1835 thus: "[Smokers inhale] the full volume of smoke directly into the lungs, retaining it there as long as breath can be held. Individuals have been killed by its effects, and how much disease may have been induced or exacerbated thereby remains to be ascertained."[36] Tobacco and alcohol abuse became common throughout Polynesia.

KAVA

Except for fresh and salt water and coconut liquid, the only indigenous Polynesian beverage was kava *(Piper methysticum)*. In its several cultivated and wild varieties of differing quality and potency, it was an integral part of Hawaiian culture, and it was gathered, prepared, and used with reverence, ritual, and prayer.[37] Its sacredness came from the gods Kāne and Kanaloa, who had brought it from Kahiki. Kāne, the god of procreation and the water of life, used his digging stick, the active symbol of fertility, to open up freshwater springs in the earth, the symbolic womb, in order to mix the water with the macerated root. Like their human descendants, the two gods often drank to excess.

Kava was the most essential type of offering to any god or spirit—to the four great gods in communal ceremonies, to a kahuna's familiar spirit, to a sorcerer's god, and to Lono, the god of rain, abundance, and freedom from trouble and illness, to whom the head of a household prayed twice daily. Kava, it was believed, soothed and propitiated the supernatural beings who craved it as their means of sustenance; as with all offerings, they consumed the essence, the people drank the material substance. Spirit mediums drank kava as part of their ritual to invite the gods to possess them. A kahuna treating a patient ill from a sorcerer's "sending gods" drank the kava himself, an act that somehow pacified the patient's demons, whom he then asked to leave his patient. Medical priests also used kava extensively, not only as a medicine for numerous ailments afflicting men, women, and children but as a means of divination to determine the patient's prognosis. Chiefs and commoners drank it before meals and at night to ease muscular fatigue and soreness, and to induce sleep.

Chiefs, having more access to it than commoners, drank it for pleasure, sociability, and hospitality, and they combined it with diet and prayer as part of a strict regimen to lose weight. Both the chief honored by being chosen to prepare the kava at a ceremonial gathering and the sequence of offering the cups demonstrated the rank of each participating chief, and a change in this ceremony might be the first signal of a chief's rise or fall in political importance. Chiefs who drank kava often and to excess aged prematurely, suffered from debility, and had scaly, cracked, and ulcerous skin, as well as blood-shot, inflamed eyes; and they experienced difficulty in walking. Their minds, however, remained clear. When they discontinued the habit they recovered fairly well unless they had been drinking excessively for many years.

A modern pharmacological study on moderate use states the following:

> The effect of drinking 15 grams of kava rootstock in a half pint of water is to pleasantly paralyze, at the cord level, sensory transmission, then the innervation of striated musculature. A euphoria develops during which the mind remains clear; the drinker is tranquil and friendly, and refuses to be annoyed; and finally, if the dose is enough sleep ensues. Several hours of dreamless sleep follow; the drinker awakes feeling marvelously well, and no hangover occurs.[38]

Although mission doctors sometimes used kava as medicine and it soon became part of Western pharmacopoeias, American Protestant missionaries sought to eradicate Hawaiian cultivation and use because of the connection with the indigenous religion and, after the abolition of the taboo system in which kava had been a sacred substance, because of its excessive use by all classes. The growing commercial value of kava later made control of its cultivation difficult, and when the kingdom acquired a monopoly on its sale a permit was required in some places even for medicinal use. Meanwhile alcohol abuse continued to rise and thus helped limit the use of kava. Hawaiians say, "The man who drinks kava is still a man, but the man who drinks liquor becomes a beast."

Kava was unimportant in the rest of eastern Polynesia, but in the western region kava ceremonies and the use of a special kava bowl were dominant cultural features. In Samoa, for example, a kava ceremony of varied importance and formality initiated and concluded every major activity. But unlike Hawaii, religion figured in only two or three of the ceremonies. A religiously oriented village ceremony using kava was held during widespread illness or loss of crops. Members of a paternal kin group gathered when an important male member was ill; an officiating elder offered a kava root and a cup of kava to the family god, and each participant confessed any ill feeling toward the patient that may have angered the family god. Also, each evening the family's titled male member, officiating as the family priest, made a kava libation to the family god and prayed then and again in the morning for the family's protection and welfare.[39]

Care for the Sick

Early Western reports on care or lack of it for the sick and disabled provide no basis for generalization. Undoubtedly epidemics and cultural change worsened indigenous nurturing practices. During smallpox epidemics Western visitors saw dying children and adults, abandoned either because others in the family had died or because they had fled in terror. The disabled and nearly helpless were not always killed as sometimes claimed; on the contrary, both Cook's expedition in 1778 and Arago's in 1819 reported altogether some dozen cases of adults and children whose disabilities had not led people to kill them. Also, skeletal remains in an indigenous cemetery at Mokapu, Oahu, were found to include many examples of progressively developed, long-term, and handicapping deterioration of the spine and other anomalies.[40]

The group most concerned for individuals who were ill, dying, or undergoing some other life crisis was the tribelike community. It was composed of members in their bilateral extended family and its branches by birth, marriage, and adoption and was dispersed from sea to mountain. Kinfolk assembled to give practical and psychological assistance and, through their combined mana and affection, to spare the patient from feeling lonely and unloved. If the afflicted person were a chief, forty or more friends and relatives might gather to assist a kahuna, himself a chief, in administering a drastic remedy reserved for chiefs, from which the patient might not recover. When a great chief or chiefess was ill or dying, commoners and members of the patient's kinship group assembled from all islands to camp nearby to offer solace and aloha, that is, love. Missionaries deplored these gatherings as idolatrous, yet one of them when alone and ill wrote yearningly of the comfort and affection of his kin across the sea. Thus familial and societal aid in illness was greatly valued; but, while both commoners and chiefs cared about an elite person's welfare, and a community cared about a commoner's, no one cared what happened to a *kauwā*, a tabooed outcast, except another *kauwā*.[41]

An individual's social class, birth order, and amount of mana (if any) determined the significance of ceremonies held for that person. Polynesian gods and people were ranked among themselves, with the highest having the most divine power. A small group of Hawaiian chiefs and chiefesses were regarded as earthly representatives of the gods because they were the firstborn sons or daughters of parents who were brother and sister in the senior lineage of their kinship group and they traced direct descent from the primal forces shaping the universe. Worship by the senior male in the senior lineage of this elite group was believed, therefore, the most effective in gaining his divine ancestors' support through temple ceremonies for his family and chiefdom. As the religious head of his chiefdom, the sacred chief officiated with his high priest (kahuna nui) at the national temples in long, very exacting, and frequent calendric and special ceremonies necessary for the health, fertility, and abundance of nature and people and the removal of afflictions. When commoners experienced widespread illness and famine in their domain, they interpreted these as divine punishment of an irreligious chief and abandoned him to seek a more righteous and religious chief favored by the gods. Because the highly elaborate ceremonies conducted for sacred chiefs and chiefesses in times of their life crises from conception to death affected everyone's welfare, they had a semipublic character, with the populace assembled at a respectful distance.

Primogeniture was also important among petty chiefs and commoners. It was an important principle in most of Polynesia except perhaps in Samoa. All ceremonies for a firstborn son or daughter were more complex than for the later children, and the blessings of a Hawaiian "path clearing" ceremony (māwaewae) held soon after the first child's birth were believed to protect the welfare of all later children. The senior male of a household, the family priest, prayed twice daily for the bodily health and well-being of his dependents, commoners, and chiefs and made offerings to Lono, symbolized by a sacred gourd in the men's eating house (mua), which had an altar. During illness and misfortune the head of the household and other men of the family prayed to the family god at another family altar, a conical Pohaku-o-Kāne (Stone of Kāne), and ritually ate their offerings. After absolution by the god, "no medicine need be given to cure sickness," wrote Kamakau, and thereafter the family had health, many births, abundant food, and freedom from accidents.[42]

Taboos—prohibitions and restrictions—protected the mana of sacred chiefs and chiefesses, and whatever else was sacred, from defilement and loss of mana. Someone or something was taboo because it was psychically dangerous. First, it might be divine, and consequently its mana required protective isolation from the corrupt and polluting (haumia), as well as from the common and unsacred (noa), to which in turn it was psychically harmful. Second, it might be contaminating to both the sacred and the common, both of which required isolation from it. The kauwā, or social outcasts, were tabooed; they were so defiling that a commoner who was polluted by trespassing in their segregated area was killed.

Other major sources of defilement were corpses, food, and blood, particularly that of female reproductive functions and war wounds. Women were forbidden, unlike men, to eat any foods acceptable to the gods as sacrifices, except on rare ritual occasions. To prevent his wife from defiling his food a man prepared two ovens, one of tabooed food for himself, one of *noa* (nonsacred) food for his women and little boys. Men ate in their eating house, which no woman dared enter. Women had their own eating house, which was taboo to men. Men, women, and children gathered in the common sleeping house. A chiefess's personal male attendants who cooked her food and ate with her became *noa* like little boys, were excluded from the men's house, and observed women's food taboos. If the chiefess and her male attendants were caught eating tabooed food, the men were sacrificed. A woman was not suitable as a sacrifice to the gods, but she might be punished physically despite her rank, and a low-ranking man might be sacrificed in her place. The gods might also punish her; one chiefess attributed her severe spinal deformity to her having eaten a tabooed fish. Eating taboos symbolized the taboo system, and when Kamehameha II abrogated the system he signaled it by eating in public with Queens Ke'ōpūolani and Ka'ahumanu.

PURIFICATIONS

Throughout Polynesia rites of purification were performed to release persons, places, or things from psychic influences connected with a condition of taboo, which might result from a surcharge of sanctity as well as of pollution. The rites then created a condition of *noa*, freedom from the former restrictions. Rites, often complex, included prayers and either total immersion in the ocean (in New Zealand in streams), perhaps a ritual number of times, or sprinkling with sacred water. Hawaiians used salt water for sprinkling, to which they added turmeric and sometimes a sea rush or red ochre. Under a priest's directions, members of an entire Hawaiian community annually immersed themselves in the sea from midnight to dawn for purification, and afterward they feasted. Tahitians also had a comparable ritual, wherein all plunged into the "trackless ocean," "the supreme temple," to pray and wash off all spiritual and temporal crime and pollution. Individuals such as women after menstruation and childbirth, the sick, warriors, or corpse-handlers had their taboo of defilement removed by immersion or sprinkling. On leaving a temple men had their taboo of sanctity removed to protect themselves and the sanctity of the temple. In Polynesian life there were innumerable occasions calling for cleansing and purification from psychic influences.[43]

OBSERVANCE OF DUALITIES

Like other Polynesians, Hawaiians applied the principle of duality, the source of the taboo system, to the cosmos through a series of complementary, paired, and balanced antitheses. In equilibrium the sacred and the common constituted a unity; in disequilibrium nature and people fell into a middle ground where they were subject to misfortune and death. Among the numerous paired natural forms and abstractions besides the male and female, sacred and common, were life and death, light and darkness, occult knowledge and ignorance, the world of the living (Ao) and the world of the dead (Pō), day and night, east and west, above and below, sea and land, strong right and weak left. In sorcery Ma'iola paired with Kālaipāhoa, self-confidence with fear. In therapy, Kū the Erect, the generative power, and his sister-wife Hina the Supine, the reproductive and developmental power, were invoked as a pair in pregnancy, childbirth, lactation, weaning, and in most daily work. Benevolent and approachable, they were the parents of the Hawaiian race, and they brought health and fertility to people and land. In gathering medicinal plants for a woman in labor, for example, a kahuna faced east to pray to Kū before picking five specimens with his right hand, then to the west to pray to Hina before picking five more with his left. From the right-hand, masculine, and stronger plants came the potion to make the baby "slippery" and easily born; from the left-hand, feminine, and weaker came the ointment for rubbing the woman's abdomen. A preferred time for administering medicines for certain ailments was high noon, the time of greatest mana, because Kū of the sunrise and morning united then with Hina of the afternoon and declining sun. Midnight was also a time of great mana.[44]

The medical profession itself was considered dual-natured because the spiritual and the physical combined to treat a patient holistically. Certain ailments were classified dualistically, particularly those relating to conditions believed inherited or dormant in children. 'Ea (now the word for "thrush"), encompassing various illnesses from dizziness to osteomalacia, was male and above; pā'ao'ao, encompassing weaknesses of children (mothers still diagnose "hair stomach" as one manifestation), was female and below; but both were so entwined that it was considered best to treat them at the same time. A kahuna's first treatment for an adult illness or injury was salt water (for shock) and a purgative followed by an enema. The concepts of above and below also operated in treating prostate gland disorder: a kahuna first gave the patient a beverage of 'ala'ala-wai-nui, an upland plant, and formally closed the treatment with 'a'ala-'ula, a seaweed. These plants, like several others, are matched in the genealogical prayer chant "Kumulipo," which dedicated a firstborn royal son to Lono: "Born was the 'a'ala-'ula living in the sea/ Guarded by the 'ala'ala-wai-nui living on earth."[45]

Besides the dualities, a kahuna learned the proper substitutes for a particular offering or sacrifice. If the rules were not followed, the ceremony was incomplete, and trouble would follow. "Fish" was the common Polynesian euphemism for a sacrificed man, but the reverse might occur in a certain Hawaiian rite that required an ulua fish *(Carangidae);* if unable to catch one the fisherman hooked a man as a substitute because the word *ulua* can also mean "man." Natural phenomena, plants, and animals were classified according to their resemblances of form, color, notable detail, or habit. The multiple visible embodiments of a god or spirit were recognizable on the basis of resemblances of particular sorts. *Pōpolo* (black nightshade, *Solanum nigrum,*) a very important medicine, was a proper substitute for kava because Kāne had introduced kava and *pōpolo* was one of his visible embodiments. A black pig was the best sacrifice to Lono but a sometime substitute was a grass eaten by pigs and named *kūkae pua'a* (pig dung, *Digitaria pruriens.*) In a *māwaewae* ceremony for a firstborn dedicated to Lono, the god's plant embodiment was a taro leaf shaped like a hog's ear; his ocean form, a fish with a hoglike snout; and his animal form, a hog's ears.[46]

THE KAHUNA'S PREPARATION

A kahuna was either a commoner or a chief according to his inherited class, and, unless he belonged to the two highest orders serving the king and the national temples, he usually worked only part-time as a priest. Whatever his occupation, be it hula or medicine, he was chosen by the gods and dedicated to them. During training he was in religious seclusion and had to observe all of his instructors' ordinances, or his efforts were wasted. At graduation *('ailolo),* when he was to eat *('ai)* part of the head and brains *(lolo)* of a sacrificial fish, dog, or pig, any serious mistake *(hewa)* in the ceremony was a bad omen and meant that the individual should not become a kahuna. If all went well, after ritual purification *(huikala)* and release from the powerful psychic influences of his tabooed period the student became *noa,* no longer sacred, and free to join others.[47]

Evidence to a diviner and a family head that the gods had chosen a boy to become a medical priest *(kahuna lapa'au)* included his name or genealogy, his mother's pregnancy cravings, omens at his birth, and family visions or dreams; and, on the boy's part, his possession of a good memory, consideration for others, interest in medicine, eagerness to observe and learn, generosity, and carefulness and reverence in ceremonial duties. His training usually began in childhood, undoubtedly after his admission at about the age of five or six to the men's eating house (which marked the formal end of his infancy) and after his prospective teacher had received a favorable omen.

In a departure from this tradition, however, many adult chiefs began to study medicine after the devastating *'ōku'u* (Asiatic cholera?) epidemic

of the early nineteenth century. Among the chiefs trained by Kua'ua'u of
the Lono-pūhā order and one of Kamehameha's medical men, were Boki,
governor of Oahu, and his elder brother Kalanimoku, Kamehameha's
commander in chief, treasurer, and later prime minister. In order to protect themselves and the king from sorcery, some chiefs of the royal court
studied the sorceries of praying to death and causing illness by gesture.
In addition to these adult students of medicine there were male and
female mediums untrained in medicine, called "wind kahunas" (*makani*,
"wind" or "spirit"), who claimed that during possession their god
revealed the nature of the sufferer's illness, the cause, and the prognosis.
Women, although excluded from formal medical training, learned from
family kahunas to treat ordinary illnesses and those of women and children. Tahitian women taught by a parent became doctors, but nothing has
been reported of the rituals of training for either sex.[48]

CENTERS OF HEALING

A Hawaiian boy chosen to become a medical kahuna served as an
apprentice to his father or another older relative who was a kahuna, or at
a temple for healing *(heiau ho'ola)*, a type of temple also found in Tahiti
but unreported for the rest of Polynesia. The islands of Oahu and Hawaii
had numerous temples for teaching and curing during the early nineteenth century, and an occasional temple of that kind still functioned up
to the end of the century. *Heiau ho'ola* were built to Lono-pūhā, god of
wounds and chronic diseases, and to Kōlea-moku, god of acute diseases,
by chiefs after their recovery from illness and by medical priests after fin-
ishing training. Papa, also one of Kamehameha's medical men, owned
several *heiau ho'ola* in Honolulu dedicated to these founders of medical
arts and to others. During special temple services to ask the gods' blessing
on medical work, priests prayed continuously on the second night until
morning, and during the taboo-lifting prayer absolute silence was
required under penalty of death.[49]

Traditions state that on the island of Hawaii, medical centers grew up
at Kukuihaele and in the Waimanu and Waipio valleys, where the deified
founders of medicine had practiced. The Pele'ula district of Honolulu, a
medical center, had a great number of heiaus. The Keaiwa heiau in the
Ewa district of Honolulu, partially restored in 1951, was named, it has
been said, for its first priest (perhaps later deified) and built during the
rule of the learned, peace-loving King Kakuhihewa around the sixteenth
or seventeenth century. After learning prayers for compounding medicines and healing, Keaiwa apprentices were sent to other heiaus for
advanced training. Like most medical heiaus Keaiwa had a large herb garden outside the walls, tended by apprentices. No matter what a medical
kahuna's specialty he had to know something of the pharmacopoeia,

which included over three hundred land and sea plants, twenty-nine animal elements, and over a dozen mineral elements—a very conservative estimate. Herbalists *(kāhuna lā'au lapa'au)* were, of course, the experts who knew the most about where to find what was needed and what was its preparation and use.[50]

Hawaiians also had a category of consecrated medical "houses," small huts to which the sick or convalescent were moved for special prayers and treatment. A white taboo flag bound with protective ti leaves (to keep evil spirits away) stood at each corner of the house and the patient's mat. During his last illness Kamehameha's kahunas built two houses dedicated to his Kālaipāhoa gods, who had cured a previous illness, but since he did not improve in either of these houses he was returned to his sleeping house and moved again as needed to his eating house. Ka'ū district, Hawaii, formerly had Hale Ola (houses of healing), small huts to which the sick were moved to be prayed over. The general term *moku hale* refers to any small house consecrated to a special purpose, but it might have an individual name derived from a deified medical personage or the particular kind of thatch or wood used in its construction. Thus, a Hale Lama for a sick or convalescent chief was a small hut of lama wood *(Diospyros)*, which contained additional mana because it was built by daylight *(lama)*. Such a hut might be built for a high chief to occupy during his religious seclusion in a temple area, or he might fill such a house with offerings in order to atone for wrongs to his god. The extremely taboo *'alaneo* houses, where sick chiefs went to pray, were named for the 'Alaneo, a group of four or twelve healers, hermaphrodites, who came from the mythical land of Kahiki to Waikiki.[51]

MEDICAL TRAINING

A medical apprentice consecrated to the gods of medicine lived in a *moku hale*, was celibate and guarded against homosexuals, could not cut his hair or beard (sometimes for the rest of his life), avoided defilement from women and the dead, and forever after, like the mediums, permitted no one to touch his food or possessions. He was expected to be upright, pious, and pure if the gods were to help him and evil spirits avoid him. He learned about the gods of medicine, including Ma'iola and Mauli-ola, and about the goddesses; he memorized the prayers; he learned about the body, its illnesses and their remedies. He also studied sorcery and how to counteract it. Every patient, he learned, was different, so each treatment and each medicine must be different. Each teacher had his own methods, usually secret, and he did not impart all of them to his student until he was near death. (Some teachers, however, imitated Lono-pūhā's teacher, who spat his mana and knowledge all at once into his pupil's mouth.) Training did not last a set number of years; after graduation a student might start to practice or might visit other heiaus to learn more.[52] A student might be a general practitioner or have one or two specialties, and also he might be a kahuna of nonmedical specialties, such as canoe-making, fishing, or architecture.

Hāhā (palpation, feeling with the fingers) was perhaps the most highly respected nineteenth-century specialty, and its practitioners were admired for their insight, questioning, and critical observation as well as for their special training in diagnosis. Kua'au'u and Papa were two members of the Lono-pūhā order who were renowned for *hāhā*. The unique feature of training in diagnosis was the apprentice's touching of red, white, and black pebbles (as many as 480) arranged in the shape of a human body. The student, developing an ever more sensitive touch (some said he could distinguish the colors), progressed from the feet to the head while his instructor lectured. The student "felt" prescribed points identified according to an established system as his instructor described the initial symptoms of each disease and its development as associated with these points. The student learned about the remedies and expectable results for each disease as well as about the island where a disease was first discovered. Much of the knowledge was in the form of a very long formulaic chant, which the graduating student, if satisfactorily educated, recited unhesitatingly in front of a *heiau ho'ola;* and at that time, too, his instructor confirmed his diagnosis of a man with many ailments.[53]

To become a kahuna in the beneficent branch of *'anā'anā* that divined, saved, and avenged victims being prayed to death and that performed *kuni* ceremonies in the open to identify the sorcerer was a long process. A man whose gifts had been accepted by an older practitioner went through ten or even twenty *'ailolo* graduation ceremonies as he progressed in knowledge. He finally demonstrated his accumulated mana and control by shattering a hard rock or drawing fire from a green tree, and by eating, unharmed, poisonous concoctions and loathsome things like earthworms. If he later became a "filth eater," that is, one who betrayed honorable training by seeking wealth through praying innocent people to death, the gods, particularly the sorcery goddess Uli, would punish him, and his human enemies kill him.[54]

A patient's protracted illness could use up a family's property, especially if the patient had more than one disease and each required a different treatment. But once all diseases were cured, an ethical kahuna added no unnecessary treatments. Fees and offerings to the gods depended on a patient's rank and wealth. A messenger going to call a kahuna typically brought a pig for the god Ma'iola—really a fee, in that the kahuna ate the pig after Ma'iola consumed the essence. Because a kahuna consulted so many omens as to whether to accept the case, his decision took time. Perhaps the messenger came at an unpropitious time, or the kahuna's dreams showed that the case would end in death; even on his way to the patient any number of unlucky signs might lead him to go back home.

"Pig-eating kahunas" were those experts in aumakua sickness (discussed earlier in this chapter) who required a very large number of pigs, which the wealthy gladly paid. A rich chief might have to give several hundred pigs for the altar, but after the god had the essence, the chief and those friends who had rallied around him feasted on the roasted pork, and the chief might invite the kahuna and his relatives to join them. Each aumakua had its own rules; offerings to a shark aumakua went into the ocean; those for a water spirit *(mo'o)* landed, for the most part, in a fresh-water pond.[55]

Hawaiians distinguished between false and genuine healers. The genuine practitioner healed a patient because he had mana, experience, training, maturity, and the support of the gods. The false failed to heal a patient or was an extortionist. These extortionists had a "pig's gravy" of a life (that is, "a gravy train"). Numerous examples are recorded. One of them told a healthy man he was ill whereupon the man gladly paid him for an enema, but, when it caused much suffering, the unfortunate man had to send to the kahuna for a soothing potion. Or a dishonest kahuna would tell a man that while his soul was wandering it had come to the kahuna and beaten him. Now the man's aumakua was angry with him and would punish him if he did not hold a ceremony of atonement, which, of course, the kahuna found profitable. Or a kahuna with no medical training would tell a patient—without seeing him or by touching only his toenails or his head—the nature of his illness, the cause, and the prognosis. Other "lying kahunas" claimed to cure certain diseases known— by two reputable kahunas trained by Kua'au'u himself—to be incurable. These braggarts, the two said, claimed to cure dropsy, which was impossible. They themselves had identified five kinds of edema and experimented with seventeen kinds of medicine as well as diet and physic, and they knew that for dropsy there might be some alleviation, but no cure.[56]

In 1868 a formal attempt was made to distinguish between the false and the genuine. Kamehameha V, sympathetic to many traditional customs, signed an act to establish the Hawaiian Board of Health, composed of three Hawaiians who would examine the qualifications and moral character of kahunas. Those who were licensed had to keep detailed written records about each patient (some records have been preserved); they would lose their licenses if they practiced any black magic, whether *'anā'anā, ho'opi'opi'o, ho'oūnauna,* or *ho'omanamana.* Kahunas practicing for pay without a license were fined by the police or a district judge if found guilty. Guilt was difficult to prove because recovered patients and the kahuna claimed that the treatment was done only for aloha and not for material compensation. Dissatisfied relatives of dead patients appealed to the circuit court, where Judge Abraham Fornander heard sev-

eral cases. Probably the unlicensed kahuna's claims of working only for
aloha have led to a present-day belief that kahunas were not paid for their
services. As a reaction to the licensing of kahunas, the opposition led by
foreign doctors rallied to establish a medical school to teach Hawaiian
men Western medical practices. Ten received their licenses after two
years, 1870 to 1872, with Dr. Gerrit P. Judd as their teacher. Yet despite
the good results the kingdom did not continue the school after Dr. Judd
retired.[57]

Hawaiian precontact conditions (i.e., prior to the arrival of Europeans)
have been partially revealed by the study of 1171 individuals, not all complete skeletons, excavated at a cemetery in Mokapu, Oahu. In this homogeneous coastal population the average age of an adult male at death was
32 years, that of an adult female 3 years less. (In 1910 Hawaiians had an
estimated life expectancy at birth, combined sexes, of 32.58 years, only
slightly more than that for Mokapu. By 1980 this had increased to
74.01.)[58] Over half of the children had not survived their fifth year, and
most had died before their third. There was no evidence of venereal disease.[59] Like skeletons excavated in New Zealand, most at Mokapu showed
degenerative arthritic changes that had begun early in life and advanced
with age. A similar frequency of arthritis, rheumatism, gout, and spinal
deformities was also seen in Tahiti and Hawaii in the early nineteenth
century among the living.

Among the excavated remains, three Mokapu children between five
and twelve years of age were found to be microcephalic. Nineteenth-century Hawaiians took great care to prevent premature closure of the ante-
rior fontanel (manawa), regarded as the site not only of affection and feeling but the place from which the goddess Haumea bore children.
Mothers, believing that food could be absorbed through it, placed raw,
grated sweet potato on it as an infant's first solid food.[60]

Mokapu dentition refuted the frequent assertion that all ancient
Hawaiians had perfect teeth—some did, but many suffered from tooth-
aches. The record of broken bones showed the Mokapu apparently had
some skilled bonesetters (kāhuna ha'iha'i iwi). Separated ends of broken
bone were well aligned, and sites of healing were usually small, compact,
and well formed. Mokapu had many skulls molded to the admired bullet
shape; the practice survived in Hawaii until the late nineteenth century.
Although Melanesians practiced trepanning (the removal of circular sections of the skull) into modern times, researches among Polynesians,
including Hawaiians, lack adequate bone evidence to support the frequent reports of its practice. However, the Musée de l'homme, Paris, has
informed me that it has a skull, said to be trepanned, from Nukuhiva,
Marquesas, in its Chauvet collection (no. 19210).

During the excavation, a Mokapu adult was found with above-the-
elbow arm amputation, but whether this was surgical, traumatic, or con-

genital is uncertain. No postcontact kahuna is known to have amputated on the living, and patients of Western surgeons resisted amputation because a sorcerer might steal the separated part. Mission doctors, however, performed a few amputations. That an eighteenth-century explorer in Tahiti saw a man with a perfectly healed amputated arm raises the possibility that early Hawaiians may have also done some surgery, especially since they were very skilled in severing bones of the dead, for which they probably used thin, knifelike basaltic flakes such as Mokapu grave-robbers left behind. Bones were material for tools and the creation of a familiar spirit. It was also customary to dismember a chief's corpse and hide the cleaned bones to prevent their desecration by toolmakers. Bones were also kept as relics. One of Kamehameha's queens slept with the tapa-wrapped bundle of her father's bones, and when she was absent they were laid on a featherbed purchased for that purpose. Her explanation: she loved her father very much.

Postcontact records praise the Hawaiian ability to treat most fractures, dislocations, sprains, and bruises. However, an occasional Western physician has noted deformities from treatment by poorly trained kahunas. Unlike other Polynesians who used splints, Hawaiian kahunas, after setting a fracture, soothed it with a plaited web of cool ti leaves and immobilized it with a tapa-binding. A saltwater drink warded off shock, but if the patient vomited, the kahuna expected him to get worse within twenty-four hours. The kahuna eased severe pain with the narcotic juice of prickly poppy, herbal concoctions, or kava. If he were trained in "calling medicine" *(lā'au kāhea)*, a kind of faith healing, he was said (even by Western doctors) to have produced miraculously successful cures. He could also drive out a sorcerer's familiar spirit who had caused the accident. In his healing prayers he commanded each part of the body connected with the injury to return to its proper function and health. Bone-setters used various salt and herbal poultices combined with prayer for fractures; and for these, as well as for arthritis/rheumatism and other injuries and deformities, they also used hot packs, manual manipulation, solar therapy, massage, and exercise.[61]

The Life Cycle

RULES CONCERNING WOMEN

The kahuna's practice related directly or indirectly to birth and death. Few, if any, religious rites occurred for an ordinary marriage. Couples were free to change mates and each was free to have more than one spouse at a time. Much religious ceremony, however, attended the mating of a couple of the highest rank who were siblings or part-siblings because their firstborn son or daughter would inherit more mana and rank than either parent, and be considered an earthly representative of the gods, concerned with their worship so that the kingdom would prosper. The couple lived apart until the "child-begetting" ceremony (ho'omau keiki)— which is clear evidence of knowledge of the relationship between intercourse and conception. When the princess's menstrual period and taboo-removing bath were over she was escorted to a tapa tent in an open area in view of the populace. Conception, Hawaiians believed, was most likely to occur after the end of menstruation. While priests chanted prayers of fertility, the prince left the stick image of his god at the entry and joined the princess, remaining with her until evening, when they separated. Neither had intercourse with anyone else until the birth of their child. People rejoiced at news of the pregnancy, and bards composed name chants honoring the expected child and taught them to hula companies to perform until the birth.[62]

A woman's usual customs at menstruation, pregnancy, and birth were ceremonially complex and elaborate if she were a high-ranking chiefess. Any menstruant was considered unlucky and defiling, vulnerable to hostile spirits, and contaminating to other men and women, to sacred objects and places, and to parts of nature including springs. Angry gods and villagers severely punished a couple caught having intercourse at this time. Only a woman past menopause could become a spirit medium, and any medium, man or woman, had only men or preadolescent children as attendants.[63]

A menstruant retired to a special house (hale pe'a) on the edge (pe'a) of the community or royal compound. Other Polynesians also had such houses. A ti-leaf lei protected the Hawaiian woman externally from mischievous spirits, and certain potions protected her internally. A female relative, also protected by a ti-leaf lei, brought food (cooked as usual by a man), but to avoid pollution left it outside and then took a purifying sea bath. Even to pass the house was contaminating. At the end of her stay a woman buried her pads and tampons in a special place (so defiling that not even a sorcerer would go near it for bait), took a taboo-removing sea bath (or a bath of fresh water mixed with salt), and returned to her husband.

A high chief's household had hereditary positions for persons of rank who performed certain intimate services such as the exclusive care of the private parts of a menstruating chiefess or of an ailing chief. Knowledge of when a queen was menstruating was apparently significant enough for Don Francisco Marin, who performed both business and medical services for Kamehameha, to note the fact more than once in his journal. Only a chiefess could be a royal child's wet-nurse, but to perform her services she had to be naked as evidence that she was not menstruating.[64]

Ceremonial rites for a girl's first menses were rare, except that a grandmother sang praise songs as she took the girl to the *hale pe'a*. If a woman missed going to the house, it was assumed that she was pregnant. Much ceremony, by contrast, attended women of noble birth; chiefesses attending a royal woman during pregnancy noted such signs as lassitude and lack of appetite. Even more than an ordinary woman, she was subject to malign influences and harm from ambitious nobles who might magically harm her or the fetus she carried. Unlike an ordinary woman she and her attendants went into religious seclusion, a state of taboo. She must not now live in an old house; wear old clothes or a lustrous sarong; or eat brown dogs, three kinds of white fish, or any food taboo to her and her husband's gods. To avoid being deliberately poisoned or subjected to destructive influences injected into her food, the chiefess ate no food salted by others and accepted food only from trusted attendants. Whether a chiefess or a commoner, a pregnant woman's diet was closely watched and adjusted as her time approached in order to make for an easier delivery.[65]

PREGNANCY

There was much sympathetic magic that helped to allay the anxiety of pregnancy. To prevent the umbilical cord from strangling the fetus, a woman did not wear a lei, work with cord, or sew tapa. She did not string fish to dry; if it spoiled, her child would get "strung fish" (*i'a kui*), that is, ozena, a smelly nasal disease. Food cravings must be satisfied. Numerous Polynesian myths tell of a father's disappearance while seeking the desired food. To Hawaiians the cravings were not the mother's, but the child's. The child was thereby expressing its personality. A craving for *hilu*, a shy reef fish, meant that the child would be well behaved and quiet (*hilu*). Kamehameha's mother Ke-ku'i-apo-iwa (or her unborn child) is said to have craved the eye of a *niuhi*, a very large, grey man-eating shark whose eyes are luminous at night. Parents' behavior also influenced the child's character: lazy parents, lazy child. To satisfy parental curiosity about the unborn child's sex, kahunas depended on dreams, visions, trances, clairvoyance, or a woman's response on being asked to raise her hand—if she raised the right, there would be a boy; if the left, a girl.[66]

Midwifery was often a family's specialty among its male and female members for generations. The *kahuna ho'ohanau* who was to deliver the child examined the woman frequently, determined by external palpation when labor would begin, and if necessary manipulated externally (some were expert enough to do it internally) the position of the fetus. Complications before or during parturition were believed due to the family aumakua's displeasure with family disharmony, which then had to be adjusted and the aumakua appeased with prayer and offerings. An exceptional kahuna, perhaps through powerful suggestion or hypnotism, could transfer severe labor pains caused by hostile influences to another man or woman or to an animal. His supernatural helpers might include Haumea, goddess of childbirth and fecundity, who was the first to teach natural childbirth. (Like most Polynesians and other Pacific islanders, Hawaiians believed that, until the arrival of such a goddess or god, women were cut open to remove the child and then died.) As labor pains increased, the woman squatted or knelt on mats with her knees apart in typical Polynesian fashion. Her husband or a female relative, who sat behind her to support her back, lightly massaged or pressed her upper abdomen while the kahuna sat in front to receive the infant.

DELIVERY

Among commoners birth was usually at home. The use of the menstrual house, as among some Polynesians, has not been reported. Well-to-do commoners and lesser chiefs often went to special medical heiaus, or, as in Tahiti, to a newly built house to prevent contamination of other structures. Hawaiian high chiefs aspired to have their children born at a sacred birthing place like Kūkaniloko, Oahu, or Holoholokū, Kauai. These were also places of refuge. At Kūkaniloko, which was established as a royal birthing place around the twelfth century CE, the accumulated mana and prestige of the site passed to the newborn. Kamehameha, it is said, regretted that his sacred wife Ke'ōpūolani was too ill to have their first child Liholiho born there.[67]

Little has been reported about the manner of delivery at Kūkaniloko. A chiefess may have lain within a framework of two parallel rows of stones, eighteen on each side, with a mound to support her back. Thirty-six chiefs, eighteen on each side, stood by her, perhaps in order to add their mana, assist at the birth, and see that the infant was not stolen or replaced by another. One can only guess at their duties. The infant was immediately taken to a house in the temple precincts nearby, where the king consecrated his child to his gods and participated with forty-eight other chiefs in ceremonies relating to the naval cord. Two sacred drums announced the birth of a sacred chief to the waiting multitude.

Other chiefesses and queens were attended by midwives, all of them chiefesses. When labor began, a priest set up an offering before an image of Hulu, a patron of childbirth, and after delivery brought in the stick image of the child's father's god. During labor, priests—and the waiting populace outside—chanted prayers, and the high priest offered a pig to the king's god at the temple, hoping that the god would send rain, a favorable omen. After delivery he presented a malo (a loincloth) to the king's goddess. The firstborn, if male, was identified with Wākea, ancestor of chiefs, from whose son Haloa a genealogy continued in an unbroken line down to Kamehameha's mother and Kamehameha himself. The identification reflected the continuity of birth and rebirth from the origin of the world to the present.

If the firstborn was a girl, the kahuna cut the navel cord in the birth house. If the firstborn was a boy, the kahuna cut the navel cord in the heiau with a sacred bamboo sliver, cut from a grove planted by the god Kāne, and dressed the wound. The father, holding up offerings of tapa, coconuts, and a live pig, prayed—after killing the pig—to Kū, Kāne, Lono, and Kanaloa, whom he begged "to deal gently with the new chief," and grant him long life and a vast kingdom. A lower-ranking chief or commoner who did not have his own temple took his son to Lono's altar in the men's eating house for the consecration.[68]

Regardless of the parents' rank, it was customary for girls to be reared by the maternal grandparents, boys by the paternal; or in the case of the children of high chiefs, by other chiefs who had asked for the privilege of rearing the child and had been present at birth to prevent any exchange of children.[69] These responsibilities continued through the lifetime of the caretakers, but it by no means signified that the child was not loved by its parents. They continued to oversee the caretakers and if necessary remove them.

Specialists or knowledgeable family members treated women who had never borne children, had stopped bearing or wished to stop, had only miscarriages and stillbirths, or had lost infants soon after birth. For a barren chiefess or one who had stopped bearing, kahunas chanted prayers and sometimes sacrificed a man to the gods. Herbalists entreated Kū and Hina while giving a childless couple certain foods to eat along with prayer to make them fertile. Some women spent a night praying and making offerings at mana-filled phallic rocks. A child brought by earnest prayer was regarded as a gift from the gods, who became his aumakuas. A deformed child was considered the offspring of a spirit or god and a human mother.[70]

A sterile husband might have his wife get a child by another man. The husband became the permanent father, but both men accepted the child, who benefited from additional sets of relatives. Such a child was "double-headed" *(po'o lua)*. In later life Kamehameha proudly identified himself as *po'o lua*, when he learned that King Kahekili of Maui had sired him rather than Chief Keoua of Hawaii as he had always thought. A kahuna might advise a woman with repeated stillbirths to have a child by another man, after which she would bear live children. Or he prescribed herbal remedies, and for a great chiefess, a human sacrifice. It is recorded that a twentieth-century woman bore a live child after eight stillbirths when her uncle had himself prayed to death as a sacrifice for the family's sake.[71]

Punishment of parental taboo violations was sometimes given as the reason why an infant became sick and died. The parents may have ignored a promise to a god or a relative to give the child a certain name. However, if a sorcerer's familiar spirit had killed the child, the next child was given such a repulsive name that the disgusted spirit left it alone. Once the danger was past the child was renamed.

ABORTION AND INFANTICIDE

Hawaiians did not institutionalize abortion and infanticide as did Society Islanders, who required members of the lower grades of the Arioi Society, a hierarchical organization of entertainers serving the gods, to be childless or leave it in disgrace. On the other hand, the Ariois in the highest grades, being regarded as gods, wanted children who would inherit their Arioi positions and titles. Infanticide was prevalent in Tahiti and led Captain Cook to protest to the king about it; females especially were singled out for death. Chiefs in Hawaii and Tahiti rarely destroyed their children if both parents were of equal rank. However, mating with a lower-class person, or worst of all with a *kauwā*, an outcast, marked the offspring for death.

Hawaiian abortifacients, generally similar to those elsewhere in Polynesia, included rolling weights on or beating the abdomen, herbal concoctions to poison the fetus, douches of poisonous mixtures with a bamboo or gourd syringe such as used for enemas, steaming of certain harmful leaves directed into the vagina, and stuffing the vagina with kava leaves. The most drastic method killed more than one woman. The fetus was pierced with a sharpened stick or bone. Archaeologists have found the skeleton of a young woman with such a stick embedded in the skull of the fetus.

If abortifacients failed, a woman, sometimes aided by her husband, parents, or a kahuna, killed the infant by strangling it, drowning it, or burying it alive. Reasons included poverty, advanced age (which made child care wearying), fear of childbirth pains and losing one's looks, dislike of children, jealousy, and concealment of unapproved relationships. While infanticide seems to have been common or at least acceptable in precontact times, its extent is impossible to determine. In 1823 missionaries persuaded some chiefs (already concerned about depopulation which meant a declining labor force) to disapprove of the practice, whereas formerly these chiefs might have been surprised that anyone should disapprove. Infanticide was not outlawed until 1835, although the effects of the declining birth rate and the high rate of infant mortality, with few children surviving their second year, had long been apparent. The law against induced abortion that the kingdom passed in 1850 was repealed in 1970 by the state of Hawaii, the first to do so.[72]

MALE INITIATION

The three major traditional rites of passage into manhood were, sequentially, a boy's entry into the men's eating house and sanctuary (*mua*), his receiving of the subincision called "slit penis" (*kahe ule*), and the privilege of eating pork. Until he was three or four years or even older he was *noa*, nonsacred, eating with women and eating women's food, and going naked. The ceremony of entering the *mua* marked the end of his infantile period. He was dedicated to Lono, wore a malo, and forever after ate only with men. Some formerly tabooed foods were now available to him, but not pork. His father conducted a highly ritualized ceremony of initiation in the presence of other men and then rendered the occasion *noa* so that the company could feast on whatever was left after he had ceremoniously eaten first.[73]

The operation of subincision was performed when the boy was about eight years old; the purpose was to facilitate intercourse and increase pleasure. (Many boys and girls had become sexually active even before this ceremony.) Social class and birth order determined how complex the ceremony was. Christianized families gave social but not religious significance to it, using, nonetheless, a bamboo knife cut from the sacred grove of Kāne, god of procreation. The traditional ceremony, on the other hand, was usually in the *mua* with many prayers and offerings, including a pig for Kāne. The operation was by a kahuna who was a specialist in this rite; he was assisted by another kahuna while men held the boy. Sometimes the operation was performed at one of the sacred stones consecrated for that purpose. The ceremony for a king's firstborn son involved the studying of the auguries by the high priest the night before, and if they were favorable the boy was brought before him and the god in the heiau. After his usual blessing of the bamboo knife he handed it to the kahuna who subincised the boy while a man held him. Nature's immediate response of approval was lightning, thunder, and rain, good omens that the boy would become rich. The kahuna then reminded the boy not to forget him. After more prayer the boy was taken to a heiau of the type called *kūkoa'e* for ceremonial purification. Although a former priest stated that the boy "then ate of the pig," it is likely that a high-ranking boy required a special ceremony for the privilege.[74] According to David Malo, the king's firstborn son was not consecrated for the eating of pork until he "showed signs of incipient manhood" and had been tutored in religion and other subjects essential for his future role as religious head of the kingdom. Kamehameha himself took part in tutoring Liholiho, his firstborn son, in the duties and behavior of a good king. A royal youth first underwent purification (*huikala*), had a heiau built for him, and became a temple worshiper on his own account. He was then permitted to eat pork, but the pig, unlike usual custom, had been ritually killed and baked outside the heiau. And, as Malo wrote, the boy's initiation into the eating of pork was with prayer. Nothing is reported of a ritual for other youths, but permission to eat pork signified that they could now share completely in temple and *mua* feasts that included pigs consecrated to the gods. As for the commoners who raised the pigs, they seldom had the opportunity to eat pork.[75]

DEATH AND DYING

Polynesia has numerous orally transmitted narratives of the resuscitation of the dead and the quest in the spirit world for a soul to be returned to earth. The Hawaiian demigod Lōlupe, embodied in a stingray or a man-made fish-shaped kite, was sent, after receiving prayers and offerings, to recover the soul of a stillborn child or some other individual, or to escort a royal soul to the spirit land. More than one twentieth-century Hawaiian man or woman has described a reunion with the dead before returning to life. Usually, for instance, after leaving her body (*kino*) through her lachrymal glands, a woman's soul wanders on earth or in the afterworld until a spirit who is a dead relative or an aumakua tells her that her time to join the dead has not yet come. The spirit, despite the soul's resistance, takes it to the abandoned body, forces it through the big toe and up into the torso until a faint cawing sound emerges. Then her family, who had thought her dead, pray and purify her to complete her resuscitation.[76]

Hawaiian customs and beliefs relating to the dead greatly resemble those of other Polynesians. Because of the extremely defiling nature of a corpse, all but blood relatives left the house and restricted their activities, including work, to prevent contaminating other people and nature. Uncertainty that an individual was really dead, as well as deep love, often led a family to keep the corpse several days before burial, with efforts made (if thought necessary) to slow the decomposition. Some twentieth-century Hawaiians still use salt for that purpose. In earlier times attempts at longer preservation included evisceration, with the insertion of salt or plant material, and superficial washes of salt and vegetable materials. The corpse, dressed in its customary clothing and wrapped in tapa, was buried with its possessions, even its pet dog, pig, or chicken, and with supplies either for its transition to the spirit world or for its revival of consciousness. Burial of possessions, regardless of the owner's social class, lessened sorrowful reminders, avoided pollution from them, and kept the soul from returning to complain of something forgotten.

When word came that the soul had indeed left the body, wailing began and continued intermittently until after the nonritualized "feast of lamentation" following the burial; anyone absent was suspected of having caused the death. Chants, either impromptu or stylized, that referred to the deceased were interrupted only by long wails of "a-a-a." The practice sometimes occurs in the present. Like other Polynesians, Hawaiian mourners expressed ambivalent emotions about the deceased. Along with genuine grief there was hope of strengthening rapport with the departing soul, who might return to assist its living kinfolk, as well as fear that the soul, if not propitiated with offerings and demonstrations of grief, would linger about to harm the living. Also the malicious spirits and influences that had caused the death still lurked about seeking more victims. A *kuni*, or "burning," ceremony, particularly for the souls of great persons such as a chief or king, was essential in order to drive them away and identify their controlling sorcerer.[77] An object taken from the corpse was burned to discover and kill the evil sorcerer who had caused the death.

Fear was greatest when a sacred chief or chiefess died. Since even superior mana and kinship with the gods had not protected such a person, everyone and all nature was now in danger. In Hawaii, as in some other Polynesian islands, violent demonstrations of grief frequently resulted in temporary insanity and anarchy, which ended only with the lifting of the tabooed mourning period. Mourners gashed themselves, burned spots on their skin, knocked out their teeth, ran naked, cut their hair in bizarre patterns, sought to be killed as "companions in death," engaged in prostitution (queens excepted), plundered, burned property, and murdered. To disguise themselves from dangerous spirits and exhibit humility, nobles would wear dirty fragments of old fishnets. A noble woman might have her tongue tattooed. After Kamehamalu, Liholiho's wife, had her tongue tattooed when her mother-in-law Queen Ke'ōpūolani died, the Reverend William Ellis asked her if it had not been painful. Kamehamalu's reply: Great the pain, greater the affection.[78]

When an entire corpse was buried secretly at night in a garden or a communal cavern, cave, sand dune, or other natural area, it might be in a flexed, extended, or semiextended position. Earth burials, some marked with a stone platform or border, were often near or under a dwelling. Priests and lesser chiefs were sometimes buried in similarly marked sections within temple precincts. Interment might also be in a stone cist. The most elaborate form of interment was in royal mausoleums on the island of Hawaii; Hale-o-Līloa (House of Līloa) was built around 1575; Hale-o-Keawe in 1740.[79]

Hawaii had a custom, unique in Polynesia, of disinterment and secondary burial of the cleaned skull, long bones, and occasionally other bones. The custom was practiced by royalty and higher nobility as well as by families whose aumakuas lived in a special realm, such as a volcano, freshwater pond, ocean, or the like. A special kahuna directed the rituals and offerings accompanying the deposition of the tapa-wrapped bundle of bones in the aumakua's realm; if the aumakua returned the tapa-wrapped bundle to the sender it meant that it denied the relationship or was angry for some reason. The bones of a high-ranking person that remained after other bones had been given to family members who wished to have such relics in their dwelling were secretly deposited with offerings and the deceased's possessions (tended by a trusted retainer) in the family cave, often in a nearly inaccessible cliff above the sea. Instead of a bone, a mourner might preserve a beloved person's dried palm, head hair, teeth, or fingernails to wrap in tapa and sleep with them. Such a relic was called an 'unihipili, as was whatever a kahuna had taken to convert into a controlled familiar spirit and to endow with ever-increasing mana by his chants and offerings. The spirit was as good or bad as its caretaker, who could, if dissatisfied with it, perform a "cutting" ceremony ('oki) to exorcise it.[80]

The corpse of a king or paramount chief received special attention, particularly if he had been much loved and was to be deified. His leaf-wrapped corpse was laid in a shallow grave over which a fire burned for ten days while Lōlupe-worshiping kahunas chanted continuously. When the remains were removed, the flesh and soft parts were deposited in the ocean on a tabooed night. For the skull and bones of a king, Hawaiians invented a casket plaited of sennit, shaped to have a head with shell eyes, a short neck, and a somewhat cylindrical torso without arms or legs. Two caskets found at Hale-o-Līloa, now kept in the Bernice P. Bishop Museum to prevent further deterioration, may be those for King Līloa and King Lono-i-ka-makahiki. The completed casket was probably taken to the chapel in the *mua* or to a heiau, where a priest's prayers transformed the spirit into a real god. The taboo imposed when the king died was then lifted, and the king's successor returned from the exile imposed on him to prevent his pollution. A shrine was built for the casket, and the new god was worshiped with prayers and offerings. A commoner could be deified, but the ceremony was longer and more arduous.[81]

Those who had secretly buried a corpse at night bathed in the sea on their return and then sat in a row before the house where the corpse had been. After a long prayer, the priest, a kahuna trained in the correct *hui-kala* purification ceremony, sprinkled the men with seawater containing turmeric and *kala* seaweed to cleanse them, enabling them to return to normal life. Perhaps it was not until postcontact times that it became the custom also to sprinkle and purify the house and yard, the pallbearers, and everyone who had attended the funeral. A year later the formal mourning period ended with a memorial "feast of tears," attended by all who had been at the funeral; they now rejoiced that the one who had died was at rest and the living were freed from the burdens of mourning. After laying bits of the festive food and gifts on the grave, the hosts feasted with their guests as long as the food lasted.[82]

Accounts vary as to the soul's journey after its separation from its body, but it was generally believed that it continued to live and seek its place in the compartmentalized land of spirits, unless survivors had ritually transferred it directly to its aumakua's special realm. Life in the spirit world was shadowy and vaguely like that on earth. Hawaiian accounts of life after death have little elaboration and consistency compared with those from other Polynesians but nevertheless share many familiar elements. Each Hawaiian island had several leaping places to the spirit world at cliffs above the sea; a district might have its own. An Oahu entry to the spirit world, according to one description, was guarded by a giant caterpillar and a dragonlike water spirit *(mo'o),* but once safely past them the soul reached a two-branched tree, the roadway to the spirit world. One branch faced east, the other west; one was green, the other dry. If the soul grabbed the green branch, the branch broke and plummeted the soul into Milu, a land of darkness (Pō) and unpleasant spirits, ruled by a mythical deified chief for whom the place was named. These spirits were responsive to sorcerers' incantations to harm the living. Milu was not a place of torture except in Christianized versions, which equated it with hell. The soul that grasped the dry branch safely reached the land, in one part of which lived the spirits of its ancestors. Although called the Realm of Aumakuas, the active aumakuas usually hovered near the families who worshiped them. The soul that had no trouble in reaching the Ao Aumakua was one that had been protected and guided by its family aumakua; a soul without an aumakua, or rejected by one, or with a family that scarcely grieved or prayed for it was doomed to become a *lapu,* a homeless, cranky spirit who frightened and harmed people at night and lived on spiders and other insects.[83]

The spirit world as a whole is often called Pō, which in the genealogical prayer chant, the "Kumulipo," refers to the era of darkness and the emergence of the first forms of life. Then follows Ao, the era of light, the birth of gods, and the appearance of their descendants. Life emerges from Pō and returns there. Continuity exists between Pō and Ao, for spirits return from Po to watch over their living kin in Ao and to appear to them in dreams, visions, and through trances when they possess their human mediums. Gods and spirits also send messages to their worshipers through their embodiments in nature.

The belief remains strong even yet that the spirits of the dead and the gods return to visit the land of the living. Also, people still claim to have seen and heard, on certain sacred nights, processions of spirits among whom they have recognized their relatives, or processions of gods and goddesses, or processions led by spirits of dead chiefs, including Kamehameha, followed by his retinue and soldiers. The visits may be due, it is thought, to the spirits and gods escorting the soul of one of their own class to the afterworld. People still know that if one cannot hide one must either observe the traditional positions of respect (squatting or lying face down) or expect to be killed.

The continuity of the cycle of life and death is expressed in all Polyne-

sian philosophy and mythology. Human beings rise from the spirit world
and return there only in old age unless their offenses against their
aumakua have disturbed the natural equilibrium and made them vulnerable to an evil sorcerer's incantations and rituals. According to Martha
Warren Beckwith, "the broken law is the fundamental idea in all
Hawaiian thinking about accident or early death."[84]

Notes

1. Western Polynesia (Samoa, Tonga, and islands to the north of them,
   including Tūvalu [Ellices]) is distinguishable as a cultural subarea from
   eastern Polynesia (Hawaiian Islands, Marquesas, Society Islands, Cook
   Islands, Tuamotus, New Zealand, Easter Island). Unless otherwise indicated, "Hawaii" refers to the group as a whole, "Tahiti" to the Society
   Islands.
2. David Malo, *Hawaiian Antiquities (Moolelo Hawaii)*, Bernice P. Bishop
   Museum Special Publication no. 2, 2nd ed., trans. Nathaniel B. Emerson
   (Honolulu, 1951), p. 107.
3. Robert H. Heighton, "Hawaiian Supernatural and Natural Strategies for
   Goal Attainment" (Ph.D. diss., University of Hawaii, 1971); Mary Kawena
   Pukui, E. W. Haertig, and Catherine A. Lee, *Nānā i ke Kumu (Look to the
   source)*, 2 vols. (Honolulu, 1972); Karen Ito, "Symbolic Conscience: Illness
   Retribution among Urban Hawaiian Women" (Ph.D. diss., University of
   California, Los Angeles, 1968); Patricia J. Snyder, "Folk Healing in Honolulu, Hawaii" (Ph.D. diss., University of Hawaii, Honolulu, 1979).
4. E. S. Craighill Handy, *Polynesian Religion*, Bernice P. Bishop Museum Bulletin no. 34 (Honolulu, 1927), pp. 3–8, 25–26; E. S. Craighill Handy and
   Mary Kawena Pukui, *The Polynesian Family System in Ka-'u, Hawai'i*, (Wellington, New Zealand, 1958, reprint Rutland, VT, 1972), pp. 27–39, 116–
   159.
5. Heighton, "Hawaiian Strategies," p. 21.
6. Samuel M. Kamakau, *Ka Po'e Kahiko* (The people of old), ed. Dorothy B.
   Barrère, trans. Mary Kawena Pukui, Bernice P. Bishop Museum Special
   Publication no. 51 (Honolulu, 1964), pp. 28–30, 63–91; Handy and Pukui,
   The Polynesian Family System, pp. 40–74.
7. Abraham Fornander, *Fornander Collection of Hawaiian Antiquities and
   Folk-lore*, trans. and ed. Thomas G. Thrum, Bernice P. Bishop Museum
   Memoirs, vols. 4–6 (Honolulu, 1916–1919), vol. 6, pp. 56ff.; Kamakau, *ka
   Po'e Kahiko*, pp. 7–8, 98–115, 122–141.
8. Handy, and Pukui, *The Polynesian Family System*, p. 142; John H. Wise
   and Nils P. Larsen, "Medicine," in *Ancient Hawaiian Civilization*, eds. E.
   S. Craighill Handy et al., rev. ed. (Rutland, VT, 1965), pp. 257–267; June
   Gutmanis, *Kahuna La'au Lapa'au* (The practice of Hawaiian herbal medicine), trans. Theodore Kelsey (Norfolk Island, Australia, 1976).
9. Kamakau, *Ka Po'e Kahiko*, pp. 95–98.
10. Malo, *Hawaiian Antiquities*, pp. 95–96; Laura C. Green and Martha W.
    Beckwith, "Hawaiian Customs and Beliefs relating to Sickness and
    Death," *American Anthropologist* 8, no. 2 (1926): 201–204; Handy and
    Pukui, *The Polynesian Family System*, pp. 142–145; Pukui, Haer-
    tig, and Lee, *Nānā i ke Kumu*, vol. 1, pp. 60–70, vol. 2, pp. 145ff.; see also

Gutmanis, *Kahuna La'au Lapa'au;* Claire D. F. Parsons, ed., *Healing Practices in the South Pacific* (Laie, Hawaii, 1985).

11. Mary Kawena Pukui, *Hawaiian Beliefs and Customs during Birth, Infancy and Childhood,* Bernice P. Bishop Museum Occasional Papers vol. 17, no. 17 (Honolulu, 1942), pp. 372–374; Kamakau, *Ka Po'e Kahiko,* pp. 101–105; Gutmanis, *Kahuna La'au Lapa'au,* pp. 39–42.

12. Peter H. Buck, *Regional Diversity in the Elaboration of Sorcery in Polynesia,* Yale University Publications in Anthropology, no. 2 (New Haven, CT, 1936). For Hawaii see especially Kamakau, *Ka Po'e Kahiko,* pp. 117–41.

13. Kamakau, *Ka Po'e Kahiko,* p. 139.

14. Harold M. Johnson, "The Kahuna, Hawaiian Sorcerer: Its Dermatologic Implications," *Archives of Dermatology* 90 (1964):530–535.

15. Kamakau, *Ka Po'e Kahiko,* p. 131; Martha Warren Beckwith, *Hawaiian Mythology* (New Haven, CT, 1940, reprint Honolulu, 1970), pp. 105–121; John Papa Ii, *Fragments of Hawaiian History,* ed. Dorothy Barrère, trans. Mary Kawena Pukui (Honolulu, 1959), p. 47; William Ellis, *Polynesian Researches,* 4 vols. (London, 1853); see vol. 2, pp. 335–336.

16. Kamakau, *Ka Po'e Kahiko,* pp. 128–139 (reference to Kamehameha, p. 136); Ii, *Fragments of Hawaiian History,* pp. 123–125.

17. Malo, *Hawaiian Antiquities,* pp. 100–104; Kamakau, *Ka Po'e Kahiko,* pp. 122–128.

18. Malo, p. 103, note 3 by N. B. Emerson; Pukui, *Hawaiian Beliefs and Customs,* pp. 379, 381.

19. Joseph S. Emerson, "The Lesser Hawaiian Gods," *Hawaiian Historical Society Paper* 2 (1892): 1–24; John F. Pogue, *Moolelo of Ancient Hawaii,* trans. Charles W. Kenn (Honolulu, 1978), p. 51.

20. Pukui, Haertig, and Lee, *Nānā i ke Kumu,* vol. 1, p. 48.

21. Louis Freycinet, *Hawai'i in 1819: A Narrative Account by Louis Claude de Saulses de Freycinet,* trans. Ella Wiswell, Bernice P. Bishop Museum Pacific Anthropological Records, no. 26 (Honolulu, 1978), p. 58; J. Gilbert McAllister, *Archaeology of Oahu,* Bernice P. Bishop Museum Bulletin no. 104 (Honolulu, 1933), pp. 84–85.

22. Ellis, *Polynesian Researches,* vol. 3, p. 40.

23. Samuel M. Kamakau, *Ruling Chiefs of Hawaii* (Honolulu, 1961), pp. 197, 315; Ii, *Fragments of Hawaiian History,* pp. 99–100.

24. Kamakau, *Ka Po'e Kahiko,* pp. 32–33; Pukui, Haertig, and Lee, *Nānā i ke Kumu,* vol. 1, pp. 133–134; Abraham Fornander, *An Account of the Polynesian Race: Its Origin and Migration and the Ancient History of the Hawaiian People to the Times of Kamehameha I* (1878–1885; reprint, 3 vols. in 1, Rutland, VT, 1969), vol. 1, p. 108, vol. 2, pp. 104–106; Fornander, *Fornander Collection,* vol. 4, pp. 232–234; Kamakau, *Ruling Chiefs,* pp. 215–218.

25. Kamakau, *Ruling Chiefs,* pp. 206, 213–214, 255.

26. Robert C. Schmitt, "The *Okuu*—Hawaii's Greatest Epidemic," *Hawaiian Medical Journal* 22, no. 5 (1970):363; same author, *Demographic Statistics of Hawaii: 1778–1965* (Honolulu, 1968), pp. 158–159; Ross M. Gast, *A Biography: The Letters and Journal of Francisco de Paula Marin,* ed. Agnes C. Conrad (Honolulu, 1973); Kamakau, *Ruling Chiefs,* pp. 189–190, 380.

27. James Bicknell, *Hoomanamana—Idolatry* (n.d.), p. 7; Ellis, *Polynesian Researches,* vol. 4, p. 310.

28. William Davenport, "The 'Hawaiian Cultural Revolution': Some Political and Economic Considerations," *American Anthropologist* 71, no. 1 (1961):1–20.

29. E. S. Craighill Handy, "Cultural Revolution in Hawaii" (New York, 1931), p. 3.
30. Robert C. Schmitt, "How Many Hawaiians?" *Journal of the Polynesian Society* 76, no. 4 (1967):474; same author, *Demographic Statistics of Hawaii*, 1968.
31. Francis J. Halford, *9 Doctors and God* (Honolulu, 1954).
32. See Heighton, "Hawaiian Strategies"; also Ito, "Symbolic Conscience."
33. E. S. Craighill Handy and Elizabeth Green Handy, *Native Planters in Old Hawaii: Their Life, Lore and Environment*, Bernice P. Bishop Museum Bulletin no. 233 (Honolulu, 1972), p. 224; E. S. Craighill Handy, *The Hawaiian Planter*, vol. 1: *His Plants, Methods and Areas of Cultivation*, Bernice P. Bishop Museum Bulletin no. 161 (Honolulu, 1940), pp. 150–151; Kamakau, *Ruling Chiefs*, p. 299.
34. Archibald Campbell, *A Voyage round the World from 1806–1812* (1822; reprint, Honolulu, 1967), p. 155; Ralph S. Kuykendall, *The Hawaiian Kingdom*, vol. 1: *1778–1854: Foundation and Transformation* (Honolulu, 1938), p. 161.
35. Kuykendall, *Hawaiian Kingdom*, pp. 161–163.
36. Halford, *9 Doctors*, p. 294; Campbell, *Voyage round the World*, pp. 133, 134.
37. Margaret Titcomb, "Kava in Hawaii," *Journal of the Polynesian Society* 57, no. 2 (1948):105–171.
38. F. L. Tabrah and B. M. Eveleth, "Evaluation of the Effectiveness of Ancient Hawaiian Medicine," *Hawaii Medical Journal* 25, no. 3 (1966):223–230.
39. Margaret Mead, *Social Organization of Manua*, Bernice P. Bishop Museum Bulletin no. 76 (Honolulu, 1930), pp. 107ff.
40. James King, *A Voyage to the Pacific Ocean . . . 1776–1780*, vol. 3 (London, 1784), pp. 125–126; Freycinet, *Hawai'i in 1819*, p. 58; Charles E. Snow, *Early Hawaiians: An Initial Study of Skeletal Remains from Mokapu, Oahu* (Lexington, KY, 1974).
41. Kamakau, *Ka Po'e Kahiko*, pp. 110–111; Ii, *Fragments of Hawaiian History*, pp. 47–48; *Kepelino's Traditions of Hawaii*, trans. and ed. Martha Warren Beckwith (Chicago, 1932), pp. 142–146.
42. Kamakau, *Ka Po'e Kahiko*, pp. 32–33; Beckwith, *Hawaiian Mythology*, pp. 46–47.
43. Handy, *Polynesian Religion*, pp. 50–54; Beckwith, *Kepelino's Traditions*, pp. 193–195.
44. Handy, *Polynesian Religion*, pp. 34–43; Beckwith, *Hawaiian Mythology*, pp. 12–13; Pukui, *Hawaiian Beliefs and Customs*, p. 361.
45. Martha Warren Beckwith, trans. and ed., *The Kumulipo: A Hawaiian Creation Chant* (Chicago, 1951), pp. 39, 188; Gutmanis, *Kahuna La'au Lapa'au*, pp. 40–41, 44–46; Kamakau, *Ka Po'e Kahiko*, pp. 102–105.
46. Malo, *Hawaiian Antiquities*, p. 172; Handy and Pukui, *The Polynesian Family System*, pp. 79–82, 122–123; E. S. Craighill Handy, Mary Kawena Pukui, and Katherine Livermore, *Outline of Hawaiian Physical Therapeutics*, Bernice P. Bishop Museum Bulletin no. 126 (Honolulu, 1934), p. 18.
47. Fornander, *Fornander Collection*, vol. 6, p. 70; Gutmanis, *Kahuna La'au Lapa'au*, pp. 13–16.
48. Kamakau, *Ruling Chiefs*, pp. 179, 291; Kamakau, *Ka Po'e Kahiko*, p. 109; Ii, *Fragments of Hawaiian History*, pp. 46–47; Fornander, *Fornander Collection*, vol. 6, pp. 74, 112–114.
49. Teuira Henry, *Ancient Tahiti*, Bernice P. Bishop Museum Bulletin no. 48

(Honolulu, 1928), p. 145; Ii, *Fragments of Hawaiian History*, pp. 45–46, 59–61.

50. McAllister, *Archaeology of Oahu*, p. 103; Nils P. Larsen, "Rededication of the Healing Heiau Keaiwa," *60th Annual Report, Hawaiian Historical Society, 1951* (1952), pp. 7–16; Elspeth P. Sterling and Catherine C. Summers, *Sites of Oahu* (Honolulu, 1978), pp. 11–12; D. M. Kaaiakamanu and J. K. Akina, *Hawaiian Herbs of Medicinal Value*, trans. Akaiko Akana (Honolulu, 1922); see also Handy, Pukui, and Livermore, *Hawaiian Physical Therapeutics*.

51. Ellis, *Polynesian Researches*, vol. 4, pp. 316, 326, 332–334; Handy, *Native Planters of Hawaii*, pp. 582, 586; Kamakau, *Ka Po'e Kahiko*, p. 706; Kamakau, *Ruling Chiefs*, pp. 210–211; Mary Kawena Pukui and Samuel H. Elbert, *Hawaiian Dictionary: Hawaiian-English, English-Hawaiian* (Honolulu, 1986), p. 18.

52. Kamakau, *Ka Po'e Kahiko*, pp. 26–27, 95; Pukui, Haertig, and Lee, *Nānā i ke Kumu*, vol. 2, pp. 145ff.

53. Handy, Pukui, and Livermore, *Hawaiian Physical Therapeutics*, pp. 11–12; Ii, *Fragments of Hawaiian History*, pp. 45–48; Kamakau, *Ka Po'e Kahiko*, pp. 106–112; Malcom Naea Chun, trans., *Hawaiian Medical Book (Te buke laau lapaau)* (Honolulu, 1986).

54. Kamakau, *Ka Po'e Kahiko*, pp. 119–128; Fornander, *Fornander Collection*, vol. 6, p. 74.

55. Kamakau, *Ka Po'e Kahiko*, p. 96.

56. Kamakau, *Ka Po'e Kahiko*, p. 111; Malo, *Hawaiian Antiquities*, pp. 112–113; Nils P. Larsen, "Medical Art in Ancient Hawaii," *53rd Annual Report, Hawaiian Historical Society, 1944* (Honolulu, 1948), pp. 32–37.

57. O. A. Bushnell, "Hawaii's First Medical School," in *Hawaiian Historical Review: Selected Readings*, ed. Richard A. Greer (Honolulu, 1967), pp. 107–121; Ellen Davis, "Kahuna Lapaau, Honolulu Herb Doctor," *Paradise of the Pacific* 58, no. 12 (1946): 49–51; Eleanor Harmon Davis, *Abraham Fornander: A Biography* (Honolulu, 1979), p. 210; *Laws of His Majesty Kamehameha V, King of the Hawaiian Islands: An Act to Establish a Hawaiian Board of Health, June 23, 1868, Passed by the Legislative Assembly at Its 1868 Session* (Honolulu: Printed by Order of the Government).

58. Robert W. Gardner, *Life Tables by Ethnic Group for Hawaii, 1980*, Research and Statistics Report (Honolulu, 1984), p. 7.

59. Snow, *Early Hawaiians*; Ivar Joseph Larsen, "Ancient Hawaiian Medicines" (Thesis, 1966, American Orthopedic Association, Honolulu).

60. Handy and Pukui, *The Polynesian Family System*, pp. 86–87; Snow, *Early Hawaiians*, p. 64.

61. Gutmanis, *Kahuna La'au Lapa'au*, pp. 26–28; Charles Davison, "Hawaiian Medicine," *The Queen's Hospital Bulletin* 4, nos. 3, 4 (1927): pages unnumbered (reprint of an 1899 article); see also Wise and Larsen, "Medicine"; also Larsen, "Ancient Hawaiian Medicines"; Campbell, *A Voyage round the World*, p. 149.

62. Malo, *Hawaiian Antiquities*, pp. 135ff.

63. Handy and Pukui, *The Polynesian Family System*, pp. 133, 182; Gutmanis, *Kahuna La'au Lapa'au*, pp. 31–32.

64. Beckwith, *Kepelino's Traditions*, p. 126; see also Gast, *A Biography*.

65. Fornander, *Fornander Collection*, vol. 6, pp. 2–4; see also Pukui, *Hawaiian Beliefs and Customs*.

66. Pukui, *Hawaiian Beliefs and Customs*, p. 358; Handy and Pukui, *The Poly-*

nesian Family System, p. 77, Gutmanis, *Kahuna La'au Lapa'au*, p. 34; Neen and Beckwith, "Hawaiian Customs Relative to Birth and Infancy," pp. 230–233.

67. Sterling and Summers, *Sites of Oahu*, pp. 138–141; McAllister, *Archaeology of Oahu*, pp. 134–137; Fornander, *An Account of the Polynesian Race*, vol. 2, pp. 20, 62.

68. Malo, *Hawaiian Antiquities*, pp. 136–137; Fornander, *Fornander Collection*, vol. 6, pp. 4–6.

69. Malo, *Hawaiian Antiquities*, pp. 138, 139; Kamakau, *Ruling Chiefs*, pp. 263–265, 309–310; Ii, *Fragments of Hawaiian History*, pp. 161–163.

70. Kamakau, *Ka Po'e Kahiko*, pp. 99–101; Gutmanis, *Kahuna La'au Lapa'au*, pp. 33–34.

71. Kamakau, *Ruling Chiefs*, pp. 68, 188, 386–388; Kamakau, *Ka Po'e Kahiko*, p. 114, note 2.

72. Robert C. Schmitt, *Population Policy in Hawaii* (Honolulu, 1975), pp. 2–5, 17–27; Gutmanis, *Kahuna La'au Lapa'au*, pp. 32–33.

73. Malo, *Hawaiian Antiquities*, pp. 87–93; Handy and Pukui, *The Polynesian Family System*, pp. 95–98.

74. Fornander, *Fornander Collection*, vol. 6, pp. 6–8; Malo, *Hawaiian Antiquities*, pp. 93–95; Handy and Pukui, *The Polynesian Family System*, pp. 94–95.

75. Malo, *Hawaiian Antiquities*, p. 138.

76. Beckwith, *Hawaiian Mythology*, pp. 144–164; Kamakau, *Ka Po'e Kahiko*, pp. 47–53.

77. Handy, *Polynesian Religion*, pp. 248–259; Green and Beckwith, "The Hawaiian Customs and Beliefs relating to Sickness and Death," *American Anthropologist* 28 (1926):176–208; Kamakau, *Ka Po'e Kahiko*, pp. 122ff.; Malo, *Hawaiian Antiquities*, pp. 96ff.

78. Ellis, *Polynesian Researches*, vol. 4, p. 181.

79. Snow, *Early Hawaiians*, pp. 129–148; Peter H. Buck, *Arts and Crafts of Hawaii*, Bernice P. Bishop Museum Special Publication no. 45 (Honolulu, 1957), pp. 573–575.

80. Malo, *Hawaiian Antiquities*, pp. 96–99; Handy and Pukui, *The Polynesian Family System*, pp. 146–153.

81. Malo, *Hawaiian Antiquities*, pp. 104–107; Buck, pp. 575–77.

82. Malo, *Hawaiian Antiquities*, pp. 97–98; Green and Beckwith, "Hawaiian Customs and Beliefs;" Handy and Pukui, *The Polynesian Family System*, pp. 157–59.

83. Kamakau, *Ka Po'e Kahiko*, pp. 47–55.

84. Beckwith, *Hawaiian Mythology*, pp. 163–164; Katharine Luomala, "Phantom Night Marchers in the Hawaiian Islands," *Pacific Studies* 7, no. 1 (1983): 1–33.

CHAPTER 13

Health, Religion, and Medicine in Native North American Traditions

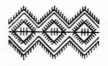

Åke Hultkrantz

Native North American beliefs closely connect health and religion in an individual. In all enterprises and life crises, Indians have turned to religion—that is, the supernatural world and its powers—in order to protect their existence and the existence of their loved ones. When serious sickness occurs, medical aid is provided by persons who, through inspiration or training, have become mediators between human beings and the supernatural powers. Life and death, medicine and health, are enclosed in a cosmic-religious context.

The following text presents the main perspectives applicable to an account of the complex of health, religion, and medicine among North American Indians. The approach that has been selected here is generally comparative, but there will be case studies whenever the context demands more palpable information. Historical arguments will occasionally be resorted to when necessary.

Concept of Health

Since the native peoples of North America represent a multitude of nations (tribes, tribelets) and are part of a great many cultures, depending on the ways these cultures are defined, it is difficult to give a unified picture of their ideas of health and illness. However, across linguistic and cultural boundaries there are certain common attitudes and beliefs that practically all of them share.[1]

The main emphasis should be placed on the concept of health. Again and again we meet concern for health in prayers, public and individual. Here is a prayer said at Christmastime (the Shalako ceremonies) among the Zuni of New Mexico:

> I have been praying for my people that they may have much rain and good crops and that they may be fortunate with their babies and that they may have no misfortunes and no sickness. I have been praying that my people may have no sickness to make them unhappy. . . . I want my people to reach old age and to come to the ends of their roads, and not be cut off while they are still young.[2]

Similarly, the Oglala Sioux in Dakota who have joined the annual Sun Dance—the greatest ceremony of the tribe, in which the participants sacrifice parts of their own flesh—cry out to the supreme powers, "O *Wakan-Tanka*, be merciful to me, that my people may live! It is for this that I am sacrificing myself."[3] At sweat baths Oglala pray to the heated stones, "O Rocks, you have neither eyes, nor mouth, nor limbs; you do not move, but by receiving your sacred breath [the steam], our people will be long-winded as they walk the path of life; your breath is the very breath of life."[4]

Today, health represents an even more important value than when hunting, horticulture, warfare, and individual prowess played more decisive roles. Many rituals once performed in connection with concerns about the annual round, access of animals, and growth of vegetation have been transformed into rituals of health. The Sun Dance of the Plains Indians is an outstanding example.

Formerly the Sun Dance was an annual renewal ceremony held when the grass had turned green and the plains teemed with buffalo, a thanksgiving ceremony to the Supreme Being for another plentiful year, and (particularly among some Siouan tribes) a sacrifice in return for a heeded prayer.[5] However, after 1890 (the year of the calamitous Ghost Dance events) when the old military pattern collapsed in a Messianistic uprising, in many areas the Sun Dance became a ritual for health and blessing. In the Shoshoni Sun Dance in Wyoming the climax is the treatment of sick persons and invalids by medicine men: they step forward in the dancing lodge to the sacred center pole—a symbol of the Great Spirit and of the path of communication with him. They stand barefoot on this sacred spot, upright before the big pole. They are swept with feather wings by the medicine man, who also prays over them. When the Sun Dance finishes, the supplicants heap blankets at the base of the pole as a token of gratitude to the Supreme Being. Similar developments in the Sun Dance have taken place among the Shoshoni-Bannock and the Ute of the Intermontane area.[6]

The theme of health dominates the religion of the Navajo in the Southwest. During their close coexistence with the Pueblo Indians from the seventeenth century onward, the Navajo adopted their ceremonial patterns. However, while the Pueblo ceremonies served the needs of agriculture and fertility, the less agricultural Navajo adapted these ceremonial patterns to the requirements of their own society in the area of health and curing. Some of the healing practices appear to have been adopted from old Navajo hunting rites.[7]

Health was a major concern also in the early history of North American Indians and, as the premise for human life, was taken to be the result of supernatural blessing. In order to establish this relationship between health and religion it is necessary to identify two separate ideological complexes in North American religions, the old hunting ideology and the ideology of "cosmic balance."[8] There is a tendency today to identify all Native American religion as furthering the perspective of cosmic balance, or cosmotheism, as it has also been called (by Horst Hartmann).[9] This is scarcely correct. Within the hunting ideology, dispersed or indigenous among the various hunting Indians but also among some horticulturists, human health is considered a gift from the supernatural powers, in particular the high god or the guardian spirits. In particular, the guardian-spirit complex is highly integrated with concerns for health. The cosmotheistic ideology has its centers among Pueblo and Prairie Indians and the descendants of the latter among the Plains Indians. It was probably originally part of the advanced horticultural civilizations of ancient Mexican design. The characteristic features of this ideology are the idea that human beings, supernaturals, and the world constitute one integrated whole and that humankind contributes to this cosmic harmony by conducting rituals intended to reflect or stabilize this harmony. The state of bodily and mental health is an integrating part of this cosmic harmony. Surprisingly, this thought has been best developed among the former hunters, the Navajo, but it appears of course among Pueblo and Prairie peoples as well.

Health is thus entirely dependent on one's relation to the supernatural. While afflictions may occur without any change in these relations, a major illness indicates that they are not in proper balance. Since health is a supernatural gift, or a consequence of correct relations to the cosmic powers, the individual's ability to improve his or her health by profane means is limited. As a rule Indians have not cared much about hygiene. To take one example, the Comanche of the Southern Plains did not wash except for certain ritual purifications. We are told that consequently parasites were a continual problem, which, however, people stoically ignored.[10] On the other hand, from childhood on boys were hardened to withstand cold, hardship, and physical pains, particularly the sons of hunting Indians. But this regimen had to do with fitness, not with health. In ethnographical monographs and native American autobiographies there are descriptions of how Indian boys, in their early childhood, were instructed by the old men of the tribe to take a dip in the river by the camp each morning. It mattered little if it was summer or winter. Among the Lakota (Dakota) there were contests of strength among young boys. In winter the contestants plunged into the icy waters to find out who could endure the longest.[11] It was customary among the same Indians that when a boy was born his young brother had to jump into the water, or if it was winter, roll in the snow naked; his sister had to be immersed. "The idea was that a warrior had come to camp, and the other children must display some act of hardihood."[12]

Before they came into contact with whites, Indians suffered less from rampant diseases; but health became a major problem after the white invasion, when epidemics of smallpox, introduced (together with other diseases) by the whites, took their toll. Population geneticists have recently shown how the Indian population was radically reduced because of the new contagious diseases.[13]

Concepts of Disease

In the view of traditional Indians, injuries and diseases of a more severe nature are signs of weakened relationships with supernatural powers. Consciousness of this fact causes the Indians to react in two ways: they accept suffering as an unavoidable consequence of the circumstances at hand, and they try to find means to reestablish their relations with the supernatural world in a positive way. Among these means of restoration are measures against vicious spirits, among whom are ghosts and ogres, and against witchcraft.

Because of the often-difficult conditions of their existence, suffering, in one form or another, is something that most Indians learn to accept and endure from an early age. To take one example, the Cahuilla of southern California lived at one time under stressful conditions that caused anxiety and physical or psychosomatic illnesses. They lived in constant fear that they would be unable to gather and hunt enough food for their families, since at any time they could be overtaken by forest fires, earthquakes, flash floods, torrential rains, or drought.[14] Much suffering is culturally induced. Literature is full of references to the stoic spirit of American Indians, their capacity to withstand pain and torment. The endurance of Northeastern Indians at the torture pole is legendary, and so is the Plains Indian's emotional indifference in facing a painful death. The many cases of self-torture in the Sun Dance or in the ordeals of the vision quest also demonstrate the Indians' ability to endure pain and suffering. In these cases the suffering is not imposed upon the individuals by others, but self-inflicted in order to evoke the compassion of the powers. The spirits take pity on individuals who exhibit their humility to them.[15]

The suffering of illness is, in the long perspective, a consequence of the introduction of death into the world. There are myths about the origin of death, according to which death was instituted in order to prevent the world from becoming overpopulated by humankind. Some myths refer the original decision to a discussion between two higher supernatural beings, usually the creator and his tricksterlike companion, or to a divination arranged by these beings.[16]

The lightheartedness with which the fate of humanity is said to have been decided is often stunning. The Blackfoot myth tells us that at the beginning of time two supreme supernatural beings, Old Man and Old Woman, disputed about whether human beings should live on indefinitely or die. Old Man wanted humankind to live forever, but his partner pointed out the difficulty with this suggestion: there would be too many people. Old Man then tried a compromise, a period of death lasting only four days. Old Woman, however, objected that only if human beings died forever could they mourn each other. Since no consensus could be reached the two beings trusted the decision to chance. They agreed to divine through the throwing of buffalo droppings into the water: if these sank the humans should die forever. Old Man threw the droppings in, and he might have gained the upper hand if Old Woman had not had a strong supernatural cleverness. She transformed the droppings into a

stone that immediately sank. Thus human beings were condemned to
die.[17] It is characteristic for this male-oriented society to blame a female
divinity for the introduction of death.

Death is thus a divinely ordained fact to which humankind has to
accommodate itself. Sometimes it comes suddenly, sometimes it is heralded by disease. Disease is believed to be a gradual dying, or the beginning of dying. This is illustrated by the course of an illness that is caused
by the loss of the soul (a phenomenon that will be described in more
detail below): the soul moves toward the realm of the dead, and once
there the person is—terminologically, that is—"dead." In many North
American languages the terms for "dead" and "unconsciousness" are the
same.[18] They refer to the apparent absence of life and motion in the body
and to the absence of the spirit or soul that normally leaves the body only
in dream excursions.

So far our discussion of illness has referred to physical pain and physical ailments, injuries, and debilities. What about the mental weaknesses
that Western culture classifies as illnesses? While such a classification may
occur, the concept of normality is not the same as our own. Much of the
behavior that would appear abnormal according to our standards is integrated with shamanism and vision-related behavior. We could say, with
Henry Wegrocki, that the "abnormal" behavior of the hallucinating
Indian is analogous to the behavior of the psychotic, but it is not
homologous.[19]

However, some behavior that deviates from the norms of the tribal
culture is interpreted by some societies as inspired by bad spirits, or even
as the result of possession. A typical instance is supplied by the windigo
complex of some Canadian woodland Algonkians. The *windigo*—or
witiko, as it is called in some western areas—is a giant, cannibalistic monster with a heart of ice who is believed to roam woods and desolate places.
Windigoes are particularly active during the long and cold winters, and
the Indian people dread them. It is easy to see that these beliefs are related
to the hunger cannibalism occasionally instanced in these regions during
the winter when it is difficult to find game. Some people are said to turn
into windigoes. There are stories of men who have devoured their hunting comrades and of women who have been forced to kill and eat their
own children. They have become possessed by windigoes, or they have
by an unfortunate chance acquired spirit helpers who are windigoes.
Since cannibalism is abhorred by Algonkian Indians, these cannibalistic
windigo persons do indeed violate the norms of their society.[20]

Being deprived of one's main soul, or free-soul, may result in similar
deviant behavior. In this case the dead may have stolen the soul (as a
revenge for some insult, or to have good company), or it may be a matter
of witchcraft. It is not uncommon in North America for medicine men
who have great powers, including evil powers, to transform themselves

into evildoing wizards who then try to destroy their fellow humans.[21] People suffering from afflictions caused by ghosts and witches are usually left alone, unless the family asks for a doctor's treatment. The first step back to health may then be the destruction of the witch or wizard through the use of magic.

The line between normal and abnormal is thus difficult to draw here. Much aberrant behavior has become socialized in Trickster myths or in clown performances—epics and rituals that function as psychological outlets in culturally patterned, strained situations.[22]

A particular problem is the Indian evaluation of the use of drugs, including alcoholic beverages. Indigenous use of liquor prior to Indian contact with whites occurred in the Southeast and the Southwest, where agave, cacti, and persimmon were used in the production of alcoholic beverages. Only where alcohol was imbibed for religious purposes—to aid falling into trance or to produce rain—was drunkenness accepted in former days; otherwise it was despised and even punished.

The summer rain ceremony of the Papago in Arizona was most important, as it promoted the fertility of the corn and the cactus in this arid, sterile country. People of all sexes and ages drank the fermented juice of the sahuaro cactus. According to one ethnographer, Ruth Underhill, there was a drinking ceremony during which the rain gods of the four directions were invoked. They were expected to wet the earth to satiety, just as the bodies of the drinkers were saturated with powerful liquor. Another ethnographer, Kenneth Stewart, contends that "the ritual drunkenness induced a purification of the mind and heart, which would impel the rains to come." Whatever the exact meaning, an alcoholic beverage was consumed until complete intoxication and stupor ensued—thus ritually ensuring the good of the society.[23]

As far as I have been able to discover, alcoholism was never classed as a particular disease, but as an aberration of the mind.

Psychotropic drugs, whether narcotic in a strict sense or not, were never evaluated as a means of intoxication leading to mental disturbances. Instead they were, and are, appreciated as "doors of perception" to another reality, supernatural in quality.[24] The best example is peyote (*Lophophora williamsii*), the small, spineless cactus that has given rise to the modern pan-Indian peyote religion. Because of its hallucinogenic character, its ability to create moods of happiness, harmony, and friendship, the peyote has become a divinity identified with both Mother Earth and Saint Mary. Indulgence in peyote produces no harmful medical consequences, as far as we now know. To the Indians it is helpful "medicine" for all sorts of afflictions and thus is used against all types of disease.[25]

Not long ago on the Southern Plains and in parts of the Southwest the "mescal bean," which contains a very toxic alkaloid, was consumed on ritual occasions.[26] It produced nausea and convulsions, indeed, even

death if taken in a large quantity. To the Indians, however, both the peyote and the mescal bean led into the world of mysteries, the supernatural
world. A person who had taken these drugs was not physically or mentally deranged but simply blessed by supernatural power.

The Medical Practitioner

The American Indian has always, like other people, had recourse to specialists who profess to be able to relieve the community of injuries, sickness, and suffering. Since the first days of French colonialism and Jesuit
missions in *La nouvelle France* these specialists have generally been called
medicine men. Most of these doctors have healed by supernatural means,
since health is a supernaturally granted state, but simpler diseases and
fractures have often not been connected to direct supernatural causality,
and they have therefore been cured by wise men without particular divine
calling.

From a modern perspective it is possible to make the following distinctions between American Indian practitioners:[27]

1. Healers of wounds and diseases that are not believed to have a
   supernatural origin or that derive from a more general supernatural
   background ("all diseases are due to bad relations with the supernatural world") and not from direct intercession by supernatural
   agents. These practitioners are often old men and women, and they
   are experienced herbalists. Some of them may heal bone fractures.
   All these doctors base their knowledge primarily on traditional
   medical lore; they need not be further discussed here.

2. Medicine men who cure by supernatural means since the disease
   agents are supernatural. These medicine men have received their
   powers through inspirational visions, but their curing usually takes
   place in a lucid state, or—perhaps more correctly—during a light
   trance.

3. Shamans, or doctors, working in a deep trance. The shaman is a
   social functionary who with the aid of his guardian spirits may
   enter a deep trance during which he may send out his soul (or one
   of his souls) or call on the supernatural powers to give him information and assistance. The shaman may be said to be a medicine
   man (if medicine is tantamount to power), but he is not always a
   doctor. Some shamans only give advice or information to people
   or help them to find the wild game. Most shamans are, however,
   doctors who cure the sick during their trance states.

Shamans who are exclusively ecstatic diviners may be attached to the curing process: although they do not cure, they are able to diagnose, as the example of the Navajo hand-tremblers shows. Hand-tremblers are persons who have received the gift of divining the whereabouts of hidden things, the outcome of hunting and war, or the nature of diseases. Their power lies in their ability to reveal what is not known. When a person is sick and the person and attached family do not know why—it could be that a taboo has been violated, or that a ghost, a witch, or even one of the holy spirits has attacked the person—a member of the family contacts a hand-trembler, and they make an agreement as to the time of the treatment and the payment.

The divination begins as soon as the hand-trembler takes his place beside the patient. He washes his own hands and arms and then puts pollen under the patient's feet, on the patient's hands, on the top of the patient's head, and so forth. Then he decorates his own right arm and fingers with pollen, praying to the mightly spirits, the Gila monsters, to tell him from what disease the patient is suffering. There is then a compact silence in the hogan (the lodge). The hand-trembler now begins to sing, invoking the Gila monsters. His hand and arm begin to shake violently. The movements his hand is making give information as to the nature of the disease. Besides telling the cause of the disease the divination reveals what kind of ceremony can remove it, the time the ceremonial should be performed, and what practitioners (ritual singers) must be selected.[28]

Due to the uneven and sparse source material on aboriginal medicine in eastern North America it is difficult to tell how common shamanic disease healers have been on this continent. The following general statements must therefore be preliminary. The best examples of shamanism with soul excursions come from the Eskimo area and the Northwest Coast, the Great Basin, and the Algonkian tribes.[29] The primary example of calling on spirits in shamanic ecstasy is the so-called "shaking tent" or "spirit lodge" ceremony (today mostly known as *yuwipi*, a modified version of the original shaking tent). It may be instanced among the Eskimo, the Algonkians, and the Plateau tribes, and in its modified form it is represented among the Lakota and other Plains groups influenced by them. Healing is perhaps less often a part of this ceremony, but it does occur.[30] There are also ceremonies in which shamans call on spirits from the tops of poles or the top of the ceremonial lodge, but as far as I know there is no connection with healing activities in these cases.

The Northwest Coast furnishes the most convincing examples of true (psychological) possession of the acting shamans, probably a continuation of the Siberian shamanic complex.[31] In other parts of North America, for instance the Plains, shamanism has been much weakened through the growth of the vision-quest complex, which opens the ecstatic experiences to any common man (or woman, particularly after menopause, when they are no longer considered dangerous or polluting). The medicine man is there, but his role deviates only slightly from the common visionary; namely, in his having more and stronger guardian spirits and in their being specialized in curing in some form.[32]

The North American medicine man is a charismatic figure who sometimes has an in-depth knowledge of ceremonial and mythological traditions, but indeed often knows very little about such matters. His expertise consists in knowing how to approach the supernatural world. He has received his training in this knowledge through visionary contacts with his guardian spirits. There is usually one particular guardian spirit for each disease he can cure, but not always; in the shaking tent ritual, for instance, the number of present spirits is legion. One of the most potent curing spirits all over North America is the bear, for reasons we cannot identify exactly (perhaps it has to do with the bear's physical strength or a combination of this strength with the widespread bear ceremonialism or the Siberian bear shamans).[33] In addition to the bear spirit—or rather, to be exact, the spirit that operates in bear form—there are many zoomorphic spirits that may mediate curing powers to a medical candidate. The methods of acquiring these powers change with cultural areas. In California and other places, a presumptive medicine man may be born with the power. In North America west of the Rocky Mountains, the spirit makes itself known in a spontaneous dream. On the Plateau and in the eastern parts of North America, the candidate generally has to perform a vision quest, that is, induce the visionary experience of the spirit through fasting and other hardships at a desolate place out in the wilderness.

As was pointed out, the latter procedure does not deviate from the normative behavior of other vision seekers—nobody knows in advance if the spirit that shows itself will confer medical powers. The candidate may pray for such powers, but the spirit that he invokes may not be a lender of medical powers, or it may disavow the supplicant because of a violated taboo or for other reasons. Sometimes the spirit is enraged and deprives the vision seeker of his senses, or his physical health.

Two cases of the conferring of visions will be presented here, the first one illustrating the acquirement of power in an unsought vision, the second one in a sought vision. Both accounts have been taken from the Plains Indians, and both concern medical power.

The Crow Indian Bull-all-the-time had received martial powers in a vision through fasting and self-torture. Later he was also blessed with doctoring powers while he was asleep in his tipi (tent). Dr. Robert Lowie, to whom the warrior confided his dream, describes it as follows: "He saw a horse fastened to a rope, which was lengthened up to him. He heard a person sing. The horse was a sign that my informant would get horses as fees for his cures. He was told that if anyone fell sick he was to doctor him. He saw an old man decorated with red paint and holding a pipe in his hand. This man was standing over the recumbent patient and blew through a pipestem over him. The sick man rose and then sat down. Bull-all-the-time saw all the sickness come out of the patient's blood and saw him get well. Bull-all-the-time showed me the pipestem he had dreamt of; it had a horse's track incised near one end."[34]

Black Elk, the well-known Oglala Lakota holy man, had a spontaneous great vision in his very early childhood to which much attention has been paid among scholars. In this vision the Thunder spirits had prepared him for his future reception of medical powers. In 1882, at the age of eighteen, he undertook the necessary ceremonies, fasting, and purification, that prepare the supplicant to quest for a vision. With a robe and a pipe, and in the company of a medicine man serving as an instructor, he went on horseback some miles into the wilderness. He stayed at a hill where he performed tobacco offerings and executed the ritual movements between the cardinal points as prescribed by tradition.[35]

As he lamented to the beings on high (the Wakan Tanka), an eagle, a chicken hawk, and a black swallow appeared close by. Then a swarm of beautiful butterflies became visible. They seemed to be crying. The eagle pronounced, "Behold them, these are your people. . . . These people shall be in great difficulty and you shall go there." Then there was a great storm—the Thunder beings were coming. Two men descended from the clouds, cheered by voices in the thunderclouds. Riding on sorrel horses they aimed with bow and arrow at a dog appearing among the swarm of butterflies. An arrow pierced the dog's head which glided upwards and was transformed into a man's head. Black Elk was crying with fear and asked the supernatural grandfathers to spare him. He wrapped the robe around himself while large hailstones fell around him; the thunder was booming and lightning flashes were lighting up the night sky. When the storm had passed eastward he observed that although much rain had fallen it was dry within the sacred circle of offering where he was lying. He dozed off to sleep, and saw in his dream his people who were worried and sick. A voice proclaimed, "Your people are in difficulty. Make haste. They need you." Black Elk began to cry again. At daybreak he was meditating on what had happened during the night. "I knew what to do now because I had clarity of understanding, and I was to be a medicine man."

The advising medicine man now appeared and brought Black Elk back to the camp. The old men were informed, and they told Black Elk to help humanity.[36]

After this vision Black Elk demonstrated his powers in a *heyoka* ceremony, a ceremony in which contrary behavior patterns are exhibited. Among other things he plunged his hands into very hot water without getting burned. (This is a common shamanic feat in the Old World.) In this way Black Elk proved his powers. Some time afterward, a man by the name of Cuts to Pieces approached Black Elk's tipi and asked him to cure his son. Cuts to Pieces had witnessed Black Elk's display of mysterious power at the *heyoka* and said that this demonstration had convinced him that Black Elk would have the power to cure his son. (This is an excellent illustration of the belief that the medicine man is able to cure not only because he has specifically medical power, but simply because he has power.) Black Elk had never cured anyone, but he had watched other medicine men healing, so he decided to follow their examples. He told Cuts to Pieces to bring a pipe with eagle feathers attached. He lit this pipe and offered it to the four quarters, zenith and nadir, and then he circulated it among those present. Black Elk informed John Neihardt, the author to whom he conveyed his teachings, that he had of course never received any instructions as to how to proceed, but just set a course for his curing.

He went to where the sick boy lay. He was four years old, all skin and bones. Black Elk arranged the pipe, a cup, a drum, and a magic herb as he had seen them in his vision. He drummed while sending a prayer to Wakan Tanka and sang a song about walking the good road with his people, healing all along the way. He felt something moving in the boy's breast, perhaps, he thought, a little blue man, and putting his mouth on the boy's belly he sucked out the disease. As he sucked he felt the little blue man in his mouth. This was the first cure Black Elk performed.[37]

These two cases exemplify different ways in which medical knowledge could be obtained: whereas Bull-all-the-time had a visionary preview of the curing act, Black Elk knew only that the powers had selected him to be a medicine man and that he had to discover through his own vague intuition how to proceed when curing. He was guided by the pattern set by other medicine men and by the symbols he had seen in his vision.

In most cases, however, there is supernatural instruction for the future medicine man. The spirit of the vision informs his client as to the sorts of disease he will be empowered to cure and about the methods he will use. Usually the cure is combined with ritual prescripts, such as instructions pertaining to clothing, body painting, singing, and the use of particular paraphernalia, like feathers and rattles. The spirit also informs the new medicine man of the taboos he must observe (not eating with a metal knife, for instance). Many little-understood details of a medicine man's appearance and behavior have their explanation in the visionary message.

There exist various ways of making a medicine man, but the general account and the examples given here typify a great many cases. As a rule there is no practical training of the candidate with another, experienced medicine man, although such apprenticeships do occur; nor is there a formal initiation rite. However, where the vision rituals are more formalized, as among the Sioux, festive meals may complete the trials. The new medicine man will be accepted as soon as he has accomplished a successful curing. The degree to which he is able to employ his profession is dependent on the reputation he enjoys—just as it is in Western society. Any person who has not been blessed by a spirit to be a medicine man would not dare to assume the role. It is generally believed that the powers will severely punish a charlatan. In some places a circle of well-known medicine men sit down to judge the visionary dreams that a candidate is reporting, sanctioning their legitimacy and correct interpretation.

The American medicine man does not dedicate himself exclusively to his vocation. He is also a family man, and a hunter, horticulturist, rancher, or tradesman. While the income from his medical profession is not insignificant, it is insufficient for his subsistence. Formerly, blankets and horses were common gifts to the medicine man from the members of the diseased person's family. Today his services are repaid in money, often equivalent to a white doctor's fee.

The individual medicine man or shaman is primarily a functionary of hunting cultures. His milieu is that of the hunting band, his curing arena that of his own or his patients' lodge, where the family of the sick person and other sympathizers from the band or group surround the curing drama. However, in some cultures, where horticultural pursuits predominate in economic life, there are no individual medicine men, but medicine societies that try to eliminate the disease factors through ritual performance, singing, and dancing. The Pueblo medicine societies of the Southwest offer good examples of this collective form of curing.

Among the Zuni, for instance, anyone who has been treated as a patient by one of the twelve medicine societies is requested to join the society; if he does not, his life is in danger. The societies are medical corporations with secret knowledge and esoteric rituals—in fact, we know very little of their traditions. All we can say is that their ceremonies are numerous and extremely intricate. The societies are protected by the "beast gods," as they have been called, animal spirits which are believed to be the givers of medicine. Most powerful among these animal powers is the bear, who is impersonated at curing ceremonies by officers wearing bear paws drawn over their hands—a token that they are identified with the bear in their curative functions. It is obvious that the bear and other beast gods play the same roles as the guardian spirits do in hunting societies. Each of the societies is specialized in curing a certain set of diseases, and has its own healing ritual. The most common method of healing is by sucking out a pathogenic object.[38]

From all appearances, the medicine societies have developed out of the fraternities of individual medicine men. However, in the course of development the original inspirational calling seems to have been supplanted by priestly education, and the trance-like curative operations by priestly ceremonials.

Diagnosis and Curing

When a patient falls ill, his or her relatives—usually the nuclear family—are anxious to find a medical specialist. However, if the problem is only a superficial wound or a more common problem like stomachache or skin disease, they may consult a knowledgeable person in the family (a grandmother, for instance). If the wound is more complicated or the trouble more insistent, the family calls upon an old man or woman versed in the healing art. Herbal remedies are common in such cases. Extensive knowledge of herbal medicine existed in North America, as the large source works on ethnobotany testify.[39] Patients with broken legs were treated by bone doctors who, using smoke, water, and other means, could put a broken bone right again.

Examples of this type of healer are the "medicine women" of the Cherokee of the Southeast (Tennessee and environs). While ordinary medicine men must be brought into their profession by older colleagues, these women are primarily midwives who are reputed to be particularly proficient in their calling. They have gradually extended their knowledge to include the handling of prenatal problems and other complications connected with childbirth, and have finally come to be looked upon as ordinary medical practitioners. As such they are also asked to treat ailments of different sorts. Among the Cherokee, treatment consists of the use of herbs and the recitation of sacred formulas that have been preserved in documents.[40]

In practically every tribe we hear of men and women who, like the Cherokee women practitioners, have absorbed some of the functions and abilities of the real medicine men. None of these doctors have been called to their functions by the spirits, or need to be. Only in the case of life-threatening disease is there need of specialists with divine calling, the medicine men proper.

The family usually has a wide field of selection in the choosing of a medicine man. It is difficult to know how many medicine men were available in the past when Amerindian cultures flourished, but some calculations seem to suggest ten to twenty medicine men per thousand individuals (I am here referring to a discussion I once had with Paul Radin). There may have been more, and it is reasonable to assume that the figure varied according to cultural context and social structure. Since patients and their relatives do not know from what disease they suffer (unless it is TB or another well-known disease with easily recognizable symptoms), the choice of a medicine man is generally motivated by the reputation a particular medicine man enjoys in that particular family, that particular society. Sometimes the chosen medicine man cedes his task to a colleague who is better acquainted with the disease symptoms. It may also happen that two or more medicine men are needed working together on the same patient, as they often do in the Sun Dance.

Sometimes the invitation to a suitable medicine man has to be made by a friend or distant family member and must be performed in a ritual manner. However, there are also reports of medicine men who have been admonished by their guardian spirits to seek out sick persons and attend to them.

The first duty of the medicine man is to make a diagnosis. He may do this in several ways: dream about the cause of the disease, "see" it through a looking glass or even a nontransparent object, or enter a trance to seek it out. Sometimes, as we have seen among the Navajo, there are special diviners to perform this function. The medicine man of the northern California Achomawi Indians learns the nature of the disease through his guardian spirits. Chanting quietly and swaying with half-closed eyes, he puts himself into a meditative state and gradually falls into ecstasy. After some time he perceives that his guardian spirit has arrived. Then he claps his hands and addresses his questions to the spirit in a rapid voice. The bystanders hear how he repeats the answers of the spirit. After a while he stops, opens his eyes, and begins the cure.[41]

In principle, we find that North American medicine men make two types of diagnosis: object intrusion (or, alternatively, spirit intrusion) and loss of the soul.

OBJECT INTRUSION AND SPIRIT INTRUSION

An object or damaging spiritual being of minor dimensions has entered the patient's body, creating pains, swelling, wounds, and other problems. We talk then about "object intrusion" and "spirit intrusion." Sometimes there is a sharp difference between the spirit and the object, but in other cases they tend to be identical, the one flowing into the other (just as the medicine power may oscillate between a materialistic and a personalistic interpretation). Cases of intrusion of objects are extremely well documented in the Americas from practically all quarters, whereas instances of spirit intrusion are more sporadic (they occur primarily in western Alaska, on the Northwest Coast, among Central Algonkians, Southeast Indians, and the Navajo of the Southwest).[42]

There is usually a spiritual agent behind these intruding forces, or possibly a human witch. When a spirit has caused the disease it has often been enraged because of the patient's breaking of taboos or ritual rules. For instance, a male patient might have been too close to a woman's menstruation hut. In some tribes there are particularly dangerous beings who dispatch diseases. One such being is the Winnebago "disease-giver"— according to Radin, "an anthropomorphic figure, dealing out death from one side of his body and life from the other." Thus, as a guardian spirit he confers the power of curing diseases. When prayers are directed to him he is implored to turn away his death side and show only his life side.[43]

Unfortunately, in Anglo-Saxon literature spirit intrusion has been confused with "possession," which is a psychological concept and should be understood as the suppression of a person's normal consciousness and its replacement by the personality of a spiritual being. Reports that a certain person, such as a medicine man, houses intruding spirits may imply true possessional states, but not necessarily.[44]

The intrusion diagnosis is primarily applied when physical pains are in the foreground of the disease. Often the particular aching spots can be pointed out by the patient, and are then referred to the care of the medicine man. There are also cases of this kind where the medicine man diagnoses a loss of the soul (or a soul). However, this is less common and probably not original.

LOSS OF THE SOUL

The soul, or one of the souls, has become lost, resulting in the patient's withering away. Underlying this belief is the idea that human beings have a separable soul—commonly known as the free soul—that in states of weakness and unconsciousness may distance itself from the body. Or it may be snatched away by a supernatural being, for instance, a deceased close relative who longs for company, or a witch that wants to destroy the person. Also, shocks and sudden injuries may make the soul "jump out" of the body and go astray.[45] Usually the wandering soul is drawn to the realm of the dead, and it gravitates toward this place.[46]

In order to understand this psychology, so predominant among North American hunting Indians but somewhat less clearly conceived in the southern and horticultural parts of North America, it is necessary to study their soul systems. These are crucial to the interpretation of disease concepts in most of North America. Although there are many variations in these systems, we may, audaciously generalizing, supply the following picture, which has an overwhelming representation in our sources. There are two different soul complexes in human beings, one covering the several souls or potencies that sustain individuals when they are in a lucid consciousness, the other consisting of just one soul that is the image of the person and is active when one sleeps or is entranced or unconscious—in other words, an extracorporeal soul, representing a person in his or her entirety. The first set of souls comprises the body souls that rule the heart, movements, pulses, emotions, and will power of the waking individual, while the image soul is the so-called free-soul, which can detach itself from the person and is then the carrier of the ego. There is an interchange of functions between the two soul concepts, which alternate in representing the human being.[47]

On the occasion of "soul loss" a soul (in the typical cases the free-soul) leaves the body for the realm of the dead. As long as some body souls remain with the body the person's life is not immediately endangered. However, once the free-soul has crossed the boundaries of the other world the body souls usually depart—there is no breath, no beating of the heart, no movements—and the patient is dead. Only in exceptional cases will it be possible for the shaman to rescue the free-soul from the land of the dead and thus restore the patient's life.

The diagnosis of soul loss occurs primarily when the patient suffers from fever or when mental capacities are reduced such that the patient seems to be absent, to be languishing away. The same interpretation is given when the person has become unconscious or is deeply entranced. It is thus the state of the patient's mind that determines this diagnosis. Sometimes, however, physical ailments may be explained as due to soul loss. From all evidence, this must be a late explanation in a society dominated by the soul-loss concept.

There has been some discussion among anthropologists concerning the relative age of these two diagnoses, in America and elsewhere. Because there have been more frequent instances of the intrusion diagnosis documented in later time, the general opinion has been that the intrusion idea is older than the soul-loss idea.[48] This conclusion could however be contested. It is true that in certain cultures there has been a tendency toward patterning disease theories in one direction only, reflecting historical development. However, if we look more closely into the North American data we find that the two diagnoses usually occur side by side, although one of them may be preferred. Comparative data from North Eurasia indicate that the two diagnoses correspond to two different lines of observation, which may be roughly correlated with the states of the body and the mind, respectively. The North American ethnographical evidence corroborates this conclusion.[49] The therapy used to alleviate these diseases is directly related to the diagnosis.

CURES FOR INTRUSION

The medicine man removes the foreign object or spirit by sucking it out, drawing it out by sweeping feathers over the aching area, blowing it out through his cupped hands, and similar methods. Such dramatic performances have been exceedingly common all over North America. Sometimes they have been combined with efforts of the medicine man to frighten away the intruding force.

The following account from the Chippewa of Minnesota may illustrate an advanced type of intrusion cure. A woman suffered from a sore throat and the medicine man who was called in treated her in the following way. First, he narrated his visionary dream in order to establish his authority as a doctor. Then he had the room darkened, sang for a while, and shook his rattle. This, he said, enabled him to discover the cause of the disease and its cure. He swallowed and then threw up small tube-like bones (a feat of jugglery which proved how clever he was). He placed one of the bones against the patient's throat and blew forcefully through it, again and again. This caused the disease to break up and flow out of her mouth.[50]

Some medicinal operations are combined with dramatic actions—for instance, the medicine man may appear in the disguise of his guardian spirit, imitating the noise and movements of the animal that the spirit incarnates. Such appearances may frighten the intruding spirit, causing it to flee.

A classic account of a curing ceremony of this type has been given by the painter George Catlin, who visited Fort Union at the mouth of the Yellowstone in 1832. There were Indians trading at the Fort, among them Blackfeet and Cree, who were old enemies. A Cree shot down a Blackfoot chief with two bullets from his gun, and a short fight ensued. Although the chief's wound was fatal, his kinsfolk called in a medicine man to treat him. Catlin describes how several hundred spectators, both Indians and traders, were assembled around the dying man. They formed a ring, leaving a space of some thirty or forty feet in diameter for the operation scene. At the arrival of the medicine man a hush descended on the crowd. He quietly approached the patient, assuming a crouching position. His body and head were hidden behind the skin and head of the grizzly bear. In one hand he shook a tambourine-like rattle, in the other he kept a wand, "to the rattling din and discord of all of which, he added the wild and startling jumps and yelps of the Indian, and the horrid and appalling grunts, and snarls, and growls of the grizzly bear, in ejaculatory and gutteral incantations to the Good and Bad Spirits, in behalf of his patient; who was rolling and groaning in the agonies of death, whilst he was dancing around him, jumping over him, and pawing him about, and rolling him in every direction." The medicine man worked on his patient in this way for half an hour, when death ensued.[51]

This dramatic occurrence may be explained thus: like many other powerful medicine men, this doctor had the grizzly bear for his guardian spirit. By donning the bear's fell he identified himself with the spirit, and by growling and crouching like a bear he exercised this spirit's powers. In this case, however, the evil powers of the injury could not be frightened away.

Many medicine men are able to suck and then spit out the pathogenic object or spirit, which sometimes is shown to the public as a small, quivering being with arms and legs. Such tricks confirm people's beliefs in the ability of the medicine man. The execution of such sleight-of-hand performances may be very simple, as the following example from the Kwakiutl on Vancouver Island demonstrates. The Kwakiutl medicine man who is about to heal a patient holds some eagle-down in his mouth under the upper lip, biting his cheek so that blood comes forth inside his mouth.

The singers that are present beat time on boards while the medicine man sings a song. He places his mouth on the area where the sickness is located and beings to suck. When the blood has saturated the eagle down the medicine man pulls it from his mouth. The spectators see it as a red worm. It is then displayed to a larger public that beholds it dangling from the medicine man's fingers. When he shakes his hands it looks as if the disease was running between them. Finally the disease is swallowed by the medicine man, although he pretends to throw it away to a being called the Disease-Maker.[52]

We might be tempted to judge such a performance as a hoax and consider the medicine man a humbug. However, this would be a premature opinion. The medicine man is no impostor or juggler, for he believes in his role. As anthropologists and psychologists have long realized, the medicine man simultaneously exhibits both sincere faith and deception. The "magic" element is complex.

There are also other means of removing a disease agent. For instance, a Pueblo medicine man may press a crystal against the sore spot, and let out the bad blood through a scarification with a knife—a method well known from the Old World popular medicine.

CURES FOR SOUL LOSS

The medicine man tries to recover the lost soul. This may be accomplished at a shamanic séance, where the shaman, in a state of ecstasy, dispatches his own free-soul, or in some cases his guardian spirit, toward the land of the dead. It is his task to interfere with the lost soul before it reaches its destination and to bring it back to its owner. Great shamans may even enter the realm of death, convincing the lost soul to return, or snatching it away from the dead; but such feats are exceptional. There is a rich folklore describing the dangers encountered on the journey to the other world, such as difficult obstacles, monsters, and temptation. The North American Orpheus tradition embroiders on such motifs.[53] When his task has been fulfilled an assistant of the shaman or another helper arouses him from his slumber.

This kind of shamanic treatment, which is usually highly spectacular, is illustrated by the following account from the Quinault Indians, who live on the northern Washington coast (at the Quinault River). The shaman arrived at the house of the sick person bringing a wand and his rattle, the latter painted with the picture of the guardian spirit that would assist in the cure. The shaman handed over the rattle to a helper—chosen among the bystanders—who also assisted him with the singing.

The shaman and his helper lay down on a mat spread on the floor. The shaman took up a song that his guardian spirit had taught him in his calling vision, and the helper shook the rattle. After a while the shaman went into a trance, signaling that the spirit had arrived and entered the shaman, causing him a sharp pain. From this moment shaman and spirit were one person, so that the shaman's voice was the voice of the guardian spirit—as it seems a case of true possession. The helper was also in a trance state, but only a light one.

The spirit-shaman followed the path taken by the lost soul. Between the songs he described the route and the perilous obstacles that he encountered along the way. The spirit-shaman did not dare to penetrate too far into the other world and certainly did not enter the villages of the dead—if he were to do this he would be lost. The soul of a seriously ill person traveled very quickly and was difficult to overtake. The search would go on for two days and two nights, during which time the shaman and his helper abstained from food and drink. During this period the shaman was only partly aware of things about him, and it is said that he apprehended people's voices as meaningless babblings.

If the shaman was able to intercept the fugitive soul he returned with it, holding it in his cupped hands, so the joyous onlookers could see. (This is a remarkable instance of the parallelism between events in the other world and this one.) The shaman finally came out of the trance, exhausted, and restored the patient's soul by massaging his body.[54]

In North America such séances have apparently been infrequent, and other means have been found to retrieve the lost soul. For instance, at Puget Sound the medicine man does not enter a trance but arranges an imitative trance journey. These Coast Salish Indians imagine that it is not an ordinary soul, but some kind of guardian spirit (or guardian soul) that has been captured by the dead and carried to their land in the west. Apparently the concepts of soul and power have been confused here.[55]

In other places the shaman sends out his own guardian spirit to catch the lost soul, or he makes a mimical soul expedition, another kind of imitative séance, seeking for the patient's soul by sneaking about in the vicinity of the settlement. The idea here is that the soul has stayed close to the village. When the medicine man finds the wandering soul he restores it to the body, holding his cupped hands over the crown of the patient's head. Here, at the place that in a newborn child is called the fontanel, is the entrance of the soul into the body.[56]

As presented here there are thus two principal models of medical treatment when the cause of disease is believed to be of a supernatural origin. However, it has been suggested that these models represent the ideal state, and that in practice they are often confused with each other, or one model prevails over the other. Thus, in areas of the North and West, shamanism is developed to the extent that shamanic flight is used for the curing of intrusion. Conversely, in other areas where shamanism has become weakened, soul loss is cured as if it were a case of intrusion. It is also possible that the soul-loss diagnosis falls away, and the intrusion of object or spirit then becomes responsible for the fading away of consciousness, formerly attributed to soul loss.

In modern times Indian medicine and Western medical practice have often joined forces, so that doctors of both types collaborate when Indians are taken to hospitals for treatment. The hospital expert is able to provide surgical operations and medication; the medicine man assumes responsibility for that part of the medical process that relates to the patient's faith and mental well-being.[57]

Finally, let us observe the medical attention given by the Pueblo medicine societies. As we have noted, a Zuni medicine society consists of persons who have been cured by the members of that society. It has animal spirits as its patrons, one of the most important being the bear, which members impersonate in ritual dances. In most cases diseases are removed by sucking; however, there are also reports of healing patients who have lost their souls. It is uncertain how this healing was accomplished, but it is known that after being cured patients joined the medicine society for their own protection.

The Zuni also believe, like many other North American tribes, that sickness may be a result of witchcraft. The witch is thought to inject a foreign, harmful substance into the patient, which the practitioners detect by use of a crystal or by partaking of a drug (possibly *Datura*) that renders the substance visible. It is then removed, either through sucking, or—if the witch's identity is known—through the malefactor's confession. The confession, which is implemented by the bow priests, a society for warriors who have taken scalps, deprives the witch of his or her power and thereby brings about an automatic cure.[58] Confessions of taboo infringement and witchcraft have been common in parts of North America.

The fate of the Zuni witch was formerly execution. We may understand this practice in the light of the prominent disease ideology: as soon as the disease object has been caught it is destroyed.

Observations on Caring

Unfortunately, ethnographic sources contain little information on the human care of patients, in distinct contrast to the enormous literature on mourning behavior. Probably only a careful reading of travelers' memoirs could provide us with sufficient material. Still, there are occasional notes on the subject in scholarly works. This is what John M. Cooper has to say about the customs of the Gros Ventre, or Atsina, of the northwestern Plains:

> As a rule, the sick were well looked after by their relatives and friends. Encouraging words and hopeful good wishes were expressed to an ill person and

these helped recovery. If the patient voiced a desire for any particular food this would be procured if possible. When on one occasion Singer's very ill husband expressed a wish for roseberries, an old man visiting him at the time rushed out, picked a big bunch of them, and brought them back at once.

Another friend prayed at his bedside and wished him good luck. When, finally, persons were on the verge of death, their people would dress them in their best robes and paint them so they were ready to die.[59]

The Gros Ventre and many other seminomadic tribes used to abandon their very old and infirm and the hopelessly ill. However, this custom should not automatically be interpreted as a sign of deficiency in care. For a nomadic group that must travel far in order to find food, protection from storms and cold winds, and a haven from enemies, the encumbrance of the old, decrepit, and hopelessly ill may entail a catastrophe for the whole group. Recent Western history provides examples of exploration expeditions in similar situations who have been forced to desert their weakened members on the polar ice and in the deserts.

Numerous accounts from all over North America report the abandonment of the seriously ill. However, families normally provided for their sick relatives' well-being during the days that were left to them. A Slave Indian group in western Canada was ready to move when an old woman was taken seriously ill. Her son decided to leave her and made a tipi for her, leaving it well supplied with wood. The next spring when the group returned they found the old woman's bones in the tipi.[60] Among the White Knife Shoshoni of Nevada a very sick person was placed in a small willow enclosure, made for the patient's benefit, before the group moved on.[61] There is, however, evidence of harsh treatment of sick persons who are a burden or a menace to society. A writer from the 1870s, Edward Neill, states that a young Dakota Indian is usually well taken care of when he is sick, but old and deformed persons are often neglected.[62] Gabriel Sagard, who traversed the Huron country in the 1620s, came upon an isolated conic lodge inside of which he found a man lying beside a fire. The man suffered from a painful disease in his private parts and had been separated from his community to die alone, for his tribesmen feared this disease.[63] The Karankawa Indians of southern Texas left their sick, even if they were young, in a bush, wrapped in a blanket, before moving to a new place.[64] Among the Choctaw of the Southeast, if the doctor declared that a sick person would not recover the patient was simply killed.[65]

However, that was long ago when the conditions of life were very hard. The Gros Ventre of today certainly provide their sick tribe members with the finest possible care. Other evidence of the care of sick friends and relatives may be found among the Cheyenne, who once roamed the middle plains. It is reported that at the end of the last century women often cut off joints of their fingers as a sacrifice to the powers for the recovery of a sick husband or child. George Grinnell informs us that when one of her children was sick Medicine Woman promised to sacrifice the last joint of the little finger of her right hand to the Sun provided that the child recovered. It did, and a holy man raised her hand to the Sun, said a prayer, and cut off the joint with a sharp knife.[66]

No one who has recently witnessed the disturbed situation surrounding a sick native American can avoid noticing the concerns expressed by the immediate family, kinsfolk, and friends. The bonds within a family are ideally very strong, and even the larger social units, the extended family, the village, the lineage, and the clan usually feel compelled to have their kinsman or kinswoman healed. The degree of sympathy with the diseased person naturally follows ingroup lines and may vary considerably with the type of social organization. Thus, during an illness a whole settlement is often engaged, the individuals contributing to the improvement of the patient with prayers and ritual participation. The prayers are made in sorrow, imploring the powers to show mercy on the afflicted person and his or her close family. I have witnessed this myself, on the Plains.

Ceremonies are also arranged to prevent diseases. The Blackfoot Indians have rituals for the prevention of diseases of the whole nation. Such an occasion is the sacred opening of the medicine pipe bundles that are inherited in certain Blackfoot families. The opening of such a bundle is made for the distribution of tobacco among people who aspire to long life, good health, and good fortune.[67]

In addition, according to my own observations, care for the sick is not necessarily limited to the members of one's tribe. White people may be given the same sympathy and medical treatment as tribal members, provided they are known among the natives. In the past, naturally enough, hostile conditions precluded that such aid be extended to other than tribe members and allies.

Ethics and Dignity of Life

The care given the sick reflects the ethical standard of American Indians. It has often been said that there is no immediate relation between ethics and religion, but that moral behavior is entirely a function of social structure. It is true that there is a relationship between social organization and morals, but it should be remembered that deities and spirits are organized according to social patterns, although their actions reveal the nonworldy order of the supernatural. The connection between ethics, society, and religion is clearly expressed among, for instance, the Fox Indians of (originally) Wisconsin. They claim that whoever lives a truly upright life is a person of whom the *manitous* (spirits) are fond. Ideally, the Fox do not

accept premarital relations—a girl is supposed to be chaste when she marries. This is reflected in their saying, "The man who knows nothing of the
nature of a woman, and the woman who knows nothing of the nature of
a man, is the one of whom the manitou thinks most highly."[68] The supernatural being is here presented as a guarantor of the moral order.

The point should not be overstressed—there are many aboriginal
tribal ethics in North America, and customs and norms vary—but there
is no doubt that overarching supernatural beings, such as the Supreme
Being (where this deity exists) are often closely connected with public
morals. In this light, the care of the sick and the operations of the medicine man may have both a moral and a religious value.

There is also another aspect of ethical values to be taken into account.
The Indians' attitude to nature, and to the living beings around them—
trees, plants, animals, birds—evinces their profound fellow-feelings with
all these beings. This respect for life permeates the thinking and feelings
of all those Indians who still believe in their ancient traditions. Its basis
is spiritual. Black Elk, the Oglala Sioux holy man, makes this clear when
he speaks of the Great Spirit, Wakan Tanka: "We should know that He is
within all things: the trees, the grasses, the rivers, the mountains, and all
the fourlegged animals, and the winged peoples."[69] This feeling of oneness with all living beings through the supernatural explains the caring
attitude toward animals and trees, the feelings of closeness with the spirit
animals of the visions, the creative appearance of animals in myths and
tales, the occasional expression of totemism, and animal dancing.
Humankind's participation in the same mysterious life as the animals and
the plants obliges human beings to show consideration and friendship in
their communion with all these beings.

The sanctity of life does not preclude the taking of life in certain situations. Hunters must kill animals, and gardeners must harvest plants in
order to survive. There are certain ceremonies to appease the angered animals, or their supernatural owners, after the killing. Herein may be seen,
as Christopher Vecsey has observed, a tension in humanity's relations
with the animals.[70]

The same tension is felt in the attitude toward relations between
human beings. As human beings are part of the mystery of living, they
should therefore be cared for and, within limits, loved, in the family and
the larger social unit. However, they are also individuals to be distrusted
when they break the social codes, when they rob or kill their tribe members, when they practice witchcraft against their fellow humans, or when
as members of foreign groups they turn in violent warfare against one's
own group. In such situations life must be taken. Indeed, this may even
have been ordained by the supernatural powers themselves. Among a
northeastern tribe like the Iroquois, dreams could provoke and sanction
warfare to an unbelievable extent.[71] In many tribes the killing and molest-

ing of enemies demands particular rites to propitiate the ghosts of the fallen. In spite of the fierce fighting and the desire for vengeance, the feeling of just, traditional behavior is the dominant sentiment among North American warriors, particularly on the Plains. Concern for the lives of others is just as important as the concern for one's own life.

With their very deep feelings for the dignity of life, and their high self-esteem, Indians—especially Indian men—were formerly very particular about their behavior and appearance in the face of fatal illness and death. It is well known that almost all of the Mandan tribe on the Upper Missouri succumbed during the smallpox epidemic in 1837. A young Mandan warrior decided to preclude his physical disfiguration by committing suicide while he was still in a dignified form. He asked his wife to dig a grave for him, and dressed himself in his most beautiful finery. Then he went to his grave, cut himself severely, and the grave was filled up over him.[72]

In Native American belief and practice the dignity of human beings and life are intrinsically connected with moral values. However, the rules change from tribe to tribe. While there is general agreement between researchers that norms are more binding than in European-American society, there are few studies of tribal ethics (in spite of many efforts to sort out "values"). One of the best has been written on Navajo ethics.[73] In this book the author, John Ladd, interprets the whole moral code of the Navajo. A point at issue is the attention given to disease. It has been stressed in the foregoing that the whole Navajo ceremonial system revolves around disease and healing. John Ladd rightly says that an outsider might receive the impression that the Navajo are hypochondriacs. However, as he points out, they do include under the category of sickness many conditions that are not thus identified in Western society—for instance, having bad dreams. In the 1930s about 20 percent of the time and money in a Navajo household was spent on curing ceremonies.[74]

Trangression of taboos seems to be responsible for most Navajo disease episodes. This complicates Navajo relations with nature, fellow tribe members, and the supernatural.

Approaches to curing disease differ widely among different cultural traditions. A rough division may be made between those cultures that have fixed institutional approaches and those that have not. The former primarily belong to the southern horticultural belt and include hunters in that region. Thus, Zuni and Keres Indians and a former hunting people like the Navajo have established patterns, unquestioned by tribal members. The Navajo patient who turns to a specialist knows that the song ritual ("chant") belonging to the cure of that particular disease has to be used.[75] Most hunting Indians in the north do not have such stable medical prescripts. Therapies, although usually placed within the general frame of shamanic soul excursions and extraction of disease agents, depend upon the medicine man's blessings from his guardian spirit or spirits. This cir-

cumstance gives occasion to rivalry between medicine men and to antag-
onism between different social groups who favor different medicine men.
The strength and capacity of the guardian spirits, successes in healing,
and trust in the medicine man's honesty and good nature are decisive
factors in a group's choice of healers. When competition comes to the fore
the medicine man's association to the group also becomes a crucial factor.
General opinion and shame pronounce the verdict in such cases.

The failure to bring a patient back to health may lead to a medicine
man's downfall. He may lose his reputation, his power may be considered
forfeited, or he may be judged a witch and be killed. Some medicine men
lose their powers, but regain them, to the satisfaction of their relatives and
sympathizers.

Life and Death

As has been emphasized, the involvement of supernatural power in healing is related to the idea that health and life itself are a supernatural gift.
There is evidence from many tribes that human beings existed in the other
world before birth.[76] For instance, the Ingalik of Alaska believe that the
unborn children wait impatiently in a preexistent world to be called to the
earth. When one of them is called the rest slap this soon-to-be-born one,
since they are jealous and impatient. The marks of the ill-treatment are
birthmarks.[77] A great many tribes believe that it is the Supreme Being
himself who hands the soul (life-soul or free-soul) over to the body at
birth. Indeed, among some tribes a person's soul is believed to be a part
of God's own being.[78] (There may be an association with the speculations
about cosmic harmony here.) In spite of this heavenly origin of young
children, some tribes do not hesitate to sanction the killing of girl babies
or of a twin. Among nomadic groups with precarious access to food
resources, this practice is understandable, although it may seem to con-
tradict the ruling norms of the value of life. In this case it looks indeed as
if the sanctity of life and divine preexistence, are concepts that in reality
play a minor role. Or perhaps the sacred origin has reference to the soul(s)
rather than the mortal body.

Another complication to the sanctity of life is sex. Once puberty rites
are completed, sexual intercourse is a natural thing for men in most
groups, while the code for unmarried women varies. Some men prefer not
to engage themselves in married life with women or in male occupations
on the whole. As a consequence of a supernatural dream such men have
become berdaches, or manwomen. They dress up in women's clothes,
partake in female work, and even marry men. Some women, in their turn,
dress up as men and join war parties. Because berdaches have a supernatural calling they are both feared and respected. Although some ber-

daches are overtly homosexual, such an inclination has not been the rule.[79]

There is reason to suspect that this transvestism may be related to an original shamanism. In the Old World the change of sex, biological or cultural, has been characteristic of many shamans, men and women.

Among native Americans the evaluation of sexuality is basically different from its evaluation in many Western circles. Sex as practiced by human beings is not an object of supernatural sanctions, except in certain critical situations. Thus, abstinence from sexual intercourse is a necessity in connection with hunting and some ceremonial performances. A man who has slept with a woman scares the animals away, and by draining his sexual powers such activity may cause him to be unable to concentrate on sacred ritual. Connected to this understanding is the fear of the blood and smell from a menstruating woman. A woman in this condition who approaches a ceremony may destroy it. Indeed, a meeting with her may be bad for a man—and for her.

This preoccupation with sexual danger and menstrual blood seems most pronounced in hunting societies. Anthropologists have proposed that such a concern is an atavistic survival from humanity's primeval era, which has been overcome in modern times—a victory over the primitive in us.[80] Whatever truth there is in this, it is a fact that horticultural societies in America have turned away from the fear of sex in their coupling of sexual license with fertility rituals.

Among native North Americans, religion is an institution in the service of this life. Gods and spirits and rites guard or threaten the lives of human beings. Health and prosperity for the individual, the family, and the group stand in the foreground of interest. In daily life little is said about death, and the few statements that are given are often both vague and contradictory. Death is not feared as such, but it is not quite comprehensible to a living man or woman. It is set apart, just as the realm of the dead is secluded from the world of both humans and gods and spirits. The sphere of death is avoided. Many hunting tribes, such as the Athapascans, shun the contagious qualities of a corpse, the "death stuff." They desert the lodge of a dead person, even flee from the place. However, they are not afraid to die. Their intrepidity toward death is manifest in daring warlike actions and in the preference of death in battle ("This is a fine day to die!") to the disgraceful languishing of an old, decrepit man. In many cultures there is also an ideological expectation that violent death in warfare and from lightning may secure a good place in the afterlife.

We have seen that there are shamans and critically ill persons who have visited the land of the dead and are able to tell their fellow tribe members what it is like. However, there are many persons who do not trust such reports unless they experience similar things themselves.

The land of the dead looks more or less like this world and portrays the culture of the living in an impoverished or idealized form. Thus the Plains Indians have their "happy hunting grounds" and the Navajo their gloomy underworld in the north. Most hunting Indians believe that their land of the dead is situated somewhere on earth, behind the shining mountains, on an island in the great western ocean, or in the sky. Many agricultural tribes think it is situated under the ground where the plants and seeds are hiding. Some tribes believe in a final extinction after a period of time in the world of the dead, others cherish the hope of reincarnation or even transmigration into animals. Some peoples, such as certain tribes of the Southeast, believe that their leaders will live on among the gods. Often different lines of thought exist side by side in the same individual. The chaos in ideological expressions reflects the uncertainty and also the spirituality of the other life.

There is therefore no point in planning for the next life. The Navajo, writes Gary Witherspoon, frankly admit that they really do not know whether their existence continues after death; that is a problem they will solve when they have died. Since there is no answer they believe that they should not waste their lives in worrying about these things, but concentrate on making this life happy and harmonious.[81] This is perhaps a rather extreme point of view, not quite representative of other groups. However, most native Americans might say that the main concern of human beings is to maintain their existence in this life, and here religious faith and medicine come to their aid.

Notes

1. Cf. the account in Åke Hultkrantz, *The Religions of the American Indians* (Berkeley and Los Angeles, 1979), pp. 84–102.
2. Ruth Bunzel, "Zuñi Katcinas," *47th Annual Report of the Bureau of American Ethnology* (Washington, DC, 1932), pp. 965–966.
3. Joseph Epes Brown, *The Sacred Pipe* (Norman, OK, 1953), p. 87.
4. Ibid., p. 37.
5. Åke Hultkrantz, "Prairie and Plains Indians," *Iconography of Religions* 10, no. 2 (1973):9–18.
6. Joseph G. Jorgensen, *The Sun Dance Religion: Power for the Powerless* (Chicago, 1972).
7. Karl W. Luckert, *The Navajo Hunter Tradition* (Tucson, 1975), p. 185.
8. See Åke Hultkrantz, *Native Religions of North Americans* (San Francisco, 1987), chaps. 1 and 2.
9. Horst Hartmann, *Die Plains- und Prärieindianer Nordamerikas* (Berlin, 1973), pp. 186ff.
10. T. R. Fehrenback, *Comanches: The Destruction of a People* (New York, 1974), p. 114.
11. Luther Standing Bear, *Land of the Spotted Eagle* (Lincoln, NE, 1978), p. 35.
12. Charles Alexander Eastman, *Indian Boyhood* (New York, 1902), p. 4.
13. Cf. Henry F. Dobyns, "Estimating Aboriginal American Populations,"

Current Anthroplogy 7 (1966):395–412. See also Calvin Martin, *Keepers of the Game: Indian-Animal Relationships and the Fur Trade* (Berkeley and Los Angeles, 1978), pp. 40–55.

14. Lowell John Bean, *Mukat's People: The Cahuilla Indians of Southern California* (Berkeley and Los Angeles, 1974), pp. 146, 162.

15. Suffering was often seen as a means of creating a bond with the supernatural powers; on this subject see Åke Hultkrantz, "The Contribution of the Study of North American Indian Religions to the History of Religions," in *Seeing with a Native Eye: Essays on Native American Religion*, ed. Walter H. Capps (New York, 1976), p. 95. On the other hand, suffering to save others, or suffering as a sacrifice, was not always understood. See Gladys A. Reichard, "The Navaho and Christianity," *American Anthropologist* 51, no. 1 (1949):67–68.

16. See Franz Boas, "The Origin of Death," *Journal of American Folklore* 30 (1917):486–491.

17. Clark Wissler and D. C. Duvall, "Mythology of the Blackfoot Indians," *Anthropological Papers of the American Museum of Natural History* 2, no. 1 (1908):21.

18. Åke Hultkrantz, *Conceptions of the Soul among North American Indians*, (Stockholm, 1953), pp. 280–281, 458ff.

19. Henry J. Wegrocki, "A Critique of Cultural and Statistical Concepts of Abnormality," in *Personality in Nature, Society, and Culture*, eds. Clyde Kluckhohn and Henry A. Murray (New York, 1948), p. 560. Cf. also Ruth Benedict, *Patterns of Culture* (London, 1935), pp. 191ff.

20. There is a good overview of the subject in Morton Teicher, "Windigo Psychosis: A Study of a Relationship between Belief and Behavior among the Indians of Northeastern Canada," *Proceedings of the 1960 Annual Spring Meeting of the American Ethnological Society* (Seattle, 1960). Most psychological interpretations are otherwise less convincing, including those by Raymond Fogelson and Thomas Hay. For the latter, see Thomas H. Hay, "The Windigo Psychosis: Psychodynamic, Cultural, and Social Factors in Aberrant Behavior," *American Anthropologist* 73, no. 1 (1971):1–19.

21. On witchcraft, see Deward E. Walker, Jr., ed., *Systems of North American Witchcraft and Sorcery*, Anthropological Monographs of the University of Idaho, vol. 1 (Moscow, ID, 1970).

22. On Trickster myths, cf. Paul Radin, *The Trickster: A Study in American Indian Mythology* (New York, 1956). On clown societies, see J. H. Steward, "The Ceremonial Buffoon of the American Indian," *Papers of the Michigan Academy of Science, Arts, and Letters* 14 (1931):187–207; Verne F. Ray, "The Contrary Behavior Pattern in American Indian Ceremonialism," *Southwestern Journal of Anthropology* 1, no. 1 (1945):75–113.

23. Ruth M. Underhill, *Papago Indian Religion* (New York, 1946), pp. 41ff., 51; Kenneth M. Stewart, "The Southwest," in Robert F. Spencer et al., *The Native Americans*, (New York, 1965), p. 301; Edward F. Castetter and Willis H. Bell, *Pima and Papago Indian Agriculture* (Albuquerque, 1942), pp. 222ff.

24. Cf., for instance, Weston La Barre, "The Narcotic Complex of the New World," *Diogenes* 48 (1964):125–138.

25. Weston La Barre, *The Peyote Cult*, 4th ed. enl. (Hamden, CT, 1975); Omer C. Stewart and David E. Aberle, *Peyotism in the West: A Historical and Cultural Perspective* (Salt Lake City, 1984).

26. James H. Howard, "The Mescal Bean Cult of the Central and Southern Plains," *American Anthropologist* 59, no. 1 (1957):75–87.

27. Åke Hultkrantz, "The Shaman and the Medicine-Man," *Social Science and Medicine* 20, no. 5 (1985):511–515.

28. Clyde Kluckhohn and Dorothea Leighton, *The Navaho* (Cambridge, MA, 1947), pp. 146–149; A. H. Leighton and D. C. Leighton, *Gregoria, the Hand-Trembler* (Cambridge, MA, 1949).

29. Forrest E. Clements, "Primitive Concepts of Disease," *University of California Publications in American Archaeology and Ethnology* 32, no. 2 (1932):185–252; see in particular pp. 193ff., 227, 231ff.; William W. Elmendorf, "Soul Loss Illness in Western North America," in *Indian Tribes of Aboriginal America*, ed. Sol Tax (Chicago, 1952), pp. 104–114; Hultkrantz, *Conceptions of the Soul*, pp. 448–463.

30. Cf. William K. Powers, *Yuwipi: Vision and Experience in Oglala Ritual* (Lincoln, NE, 1982); Åke Hultkrantz, *Belief and Worship in Native North America* (Syracuse, NY, 1981), pp. 61–90.

31. Åke Hultkrantz, "Ecological and Phenomenological Aspects of Shamanism," in *Shamanism in Siberia*, eds. Vilmos Diószegi and Mihály Hoppál (Budapest, 1978), pp. 27–58; on connections between Siberia and North America, see in particular pp. 51–55.

32. Cf. Åke Hultkrantz, "The American Indian Vision Quest: A Transition Ritual or a Device for Spiritual Aid?" in *Transition Rites*, ed. Ugo Bianchi (Rome, 1986), pp. 29–43.

33. Cf., for instance, S. A. Barrett, "Pomo Bear Doctors," *University of California Publications in American Archaeology and Ethnology* 12, no. 11 (1917):443–465.

34. Robert H. Lowie, "The Religion of the Crow Indians," *Anthropological Papers of the American Museum of Natural History* 25, no. 2 (1922):328.

35. Cf. Brown, pp. 56–58.

36. Raymond J. DeMallie, *The Sixth Grandfather: Black Elk's Teachings Given to John G. Neihardt* (Lincoln, NE, 1985), pp. 227–232.

37. Ibid., pp. 235–240.

38. Ruth L. Bunzel, "Introduction to Zuñi Ceremonialism," *47th Annual Report of the Bureau of American Ethnology* (Washington, DC, 1932), pp. 528ff.

39. For an overview, see Virgil J. Vogel, *American Indian Medicine* (Norman, OK, 1970).

40. James Mooney and Frans M. Olbrechts, "The Swimmer Manuscript: Cherokee Sacred Formulas and Medicinal Prescriptions," *Bureau of American Ethnology, Bulletin* 99 (Washington, DC, 1932), pp. 83ff.

41. Jaime de Angulo, "La psychologie religieuse des Achumawi," pt. 4: "Le chamanisme," *Anthropos* 23 (1928):567–568.

42. Cf. Clements, pp. 188ff., 210, 217.

43. Paul Radin, "The Winnebago Tribe," *37th Annual Report of the Bureau of American Ethnology* (Washington, DC, 1923), pp. 287, 440. Radin thinks that this type of supernatural being is unique for the Winnebago (pp. 168 n. 9; 440); however, this is scarcely so. A supernatural being with double functions, and sometimes double faces, is known from Algonkian and Siouan peoples. The Winnebago are a Siouan isolate in an Algonkian population area. Cf. Werner Müller, *Glauben und Denken der Sioux* (Berlin, 1970), pp. 229–230.

44. It seems that Kenneth M. Stewart has been too liberal in his interpretation

of instances of alleged possession in his article "Spirit Possession in Native America," *Southwestern Journal of Anthropology* 2, no. 3 (1946):323–339.

45. Hultkrantz, *Conceptions of the Soul*, p. 454.

46. Ibid., pp. 379, 453.

47. Ibid., pp. 51ff., 241ff., 255ff., 269ff., 441ff.

48. Robert H. Lowie, "On the Historical Connection between Certain Old World and New World Beliefs," *Proceedings of the 21st International Congress of Americanists* (Göteborg, 1925), pp. 546–549.

49. See Åke Hultrantz, "North American Indian Religions in a Circumpolar Perspective," in *North American Indian Studies: European Contributions*, ed. Pieter Hovens (Göttingen, 1981), pp. 11–28.

50. Frances Densmore, "Chippewa Customs," *Bureau of American Ethnology, Bulletin* 86 (Washington, DC, 1929), p. 46.

51. George Catlin, *Letters and Notes on the Manners, Customs, and Condition of the North American Indians*, vol. 1 (London, 1841), pp. 39ff.

52. Franz Boas, *The Religion of the Kwakiutl Indians*, pt. 2 (New York, 1930), pp. 8–10; Franz Boas, *Kwakiutl Ethnography*, ed. Helen Codere (Chicago, 1966), pp. 143–144.

53. Åke Hultkrantz, *The North American Indian Orpheus Tradition* (Stockholm, 1957).

54. Ronald L. Olson, "The Quinault Indians," *University of Washington Publications in Anthropology* 6, no. 1 (1936):160–161.

55. Herman K. Haeberlin, "SbEtEtdáq, A Shamanistic Performance of the Coast Salish," *American Anthropologist* 20, no. 3 (1918):249–257; W. G. Jilek, *Indian Healing* (Washington, DC, 1981).

56. Cf. Homer G. Barnett, *The Coast Salish of British Columbia* (Eugene, OR, 1955), pp. 215, 229, 237.

57. Many examples could be adduced. See for instance Fred W. Voget, *The Shoshoni-Crow Sun Dance* (Norman, OK, 1984), p. 318.

58. Bunzel, "Introduction to Zuñi Ceremonialism," p. 533.

59. John M. Cooper, *The Gros Ventres of Montana*, pt. 2: *Religion and Ritual*, ed. Regina Flannery (Washington, DC, 1956), p. 321.

60. John J. Honigmann, "Ethnography and Acculturation of the Fort Nelson Slave," *Yale University Publications in Anthropology* 33 (New Haven, CT, 1946), p. 86.

61. Jack S. Harris, "The White Knife Shoshoni of Nevada," in *Acculturation in Seven American Indian Tribes*, ed. Ralph Linton (Gloucester, MA, 1963), p. 66.

62. Edward D. Neill, "Dakota Land and Dakota Life," *Collections of the Minnesota Historical Society*, vol. 1 (Saint Paul, 1872), p. 271.

63. Gabriel Sagard, *Le grand voyage du pays des Hurons* . . . (Paris, 1632), pp. 270ff.

64. Albert S. Gatschet, "The Karankawa Indians, the Coast People of Texas," *Archaeological and Ethnological Papers of the Peabody Museum* 1, no. 2 (Cambridge, MA, 1891), p. 67.

65. John R. Swanton, "The Indians of the Southeastern United States," *Bureau of American Ethnology, Bulletin* 137 (Washington, DC, 1946), p. 725.

66. George Bird Grinnell, *The Cheyenne Indians: Their History and Ways of Life*, vol. 2 (New Haven, CT, 1923), p. 196. The sacrifice of a finger joint in times of distress was common among many tribes on the plains.

67. Unpublished notes from Blackfoot Reserve, Alberta, May 1984, by John C. Hellson.

68. Truman Michelson, "Notes on the Fox Wâpanowiweni," *Bureau of American Ethnology, Bulletin* 105 (Washington, DC, 1932), p. 17.

69. Brown, p. xx.

70. Christopher Vecsey, "American Indian Environmental Religions," in *American Indian Environments*, eds. Christopher Vecsey and Robert W. Venables (Syracuse, NY, 1980), pp. 22ff.

71. Cf. A. F. C. Wallace, "Dreams and the Wishes of the Soul," *American Anthropologist* 60, no. 2 (1958):234–248.

72. Maria R. Audubon, ed., *Audubon and His Journals* (New York, 1897), vol. 2, p. 45.

73. John Ladd, *The Structure of a Moral Code: A Philosophical Analysis of Ethical Discourse Applied to the Ethics of the Navaho Indians* (Cambridge, MA, 1957).

74. Ibid., pp. 208; 450 n. 12.

75. LeLand C. Wyman, "Navajo Ceremonial System," in *Handbook of North American Indians*, vol. 10: *Southwest* (Washington, DC, 1983), pp. 536–557.

76. Hultkrantz, *Conceptions of the Soul*, pp. 412–430.

77. John W. Chapman, "Tinneh Animism," *American Anthropologist* 23, no. 3 (1921):302.

78. Hultkrantz, *Conceptions of the Soul*, pp. 179–208.

79. Cf. Charles Callender and Lee M. Kochems, "The North American Berdache," *Current Anthropology* 24, no. 4 (1983):443–470.

80. A. L. Kroeber, *Anthropology* (New York, 1948), pp. 300–304.

81. Gary Witherspoon, *Language and Art in the Navajo Universe* (Ann Arbor, MI, 1977), pp. 189–190.

CHAPTER 14

Mesoamerican Religious Tradition and Medicine

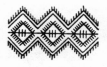

BERNARD R. ORTIZ DE MONTELLANO

Mesoamerica is defined geographically as the area comprising Mexico, Guatemala, Honduras, and El Salvador. But it may be more significantly defined as an area of historical interactions that have built up a basic cultural unity.[1] Before the Spanish conquest this unity was based on corn as a basic staple, similar technology, a common calendar, and common religious views. This essay will focus on ancient rather than on modern Mesoamerica, and more particularly on the Aztecs, for the following reasons:

1. Many of the kinds of questions (such as ethical questions in medicine) that ought to be addressed have not been asked in most modern ethnographic investigations of healers in Mesoamerica; basic information is unavailable, and gathering that data should constitute a future area for research.

2. Religion in Mesoamerica today combines elements of Catholicism and pre-Columbian religious beliefs. The Spanish conquest of America destroyed the official Aztec religion but left largely untouched the isolated Indian community, which retained a version of the official religion. L. Marie Musgrave-Portilla points out: "In many Mexican Indian communities today, the process of mutual influence between the simplified folk version of the pre-Hispanic religion and the equally simplistic understanding of Christianity which began during the colonial period has created a new syncretic religion. This new religion takes elements from both its parents and yet does not really resemble either very closely. Christian concepts are sometimes understood only from a pre-Hispanic point of view and vice versa."[2] Since the relationship between the Catholic religious tradition and medicine has been treated in *Caring and Curing: Health and Medicine in the Western Religious Traditions* (New York, 1986), I have chosen to treat the pre-Columbian Mesoamerican religious tradition in a pure form. Knowledge regarding the interaction of this tradition with medicine and health will allow us to see modern practices in a clearer light and to disentangle beliefs that are Christian from those that are not.

3. Although beliefs varied and shifted emphasis over time, a basic unity of fundamental religious outlook prevailed throughout Mesoamerica.[3] In spite of local specialization (such as belief in tutelary deities), something like a pan-Mesoamerican religious system flourished, with its roots set in the distant past.[4] This homogeneity makes it possible to generalize from the study of one particular culture to the rest of the area.

4. More information exists about the Aztecs than about any other culture in Mesoamerica, because they were the dominant power at the time of the conquest and the group whom the Spanish dealt with most extensively. The efforts of missionary friars to accumulate information about Aztec culture and religion (in order to convert them to Christianity) have furnished invaluable documentary sources, including the massive works of Fray Bernardino de Sahagún.[5]

5. The Aztecs were latecomers to the valley of Mexico, arriving there about 1200 CE. They founded Tenochtitlan in 1325 and began their independent empire in 1428. Since they absorbed the culture and religion that had developed in Mesoamerica over the course of several thousand years, the Aztecs represent the summary chapter of a very long book and validly portray the Mesoamerican cultural tradition.

The focus of this chapter is pre-Columbian religious and medical beliefs, but some practices that survive today will also be used to illustrate how a creative synthesis of historically diverse medical systems has occurred. Examples of such beliefs are the idea of "hot-cold" as a cause of disease, the loss of animating spirit as a cause of illness, and shamanic diagnosis of illness. In regard to these matters, this essay owes much to the seminal work of López Austin in this area.

In many belief systems, treatment of illness involves empirical, magical, and religious elements in varying proportions. I will not deal extensively with the empirical aspects of Aztec medicine here,[6] nor with a detailed description of Aztec religious beliefs. Instead, I begin with a brief overview of religious essentials, with particular reference to themes basic to medicine.

Survey of Aztec Religion

Aztec religion was an institutionalized state-ecclesiastical religion with priests, temples, and manifold rituals. With no separation of church and state, civil rulers performed religious functions, and high religious officials filled government offices. Aztec religion was a highly complex and ritualized belief system directed toward powers manifest in nature. Animals, plants, and natural phenomena were often the protagonists of Aztec mythology.[7] In contrast to other major religions, Aztec religion retained strong elements of shamanism (illness vocation, use of hallucinogens, and altered states of consciousness).[8]

COSMOGONY

Mesoamerican cosmological beliefs were the ground of many of the ethical imperatives guiding human action, especially medical treatment. Several of the most important beliefs merit description.[9]

1. *The Four Suns.* The Aztecs believed that the world had been created and destroyed several times. Each of these ages ("suns") possessed a distinctive set of characteristics and each ended in a different kind of cataclysm. The first sun, Ocelotonatiuh, was ruled by the god Tezcatlipoca. Giants who inhabited the world and subsisted on acorns were destroyed by voracious jaguars on day 4-Ocelot of the Aztec calendar. The next sun, Ehecatonatiuh, was subject to Quetzalcoatl, a god opposed to Tezcatlipoca. During this era, humans, whose food was piñon nuts, were destroyed by a great windstorm on a day called 4-Wind and, as a result, were changed into monkeys. The third sun, Tletonatiuh, was governed by Tlaloc, the god of rain. On day 4-Rain, a rain of fire destroyed the populations and transformed them into birds. The fourth sun, Atonatiuh, was ruled by Chalchiuhtlicue, the female counterpart of Tlaloc. The population, which subsisted on a grain precursor to corn, was destroyed by a great deluge. The sky fell, plunging the world into darkness. Humans were converted into fish on a 4-Water day.

Although details vary, this concept of several creations and destructions of humankind was present among the Maya, who predated the Aztec by many centuries.[10] This myth conveys a message that mixes fatalism with hope: the world will inevitably be destroyed, but since we are dealing in cycles, the world will be created again. Life and death are intertwined, as are so many other oppositions and dualities: Tezcatlipoca and Quetzalcoatl, the male Tlaloc and female Chalchiuhtlicue, and so on.

2. *The Fifth and Present Sun.* After the deluge, the earth lay in darkness, while all the gods met to recreate the sun. Tecciztecatl, a rich god, competed with the pauper Nanahuatzin ("the little pimply one") for the honor of becoming the sun. The contest consisted of jumping into a great fire. Tecciztecatl, who had claimed priority because of his status, balked several times. Nanahuatzin seized the honor, jumped into the fire, and changed into the sun. Although Tecciztecatl soon followed suit, his initial cowardice reduced the intensity of his light, and he became merely the moon. The sun was created in a stationary orbit, but it needed to move in order to function as a creator of vegetation and life. And it would require nourishment, if ever it were going to move. Through voluntary self-sacrifice, the assembled gods fed the sun with their own blood and set it in motion. This set an example for humankind to follow for all time. This myth conveyed the message that human beings owed a debt to the gods in payment for the divine sacrifices that created the world of animal and plant life.

The self-sacrifice of the gods proved insufficient nourishment for the sun, who needed daily feedings to continue his daily rounds and thereby to forestall the end of the world. Feeding the sun became the primary responsibility of humanity; they waged war in order to obtain captives, whose sacrificed hearts and blood would nourish the sun.[11] López Austin argues that the relationship between god and humanity was mercantile. By delivering blood, hearts, fire, incense, and quail sacrifices to the gods, human beings obtained crops and water and were freed from illness and plagues.[12] This claim finds etymological support. The word for sacrifice to the gods is *nextlahualiztli*, literally, "the act of payment." The offering of fire to the gods, *tlenamaca*, means "to sell fire."

3. *Creation of Human Beings.* The theme of self-sacrifice by gods is continued in the myth concerning the creation of human beings.[13] The Aztecs believed that Quetzalcoatl descended to the underworld to obtain the bones and ashes of previous generations from the ruler of the underworld, Mictlantecuhtli. Quetzalcoatl successfully performed the several challenging tasks imposed as a precondition by Mictlantecuhtli. He then undertook the hazardous journey back to earth, but he was chased and fell down, breaking some of the bones he was carrying. Nevertheless he delivered the bones to the assembled gods in Tamoanchan, where the goddess Cihuacoatl-Quilaztli ground them and put them into a precious pestle. Quetzalcoatl pricked his penis and dripped his blood onto the

bones; other gods also autosacrificed. After four days, a male child emerged, and after four more days a female infant emerged to join him. All humankind has descended from this pair. The etymology of the word for "commoner" reflects this myth. "Man was therefore the product of the gods' penance. With their sacrifice, the gods 'deserved men' back to life. For this reason, the people were called *macehuales*, a word which means "those deserved and brought back to life because of penance."[14]

UNITY OF UNIVERSE AND HUMANITY

In societies where mythical thought predominated, such as the Aztec, attempts were made to find the total order of the universe and to make homologies between different processes, natural as well as social. One taxonomy was projected onto another to try to achieve a synthesis. Architecture was used to dramatize cosmogony by constructing on earth a reduced version of the cosmos, usually in the form of a state capital. This symbolism was, in turn, used to legitimize the status and powers of the ruling class by identifying the rulers with the gods and the power of the cosmos.[15] The ideal city was a sacred space oriented around a particularly sacred center, a temple or pyramid believed to be the center of the world and the point of intersection of all the world's paths, both celestial and terrestrial. Thus we find the main temple of Tenochtitlan representing an *axis mundi*, which has been described as "the meeting point of heaven, earth and hell" or as "the point of ontological transition between spheres."[16]

Recent excavations of the main temple of Tenochtitlan (now in downtown Mexico City) show that the temple is an architectural reenactment of the myth of the creation of Huitzilopochtli, the solar patron god of the Mexica Aztecs.[17] Cihuacoatl conceived Huitzilopochtli through magical intervention at a place called Coatepec ("snake hill"). When her other children, the Centzon Huitznahua (who represent stars), found out that she was pregnant they were very angry, and they plotted with their sister, Coyolxauhqui (the moon goddess), to kill this child as soon as it was born. Huitzilopochtli was forewarned and was born fully grown and armed. He dismembered Coyolxauhqui and threw her down the side of the hill, and he defeated the Centzon Huitznahua—an analogy of the defeat of the stars and the moon by the rising sun.[18] At Tenochtitlan the serpents bordering the temple indicate that the temple symbolizes Coatepec; a sculpture of a dismembered Coyolxauhqui is set at the bottom of the temple, and Huitzilopochtli, the winner, is worshiped at the top of the temple.[19]

López Austin points out that the Aztecs attempted to connect the human body to the universe. For example, the most common name for the human body, *tonacayo*, was also used as a name for corn, thus establishing a metaphorical connection between people's bodies and the cereal to which they owed their existence.[20] A Quiche Maya myth states that

God made human beings out of corn dough.[21] No comparable Aztec myth is known; but Aztecs believed that Quetzalcoatl and other gods traveled to the underworld to retrieve corn as a food for human beings. A second metaphorical phrase for the body, *in tlalli in zoquitl* ("the earth, the mud") is probably based on an origin myth. We do not know the Aztec myth, but the Maya myth states that the birth of humans was due to the action of the gods on wet soil.[22] In magical rites the body was called by a third name, *Chicomoztoc* ("seven caves"), the mythical place of origin of the Aztec tribes before their migration to Central Mexico. This usage was probably due to their view of the body as having seven orifices. Thus the body itself was seen as a metaphor for the Aztec tribal origin myth.

The cosmos was conceived in terms of a corporeal model, and, in reverse fashion, human physiology was explained in terms of general processes of the universe.[23] The cosmos was divided into three levels—the superior heaven *(ilhuicatl)*, the lower heaven, and the underworld. These levels corresponded to the human body and to the animating forces ("souls") that resided in the body. *Ilhuicatl* was linked to the head and to the force *tonalli*. The lower heaven was linked to the heart and to the force *teyolia*. The underworld was linked to the liver and to the force *ihiyotl*, which resided there. For example, the word for cultivating land with a digging stick was *elimiqui* ("to harm the liver").[24] These animistic forces, which gave humans vitality and life, will be discussed later.

PANTHEON OF DEITIES

The Aztecs had a large number of deities. Nicholson has summarized and synthesized the group.[25] Deities are anthropomorphic, enlivening spirits manifest in the active cosmos; almost any aspect of nature has a deity associated with it. Many deities have animal "doubles" or alter egos called *nahualli*. Deities have dual and quadruple natures, the former associated with the concept of opposites and the latter associated with the cardinal directions. The dual nature is particularly common in creator deities but is also found in consort deities (e.g., Tlaloc-Chalchiutlicue). Particular sociopolitical groups (towns, trades, professions, and social classes) have special tutelary deities. Although there is a multiplicity of deities, Nicholson finds that they can be grouped under three major themes. Only a few of the major gods are listed here:

1. Celestial Creativity–Divine Paternalism
   Ometeotl (God of Duality) complex
   Tezcatlipoca complex
   Xiuhtecuhtli complex

2. Rain–Moisture–Agricultural Fertility
   Tlaloc complex
   Centeotl (Corn God)–Xochipilli complex

> Ometochtli (Fertility God) complex
> Teteo Innan (Earth Goddess) complex
> Xipe Totec complex

3. War–Sacrifice–Sanguinary Nourishment of the Sun and Earth
   Tonatiuh (Sun God) complex
   Huitzilopochtli complex

4. Quetzalcoatl as a deity combines characteristics of several themes. He is a prime creator but also participates in the Rain–Fertility complex.

Deities had important but varying influences and functions as patrons of the days and of the longer divisions of the Mesoamerican calendar. This aspect will be dealt with in connection with the health and illness aspects of astrology and birth dates. For our purposes it is interesting that violations of ritual or offenses against particular gods would bring about punishment in the form of diseases particularly associated with that deity. If a couple had sexual intercourse during periods of ritual abstinence, Xochipilli, god of sex and love, would afflict them with venereal diseases and hemorrhoids.[26] Xipe Totec, god of spring and of the "renewal of the skin of the earth," if offended would afflict people with blisters, eye pains, and cataracts.[27] Tlaloc's anger took the form of gout, dropsy, rheumatism, *teococoliztli* ("divine illness," usually translated as leprosy), and other ailments associated with water and cold.[28] Death due to these illnesses or death by drowning or by lightning (also considered to be due to Tlaloc) was not necessarily a misfortune since it was believed that the victims would be reborn to the pleasures of Tlalocan, Tlaloc's paradise.[29] Tezcatlipoca punished violations of religious vows or of ritual fasting by contagious or incurable diseases.[30] These diseases, being of divine origin, were to be cured by expiation and prayer. For example, patients afflicted by diseases attributed to Xipe Totec ("Our Lord the Flayed One") would vow to wear the skins of victims flayed in his honor as a penance in exchange for being cured.[31] Those who were stricken by ailments due to Tlaloc would make dough images of the gods and would offer them at shrines on the appropriate hill or mountain. It was believed that the *tlaloque*, Tlaloc's helpers, resided in hills from whence rain came.[32]

Ethical Bases

Wigberto Jiménez Moreno has pointed out a fundamental distinction between Mesoamerican religions and Christianity:

> There is a fundamental distinction between indigenous religions and that of Christ. In the latter, the major emphasis is put on the salvation of the soul and thus on the welfare of the individual in the after life. While, in pre-Hispanic

paganism, the emphasis is put on preserving the cosmic order, and the individual, as such, has almost no value in isolation except to the extent that he
contributes to collective activities that have the conservation of that order as
a goal. While a Christian thinks that one must perfect one's character and must
love others, in indigenous religions the ethical norms put greater emphasis on
the good of the group rather than that of the individual.[33]

Mesoamerican religions are prime examples of Durkheim's theory that
the function of religion is to enforce social solidarity in its members. The
Mesoamerican rulers aligned themselves with the central axis of the universe, as mentioned above, and with creation itself, setting themselves off
symbolically as a race apart from ordinary humankind.[34] Thus, duty to
the state became a religious command and was divinely sanctioned.
Going to war, particularly for the purpose of capturing warriors to be sacrificed in order to prevent the world from ending, became a sacred mission, and the Mexica Aztec considered themselves to be the "People of
the Sun," that is, God's chosen. The Aztec myths of the origin of the
human species served several purposes in this connection. The alternate
dominion of the "suns" and the death of warrior gods provided ideological support for tribes that wanted to justify their hegemonic position.
These myths were also the basis of the mechanisms of social control, of
the praise of battlefield courage, and of popular support for the militaristic
ends of the group in power. A large component of social control involved
the use of etiology of diseases whose cause-effect relationships could only
be explained by the supernatural.[35]

A person's fate in the afterlife depended primarily on the manner of
death rather than on behavior on earth; there was no doctrine of personal
salvation. Persons who died by Tlaloc's intervention went to Tlalocan, a
fertile place of abundant food, but one could not choose to die in this
fashion. People who died ordinary deaths by illness or accident went to
a place called Mictlan, where their souls underwent a series of nine hells
for a period of four years. Poems survive that demonstrate considerable
uncertainty regarding what actually happened after that.

A person's best fate was to die in battle or as a sacrificial victim, for
such souls were destined to accompany the sun in its journey from east
to west from sunrise to noon. After four years the souls of these warriors
would be reborn as hummingbirds or butterflies—thus the abundant use
of these images in Aztec poetry. These beliefs provided a powerful impetus toward death in battle. The following poem is one of many:

> There is a clamor of bells,
> the dust rises as if it were smoke.
> The Giver of Life is grateful.
> Shield Flowers open their blossoms,
> the glory spreads,

it becomes linked to earth.
Death is here among the flowers
in the midst of the plain!
Close to the war,
where the war begins,
in the midst of the plain,
the dust rises as if it were smoke,
entangled and twisted round with
flowery strands of death.
Oh Chichimec princes!
Do not fear, my heart!
In the midst of the plain,
my heart craves death
by the obsidian edge.
Only this my heart craves:
death in war . . .[36]

Women who died in childbirth, which was considered symbolic combat, would accompany the sun from noon to sunset. However, these women would not be reborn as hummingbirds.[37]

Aztec formal education as well as formalized orations and admonitions called *huehuetlatolli* ("talks of the elders") emphasized the idea of duty as a key ethic. Little value was placed on individual freedom, self-fulfillment, or autonomy. The crucial values were obedience, respect, conformity, moderation, honesty, and the good of the social group. This loyalty extended from family to *calpulli*, a territorial subdivision of the city, and to the state. This view can be contrasted with present-day recommendations of the U.S. President's Commission for the Study of Ethical Problems in Medicine on decisions to forgo treatments for seriously impaired children:

> The Commission has recommended that "the best interests of the child" should govern decision making in the neonatal nursery. Significantly such a standard would preclude any and all consideration of possible adverse effects of a child on her parents, siblings or society at large. "Burden to others" is then ruled out as a possible justification for non treatment of an imperiled newborn.[38]

Such a statement would be inconceivable in the Aztec ethical tradition of placing the interests of the group over those of individuals.

Views of the Aztecs on the use of alcohol can be tied to this concept of duty as a prime value. There were severe strictures against the overuse of the fermented sap of *octli* (*Agave* sp.). There was an apparent fear of a loss of control, of the inability to perform one's duty. Members of the nobility, the *pipiltin*, were held to a higher standard of behavior than were

the commoners, *macehualtin*. The rationale seems to be that nobles, having received greater benefits from the state, owed stricter standards of performance to it. A priest found drunk was punished with death, as were
nobles who were found drunk in the palace. Drunken commoners had
their heads shaved for the first offense, but repeat offenders were punished with death. The concept ties together ideas concerning loss of control, drunkeness, and duty to the state and is supported by the fact that
old men and women were allowed to drink and to get drunk with impun-
ity, presumably because they had discharged their obligation to serve the
state and were no longer subject to the same strictures as younger people.[39] Complete abstinence was not called for, since *octli* was used as a
food. Moderation in its use was the key, as in all other things. The effects
of drunkenness as well as the ingestion of hallucinogens were explained
in terms of the possession of the individual by supernatural beings that
inhabited these products. Drinking *octli* introduced into the body one of
the four hundred deities they called "rabbits." The large number was
used to explain all the varieties of drunkards (e.g., pugnacious, sleepy,
weepy) by attributing different types to particular rabbits. People who
were born on a day 2-Rabbit were destined to be alcoholics.

Given the shamanic tradition of Mesoamerica, which continues to this
day, the use of hallucinogens was not condemned. Speaking of *peyote*
tlapatl (*Datura* sp.) and *ololiuhqui* (*Rivea* sp.), the texts use language that
indicates that their effects were believed to be due to possession by deities
contained in the plant. This concept of "god in a plant" is expressed by
the word "entheogen" ("God within us"), which A. P. Ruck coined to
replace terms such as hallucinogens, psychotomimetics, and psychedel-
ics.[40] These drugs had a double effect. They housed the god that took possession of those who partook, and they sent the *tonalli* (one of the three
souls) on an out-of-body trip to the dwelling of the gods.[41] One of the
purposes for which this out-of-body experience was used was that of
diagnosing illness and finding the appropriate remedy. Shamanic curing
and the use of entheogens is still widespread among native groups in
Mesoamerica.[42] Today, as in the time of the Aztecs, the vocation of certain
types of healers and their power to heal are obtained in trips to the
beyond. Those who are called by God suffer a transitory death by lightning, in an epileptic attack, or during a serious illness, and obtain in the
other world the secrets of healing. Today it is believed that to refuse the
call by not exercising the profession designated by God will have grave
consequences for the defaulter.[43]

Multiple Souls (Animistic Forces)

The Aztecs believed that the human body had several animistic forces
(souls). As noted earlier in the chapter, the principal ones were *tonalli*,

which was predominantly located in the head; *teyolia*, which was located in the heart; and *ihiyotl*, which was located and emanated from the liver. Each of these souls had complex specific functions, and the health of an individual depended on the harmony that could be established between them and on the relative amount of each that was present.[44]

Tonalli was a force that determined the degree of vitality in individuals, impressing a particular temperament on them, which affected their future conduct and established a link between human beings and the divine will by means of their allocated fate. The word *tonalli* has a number of meanings. The root, *tona*, means "heat" or "warmth" and is related to the sun god, Tonatiuh, and to the basic Mesoamerican ritual calendar. This calendar, which had existed from the time of the earliest Mayas, was based on the interaction of the numbers one through thirteen and twenty day-names for a possible 260 different combinations. This astrological calendar and the patron deities of the various days determined the destiny of persons. The *tonalamatl* ("book of the days or fates") was interpreted by specialist priests, the *tonalpouhque*, who could calculate the complex interaction of omens and predict the fate of a newborn child. A birth date could determine future health, the length of a person's life, and even the type and frequency of ailments to which one might be subjected. For example, people born on a day 1-Twisted Grass would have many children, but they would all die young.[45] Those born on a day 6-Dog would be sickly and weak and would soon fall dead: "If he lived, he would live only in suffering . . . [he] would go about constantly and continuously coughing, pallid, green-faced, white with cold etc."[46] On the other hand, those born on 1-Lizard would be very strong and healthy. They would even be able to survive falls without harm, as lizards do.[47]

These fates were not absolutely inflexible. *Tonalpouhque* priests could counsel parents to shift baptism of the child by several days to ameliorate a bad omen (by making it appear that the child had been born on a different day), even though children were supposed to be ritually bathed four days after birth.[48] Many of the forecasts of the *tonalamatl* were presented in terms of temperament and behavior. This implies that the *tonalli* could interact with the other two animistic forces. Thus, different fates were possible depending on the temperament *(tonalli)* of the individual and particular circumstances. For example, a woman born on 1-Flower was destined to be an able weaver but only if she carried out penances, drew blood, and fasted on 1-Flower days. If she did not, she would harm her *tonalli* and would end in misery and poverty as a harlot and prostitute.[49]

Tonalli, as an animating force that provided vigor, was infused into the fetus by Ometeotl, the god of duality and a creator god. Similarly, *teyolia*, the animistic force that resided in the heart, was infused by deities *in utero*, expressing the Aztec belief that life existed before birth. However, after being born, the child needed stronger vital forces in order to prosper, and the corresponding rituals were followed. The sun was the best source of *tonalli*, but it was thought dangerous to expose a newborn to it without knowing whether the child's birthday was a good or bad *tonalli* (in its meaning as a fate or temperament). Therefore it was necessary to supply another form of heat. When a baby was born, a fire was lit in the room and was kept constantly burning for four days until the baby was ritually bathed, named, and assigned his or her definite *tonalli*. The bath ceremony, a rite of passage, simulated a rebirth. At that time Ometeotl was asked to give the child additional *tonalli*, and Chalchiuhtlicue was implored to provide additional *teyolia* for the baby.[50]

Tonalli was considered to be a personal link with the heavens and the deities. It seems that this link was conceived as a string extending from a person's head and connecting him or her to the heavens. *Tonalli* was seen as essential to the growth and development of children; the severing of this link would result in stunted growth. For example, if someone jumped over a child who was lying down, it was believed that the child would not grow (presumably because his *tonalli* would be bent or damaged). In order to undo the harm it was necessary to jump over the child in the reverse direction.[51] Further, stepping over someone's head was a great offense, and to protect the head was to protect the name, reputation, and fate of an individual.

Today, the Tzotziles have the concept of *ch'ulel*, a hot, vital force that closely corresponds to *tonalli*. They believe that men are born with a stronger *ch'ulel* than women.[52] This sexual difference is not mentioned in Aztec sources. Among Aztecs *tonalli* increased with age and with the performance of important duties for the state (another physiological reinforcement for the ethic of duty). Nobles were supposed to require a stronger *tonalli* than commoners because they would have to perform the arduous duties of governing. Governing would in turn increase their *tonalli*. This difference in *tonalli* came from two sources: first, nobles were born with stronger *tonalli* (the *tonalamatl* often gives different fates for nobles and commoners born on the same day); secondly, this initial difference was increased during life. *Tonalli* was strengthened by performing brave deeds in battle, by filling responsible positions, and by adherence to a higher moral standard. Aztecs believed that premature sexual activity diminished growth and intelligence, both functions of *tonalli*. Noble youth in the *calmecac*, that is, the school, were expected to remain chaste and to hoard their *tonalli*, while commoners, *macehualtin*, were allowed earlier sexual activity. This distinction again emphasized the difference and superiority of nobles, *pipiltin*, and validated their right to rule—first, through the moral authority of meeting a higher moral standard and second, by the physical superiority of a *tonalli* that had not been diminished.[53]

Tonalli could leave the body, but there was a distinction between normal and abnormal departures and between voluntary and involuntary departures. *Tonalli* was essential for life. One could live without it but only for a short time. Among today's Indian population, *sombra* ("shadow" or soul) is the equivalent of the *tonalli* of the classical Aztecs. *Sombra* can normally leave the body involuntarily when one is drunk, unconscious, asleep, or having sexual intercourse.[54] It is believed today that it is very dangerous to wake a sleeping person suddenly because this can occasion loss of the soul. The classical Aztecs believed that dreams were the perception by *tonalli* of reality in places distant from the body. *Tonalli* also left the body during sexual intercourse. There were strictures against sudden interruption of coitus, which would not allow the *tonalli* to return slowly and gradually to the body and could produce illnesses.[55] Shamans, however, could send their *tonalli* on out-of-body excursions voluntarily without adverse consequences.

Involuntary loss of *tonalli* caused illness and even death. This loss could be the result of cutting the hairs from the crown of the head or the result of a sudden scare. The most common cause was fright, as reflected in Alonso de Molina's definition of the word *netonalcahualiztli*, "fright of someone who is frightened," but literally this word means "the abandonment of *tonalli*."[56] Children were particularly prone to loss of *tonalli* because their fontanels had not closed completely, and thus they were provided with an opening through which *tonalli* could escape. Diagnosis was performed by divination. A shallow bowl of water was used and the child was placed so that the reflection of his or her face could be seen in the water. If the face had a light or clear appearance, no loss of *tonalli* had taken place. A dark image was due to loss of *tonalli*.[57] The loss of *tonalli* in the child created a physical vacuum, which manifested itself as a depression in the cranium. The *teapahtiani* ("healer of the fontanel") attempted to restore health mechanically by turning the child upside down and shaking it or by pushing up on the child's palate.[58] This "fallen fontanel" was in reality due to dehydration of the child.

Belief in the nature of this ailment presently manifests itself in two different ways and can be used to make a more general point about the synthesis of diverse medical systems. Among a number of Mesoamerican groups that have the concept of *sombra*, there is an illness called "soul loss." Here the Aztec etiology has been preserved and has suffered little change. On the other hand, the culture-bound syndrome, *caida de mollera* ("fallen fontanel"), a children's disease, is widely dispersed from El Salvador to the Chicano population of the United States. Urban and non-Indian as well as rural populations acknowledge the ailment. Standard works on folk medicine such as Foster's classical paper attribute the perception of this ailment solely to Spanish folk medicine brought over to the New World.[59] The etiology, as presently conceived, is purely mechanical, in that the sunken fontanel is attributed to a sudden withdrawal of the nipple while nursing or to a fall that caused the fontanel to sink toward the palate, causing eating difficulties in the child. The etiological connection to religion and the concept of *tonalli* has been lost. However, the preferred treatment for this syndrome—turning the child upside down and/or pushing the palate up—is identical to the classical Aztec treatment. An important datum against a purported Spanish origin is that the existence of this syndrome corresponds to the limits of Mesoamerica and is absent from other parts of Latin America where Spanish influence is even stronger.[60] This example reflects the use of therapy of Aztec origin for diseases known to the Aztecs even though the religious etiological connection has been lost. This pattern may be quite common, and it makes the analysis of modern folk medicine very complicated.

Another example is the case of the medicinal uses of two plants—*iztauhyatl (Artemisia mexicana)* and *yauhtli (Tagetes lucida)*. At the time of the Aztecs these two herbs were used extensively and exclusively in rituals of the Tlaloc Water God complex. As a natural extension these herbs were used medicinally for such diseases as paralysis, rheumatism, gout, dropsy, intermittent fevers, and fright, which were perceived as inflicted by Tlaloc or his helpers.[61] Today these same diseases are treated in Mexican and Mexican-American folk medicine with these same herbs (or their generic equivalents, rue and rosemary). However, the religious connection has been broken over the centuries, and the cause and cure are rationalized in the purely secular terms of using "hot" plants to cure diseases of "cold" origin.[62] More complete transmission does take place. William Madsen found that there was an ailment called *ehecacoacihuiztli* ("the wind paralysis") resembling rheumatism. The ailment was attributed to little dwarfs who lived in nearby mountains and caused rain (exactly analogous to Tlaloc's helpers in Aztec mythology), and it was treated with Tlaloc's herbs.[63] In this case the only displacement caused by Christianity was the loss of Tlaloc as a deity. The creative reworking of symbolic systems is also in evidence in the appearance of the Christian cross, which is painted blue (Tlaloc's color), as well as in the use of the *yauhtli* plant in the initiation rites of a guild of healers who claim the power to attract and repel hail.[64]

The second animistic force, *teyolia* ("that which gives life to people"), resided primarily in the heart. It provided vitality, knowledge, and inclination, because for the Aztecs the center of the intellect was in the heart. The heart was tied to thought, emotion, will, and memory. Thus it was said that people who had achieved distinction in the fields of art, divination, or imagination had received a divine force and were *yolteotl* (possessed of a "deified heart").[65] This force was probably thought to be given to the fetus by the patron god of the *calpulli*, the territorial subdivision of the city, but it required a ritual rebirth, as mentioned earlier. This soul was inseparable from the human body and was identified as the soul "that went beyond" after death. It is thus equivalent to the *anima* ("soul") of modern ethnographic investigations.[66]

Damage to *teyolia* and to the heart could have different etiologies. There were a group of diseases and symptoms that were believed to proceed from excess humors (phlegms) in the chest pressing on the heart and nerves:

> Accumulation of phlegms, white, green and yellow . . . penetrate the nerves, head and chest. These phlegms produce pressure on the heart, fever, pulsations of the temple and muscular and nervous trembling. The pressure on the heart proceeds from one side, injures the viscera (the organs of thought) and produces a loss of consciousness.[67]

This displacement of the heart led to mental illness and insanity, as can be seen from the etymology of some of the terms in Molina's dictionary: *teyolcuepaliztli* ("turning around of the heart") is equivalent to being dumb, out of one's mind; *teyolmalacacholiztli* ("spinning around of the heart") means to be crazy, to rave; *yolpatzmiquiliztli* ("crushing of the heart") means heart disease, epilepsy, and *yolzotlaualiztli* ("fainting of the heart") means the same. Thus, pressure on the heart, the flipping of the heart, or a plummeting feeling around the heart could lead to insanity, fainting, or epilepsy. This pressure was believed to be due to an excess of phlegm in the chest. Since the heart was believed to be the seat of the intellect, pressure on it could cause fear or make people evil, mad, bewitched, dizzy, or epileptic. Some descriptions of illness in the *Florentine Codex* supplement those given above: *alaoacquipoloa yiollo* ("phlegm destroys the heart"), *poliuiznequi yiollo* ("heart wants to die"), *motlaeltia toiollo* ("nausea about the heart"), and *patzmiqui in yiollo* ("crushed heart").[68] The development of excessive phlegm could take place slowly and produce fever and other diseases. However, it seems that a sudden, terrifying experience could precipitate a sudden accumulation of phlegm in the chest, which could then produce illnesses such as epilepsy or those attributed to "evil wind" or a "near miss by lightning."[69]

Alfredo López Austin has an alternative explanation. Since the *teyolia* of the dead was what went on to the other world, the *teyolia* of those who were chosen by Tlaloc to die became his helpers—the *ahuaque* ("possessors of water") and the *ehecatotontin* ("little winds"). These helpers provided beneficent rains as well as hail, lightning, and storms. The intrusion into and possession of a person by one of these spirits, specifically the one who had descended with the lightning, produced a progressive disease in the victim, which manifested itself in a tendency to antisocial behavior and insanity. This is the reason why a "raving maniac" was called *aacque* ("one who has suffered an intrusion"). Similarly, epilepsy was caused by the intrusion of the *teyolia* of the Cihuateteo, women who had died in childbirth and therefore had been "chosen" by the solar deity.[70]

Interpreting the diseases as a sudden accumulation of phlegm precipitated by supernatural events allows us to explain the connection between the use of the same medicines for both supernatural and natural diseases. The medicines prescribed are supposed to act by the expulsion of phlegm, which is the proximate cause of the problem whether it was caused by "natural" accumulation or as a result of supernatural intrusion. As in modern beliefs about mental illness, where physiological and psychological causative agents are not mutually exclusive, explanation of these diseases by the use of both intrusion and phlegm allows us to extend our area of explanation. In fact, analysis of the chemical constituents in fever remedies shows that 70 percent of them were either diuretic, diaphoretic, emetic, or purgative, which would in fact expel matter from the body.[71]

The heart could also be harmed by immoral conduct, particularly of a sexual nature. The goddess Tlazolteotl tempted men to sexual excesses that harmed their hearts. This constant theme of moderation and balance and the harm due to excess is reiterated in this *huehuetlatolli* directed toward young men:

Do not throw yourself upon women
like the dog which throws itself upon food.
Be not like a dog
when he is given food and drink,
giving yourself up to women before the time comes.
Even though you may long for women,
hold back, hold back with your heart
until you are a grown man, strong and robust.
Look at the maguey plant.
If it is opened before it has grown
and its liquid is taken out,
it has no substance.
It does not produce liquid; it is useless.
Before it is opened
to withdraw its water,
it should be allowed to grow and attain full size.
Then its sweet water is removed
all in good time.

This is how you must act:
before you know woman
you must grow and be a complete man.
And then you will be ready for marriage;
you will beget children of good stature,
healthy, agile, and comely.[72]

The cure for this disease was confession to Tlazolteotl in the presence of and in consultation with a priest. This is also an example of the duality concept in Aztec thought in that Tlazolteotl was the agent both of temptation and of redemption. Good and evil were not dichotomous as in Christian thought, but different facets of the same reality, as were the concepts of life and death and of creative and destructive deities. The act of confession and performing the penance that followed could be done only once in a lifetime, usually in old age, and was called *neyolmelahualiztli* ("the action of straightening out hearts"). The third method of harming hearts involved magical attacks by sorcerers called *teyolocuanime* ("he who eats hearts of people") and *teyollopachoanime* ("he who squeezes hearts of people").[73]

The foregoing demonstrates that the supposed etiology of a disease will dictate the nature of the remedy. If the cause is sin and transgression against a deity, the appropriate remedy is confession and expiation. If the illness is due to natural causes, the remedy is also natural, and magical diseases require countervailing magic. However, this is often a heuristic device for our analysis, and in reality illness was often treated on all three levels. Those afflicted with possession might be treated variously with appeals to Tlaloc, an effective diuretic to remove phlegm, and a heart-shaped flower, *yolloxochitl*, which cured by imitative magic. An analogy in our society would be patients who go to a hospital for surgery, but consult their horoscope for the proper day and stop in church to pray on their way. Although we can separate etiological classifications for analytical purposes, the members of Aztec culture did not do this. "A native might think that his rheumatic problems came from the supreme will of Titlahuacan, from the punishment sent by the Tlaloque because of the omission of a certain rite, from a direct attack of a being that lived in a particular spring, and from prolonged chilling in cold water; the native would not consider it all as a confluence of divine causes but as a complex."[74]

Ihiyotl, the third animistic force, was concentrated in the liver. It provided the force of passions—bravery, happiness, desire, envy, anger, hatred, love, and the like. *Ihiyotl* was thought of as a luminous gas, which had the ability to influence other beings and in particular to attract them to the source of the gas. For example, a magnetic stone was called *tlaihiyoanani tetl*, "stone that attracts things with *ihiyotl*."[75]

The condition of the liver affected the state of the whole person. Thus, a *cemelli* ("a united, a whole liver") meant pleasure, a happiness that was the result of harmony between contending internal forces. A virtuous person had a clean liver, while dirt was associated with an immoral life and particularly with sexual transgressions. This attitude is reflected in the metaphor for sex, *in teuhtli in tlazolli* ("the dust, the garbage"), or in the references to sexual transgressions as "covering the *tonalli* with dust" or "filling the *tonalli* with garbage."[76] The metaphor for carnal sins is *in cuitlatitlan in tlazoltitlan* ("in the excrement, in the refuse").[77] Sins affected the liver, causing it to emit *ihiyotl*, which could harm the innocent in apparently magical ways.

The group of diseases to be discussed can be divided into three categories. *Tlazolmimiquiliztli* ("filth death") caused small children to cry without apparent reason or to suffer seizures that rendered them unconscious. *Netepalhuiliztli* ("that caused by someone's fault") was characterized by consumption and progressive loss of weight. *Tlazolmiquiliztli* ("garbage illness") produced a variety of incurable diseases and could also cause a series of economic reversals such as a frozen corn crop, the death of stock animals, failure of business deals, and even undercooked meals.[78] *Chahuacocoliztli* ("disease due to a husband's adultery") and *mecatianiliztli* ("concubinage") also resemble this group. The basic cause of all these diseases was supposed to be a fundamental change in the body of the person who established an illicit sexual liaison or who desired another's wife or possessions and became sad because he could not get them.[79] A second possible consequence of adultery was that if the woman became pregnant she would die in childbirth. To avoid this fate it was necessary for mothers-to-be to confess any and all adulterous relationships to their midwives.[80] Of greater significance is that these persons would also emit *ihiyotl* involuntarily and that it could harm others, such as little children or old people. This etiology would explain *tlazolmimiquiliztli*, *netepalhuiliztli*, and *tlazolmiquiliztli*. The cause of *chahuacocoliztli* was more direct, since the adultery of the husband was the direct cause of the illness. Additional evidence of this fateful emanation was the damage that adulterers caused to crops and animals solely by their presence. The presence of an adulterer was sufficient to kill young turkeys, who were considered to be especially fragile. Mice, being more resistant, did not die but detected this emanation and would gnaw holes in vessels to show the presence of the sinner.[81]

Although the emanation produced in *tlazolmiquiliztli* is not clearly identified in the sources as an "air" or a gas, it was treated as if it were. Part of the remedy for this disease was to fan what was presumably "good" air toward the patient to displace the "bad" air.[82] The guilty parties could be cured by a type of baptism ceremony, which included incantations and a ritual cleansing with water and incense. If the offense was adultery, the wife of the adulterer had to commit adultery herself to counteract his actions.[83]

Tlazolmiquiliztli exists today in Mesoamerica and is attributed to a wide range of culprits: adulterers, prostitutes, people who have just finished sexual intercourse, concubines, thieves, gamblers, and drunkards. It is now considered a "hot" force that harms children, the spouse, pregnant women, animals, plants, and other possessions. Children are affected primarily in the eyes (*ixtlazolcocoliztli*, "sickness of filth in the eyes"). Pregnant women who are exposed suffer from chills, fevers, and headaches during labor, and an exposed wife may become sterile. Harm from this disease is primarily prevented by magical means using an umbilical cord, herbs, and salt.[84] This is a fairly direct transmission of a pre-Columbian concept. The existence of this Aztec disease has also facilitated the reimagining of another culture-bound syndrome that is very widely distributed in Mesoamerica in both rural and urban centers, *mal de ojo* ("the evil eye"). This concept is found in many cultures worldwide and was brought over by Europeans, but it fits very well with several aspects of *tlazolmiquiliztli*. People can cause harm at a distance; envy is often the precipitating factor, and the ones most susceptible to it are children. All of these elements are congruent with the Aztec model.

The cases dealt with so far are those in which *ihiyotl* is emitted involuntarily by sinners. There is another group of people, *nanahualtin* ("shaman-sorcerers"), who can voluntarily emit *ihiyotl* for the purpose of harming others. These will be discussed in the section on curers.

Concepts of Life and Human Beings

One of the best ways to understand the ideology of the Aztec is to look at the *huehuetlatolli*, speeches that were used to inculcate the values of the society by constant repetition. Other fruitful sources are *difrasismos*, two-word metaphors (see, for example, such phrases as *in teuhtli in tlazolli* in the section just concluded), and poetry. The Aztecs were very interested in language and had a theory of metaphysical knowledge, called *in xochitl in cuicatl* ("flower and song," i.e., poetry), which held that poetry was the only way to achieve truth.[85] Some preliminary examples, which deal with the nature of life on earth, follow:

> [A *huehuetlatolli* directed at seven-year-old girls:] There is no rejoicing, there is no contentment, there is torment, there is pain, there is fatigue, there is want; torment, pain dominate. Difficult is the world, a place where one is caused to weep, a place where one is caused pain. . . . the earth is not a good place. It is not a place of joy, it is not a place of contentment. It is merely said it is a place of joy with fatigue, or joy with pain on earth.[86]

> [A *huehuetlatolli* spoken to a newborn:] Verily, thou wilt endure, thou wilt suffer torment, fatigue; for verily our lord hath ordered, hath disposed that there will be pain, there will be affliction, there will be misery, there will be work, labor, for daily sustenance. There is sweat, weariness, labor when there is to be eating, drinking, the wearing of rainment. Truly thou wilt endure fatigue, thou wilt suffer torment.[87]

[A *huehuetlatolli* at a cremation:] Thou hast suffered, our lord hath been merciful to thee. Truly our common abode is not here on earth. It is only for a little time, only for a moment that we have been warm. Only through the grace of our lord have we come to know ourselves.[88]

[The same theme in a poem by Nezahualcoyotl, ruler of Texcoco:]
Is it true that on earth one lives?
Not forever on earth, only a little while.
Though jade it may be, it breaks;
though gold it may be, it is crushed;
though it be quetzal plumes, it shall not last.
Not forever on earth, only a little while.[89]

Life was conceived as a brief period in which pain was normal and natural. Suffering was frequently expressed as physical pain or as fatigue, implying that humanity must endure hunger, thirst, and work as the natural consequences of being born. Life also entailed laughter, pleasure, sex, and food, but the emphasis was on communicating to the common man, the *macehualli*, a vision that his existence was ephemeral and that he should accept his premature death in combat. This dichotomy of suffering-happiness occurred in a society where wealth was distributed very unequally. Commoners had difficulty making a living and did indeed suffer hunger, thirst, and hard physical labor. The origin of suffering was not attributed to social structures but rather to the nature of life on earth itself. Suffering was not only natural but the exclusive responsibility of the gods.[90] Social stratification was justified by the physical and moral superiority of nobles due to their stronger *tonalli* and by the arduous task of ruling the state. These concepts can be seen in the metaphors describing these strata: *cuitlapalli atlapalli* ("tail and wing") describes commoners—that is, if the state is a bird the commoners provide the motive power, but not the direction; *in itaconi in mamaloni* ("that which is carried, that which can be shouldered") describes the governed—that is, the common people are carried by the rulers. This point is even clearer in the metaphor *in tecuexanco in tememeloazco* ("that which goes in one's lap, cradled in one's arms")—that is, the governed are like babies or children being cared for by the rulers. The ruler on the other hand is *motenan motzacuil* ("your rampart, your refuge").

López Austin has explored some of the concepts involved in the word *tlacatl* (man, human).[91] The meaning literally is "the diminished man." There is no known Aztec myth to explain this, but there is a Quiche myth in the *Popol Vuh* that is applicable. The first four humans were beings who possessed such great intelligence and enormous powers of vision that the gods became jealous. These beings knew everything and examined all of the earth and the sky. The creator gods decided to change this and limit human powers. The gods blew mist into their eyes, which clouded up as mirrors do when breathed upon, and thus were lost the wisdom and knowledge of the original humans.[92] A similar point is made in the Aztec myth about Quetzalcoatl's journey to the underworld to retrieve the bones of previous humans. During his return, he fell down, and the bones broke. This explains why humans are so short, since the original dwellers were giants. There are as well several extended meanings for *tlacatl* and its derivatives that lay out some of the Aztec ideals concerning the nature of human beings. They should be benign, affable, benevolent, tender, and charitable:

> *tlacatl*—human, peaceful, benign, affable
> *tlacayotl* ("what is human")—generosity, compassion, benevolence, and charity

The quality of their life should be modest and generous and should be marked by ability and chastity:

> *tlacanemiliztli* ("human life")—a modest, generous life
> *tlacatl*—able, chaste
> *zan nen tlacatl* ("worthless man")—inept
> *amo tlacayotl* ("not human")—to sin against nature

The basic rules were equilibrium, moderation, and the execution of assigned functions. If persons deviated, they acquired the qualities of a beast, which was dangerous to their health and to that of others. Social control and performance of duty was guaranteed by holding the body hostage and punishing deviations with illness. Moderation was exalted in *huehuetlatolli*:

> Take heed. On earth it is a time for care, it is a place of caution. Behold the Word; heed and guard it, and with it take your way of life, your works. On earth we live, we travel along a mountain peak. Over here there is an abyss, over there is an abyss. If thou goest over here, or if thou goest over there, then wilt thou fall in. Only in the middle doth one go, doth one live.[93]

> They went saying that on earth we travel, we live along a mountain peak. Over here there is an abyss, over there is an abyss. Wherever thou art to deviate, wherever thou art to go astray, there wilt thou fall, there wilt thou plunge into the deep. That is to say, it is necessary that thou always act with discretion in that which is done, which is said, which is seen, which is heard, which is thought, etc.[94]

States of health or illness were closely related to states of equilibrium or disequilibrium. One must be in equilibrium physically, socially, and in relation to the deities. Excesses and transgressions would affect life or health. Disequilibrium, even if transitory, could lead to illness. It was necessary to preserve or restore bodily equilibrium. A moderate diet was essential for this. The Aztecs attributed the vigor and health of their hunter-gatherer precursors to their sparse and simple diet.[95] Work, tiredness, or long hikes created disequilibrium by overheating a person's *tonalli*. Rest was seen as equivalent to "cooling" as follows: the verb *cecelia* could mean "to relax" or "to cool hot things"; the verb *cehuia* could mean "to rest" or "to cool off a hot thing"; and *tonalcehuia*, "to rest one who walks," meant literally "to cool one's *tonalli*." Some of these concepts have persisted. Indians still believe that sin, excesses, states of anger, sexual excitement, and becoming overtired create an organic vulnerability that can lead to illness.

Since physiology and ethics were closely related, confession was simultaneously a way to restore harmony between individuals and deities and to restore the internal equilibrium of the body. The once-in-a-lifetime confession of sexual sins to Tlazolteotl and confession to a midwife in order to restore equilibrium destroyed by adultery have already been mentioned above.

Nowhere was moderation and avoidance of excess more important than in sexual matters. The Aztecs were prudish in their sexual mores. Premature sex was condemned and was thought to stunt growth and intelligence, both functions of *tonalli*. Thus, in the *huehuetlatolli* cited above, fathers urged their sons not to engage in sex before being fully grown. This was particularly important for young nobles, who would need more *tonalli* in order to be able to govern. Apparently a fixed amount of this substance was present because the longer one waited to start sexual activity, the later in life one would still be able to perform. Women, on the other hand, did not lose "semen" and therefore were potentially insatiable. Sexual pleasure for adults was condoned as long as it was moderate. Excessive sex was considered dangerous because it would "fill your *tonalli* with filth." It led to emaciation and caused coughing, a blackened body, and pus in the urethra. An extreme abuse was the use of a snake called *mazacoatl* or of a worm called *tlaomitl* as aphrodisiacs, which could lead to death by uncontrollable, uninterrupted ejaculation.[96] In line with the ideal of moderation, celibacy was condemned, and rape was punished by death.[97]

The Aztec attitude toward prostitution was ambivalent. Prostitutes were held in low esteem. In *huehuetlatolli* girls were told not to chew gum and not to paint their faces like the *ahuianime* ("the happiness producers"), that is, prostitutes. The omens for the day 1-Flower, cited earlier in this chapter, stated that those women who became prostitutes would end their days in poverty and misery. However, there are a number of references to prostitutes participating in religious festivities. There was apparently a corps of prostitutes who were made accessible as rewards to warriors who had distinguished themselves in battle. A double standard of morality applied here also; since noblewomen who prostituted themselves were killed, prostitutes were commoners or perhaps slaves and women obtained in tribute.[98]

Great value was placed on having children. In the *huehuetlatolli* they were often compared to jewels and precious feathers. Reproduction was also tied to the need of the god for worshippers and, on a more mundane plane, children were economically valuable in an agricultural society that integrated them into the labor force at an early age. Constant warfare and the need for sacrificial victims to maintain the cosmos also supported a pronatalist position. Abortion was punished by the death of both the abortionist and the woman involved.[99] A number of substances were cited as being capable of inducing abortion. One of these, *cihuapatli (Montanoa tomentosa),* has been found to be effective by modern standards and is being developed as a commercial contraceptive today.[100] The one apparent exception to the ban on abortion involved the case of a delivery that threatened the life of the mother. If birth was difficult and efforts to turn the child to make the delivery possible failed, then embryotomy was allowed, and the midwife would cut the child to pieces and remove it from the uterus. The sources state that this was done if the baby was already dead, but it seems that this could also take place when it was alive. Apparently the mother's life had priority over that of the child in cases where a choice had to be made.[101] Breech births such as these were blamed on the violation of societal rules, since they were attributed to having coitus too late in the pregnancy.[102]

Sterility, which was mostly attributed to the woman, could be used by a husband as a cause for divorce.[103] Given the number of remedies that are found in the sources for this problem, sterility seems to have been an important preoccupation.[104] Although the sources do not discuss contraception, considering the pronatalist bias cited above one may conclude that it was probably not condoned. No contraceptives as such are described in the pharmacopoeia, although substances that produce sterility might be considered as such. The flesh of the hummingbird, a symbol of the patron god of the Mexica, Huitzilopochtli ("hummingbird on the left"), was used as a remedy for pustules, but it was said to make one sterile.[105] The use of hummingbirds as pustule medicine *(nanaoapatli)* may be explained by the fact that Huitzilopochtli was a solar god, and the god who became the sun in the origin myth was Nanahuatzin, who was covered with pustules. The cure would have both religious and magical components. It is interesting that this bird, with its strong symbolic ties to Aztec religion, has been used in Mexico from the eighteenth century to the present as a magical amulet to seduce the opposite sex. The desiccated bird, which resembles a penis and thus partakes of imitative magic, is wrapped with silk threads, adorned with beads, and placed in a bag carried by the user. Women carry female hummingbirds and men carry male birds. The use of the amulet is accompanied by a prayer (together with three Hail Marys and three Our Fathers) recited every Friday before an image of Christ:

> Oh divine hummingbird! You give and remove nectar from flowers, you give life and teach women to love. I take refuge in you and your powerful emanations so that you will protect me and give me the ability to make love to any woman I want whether maid, married or widowed. I swear by all the Sacred Apostles not to cease for a moment to adore you in your sacred reliquary so that you will give me all I ask, my beautiful hummingbird.[106]

Active or passive homosexuality in either males or females was severely condemned, and it, as well as transvestism, was punished by death. Those who engaged in illicit sexual relationships were believed to emit harmful irradiations. Homosexual relations were also believed to cause physical harm to those who engaged in these practices. This relationship is expressed in the various meanings of the word *cocoxqui*, "sick, withered, lame, homosexual and effeminate."[107]

The various fates of the animistic forces after death have been discussed. The fear of death and the ephemerality of life in this world are a constant theme in Aztec poetry. There the fear of death is mostly associated with the uncertainty of what is involved in going to Mictlan, the afterlife destination of those who died ordinary deaths. The metaphors used to name Mictlan express this clearly: *in toptli in petlacalli* ("in the bag, in the box"), *poctlan, yiaiuhtlan* ("in the smoke, in the mist"), *quenamican, quenonamican* ("without a body, fleshless"). This uncertainty about death in Mictlan is expressed in the following poem:

> Given over to sadness
> we remain here on earth.
> Where is the road
> that leads to the Region of the Dead,
> the place of our downfall,
> the country of the fleshless?
>
> Is it true perhaps that one lives
> there, where we all go?
> Does your heart believe this?
> He holds us
> in a chest, in a coffer,
> the Giver of Life,
> He who shrouds people in the grave.
>
> Will I be able to look upon,
> able to see perhaps, the face
> of my mother, of my father?
> Will they loan me
> a few songs, a few words?

> I will have to go down there;
> nothing do I expect.
> They leave us,
> given over to sadness.[108]

A more optimistic view perhaps refers to Tlalocan, the more privileged destination of those who died by the intervention of the god Tlaloc:

> Truly I say:
> certainly it is not the place of happiness
> here on earth.
> Certainly one must look somewhere else,
> where indeed happiness will exist.
> Or only in vain have we come to the earth?
>
> Somewhere else is the place of life.
> There I want to go,
> there surely I will sing
> with the most beautiful birds.
> There I will have
> genuine flowers
> the flowers that delight,
> that bring peace to the heart,
> the only ones that give peace to man,
> that intoxicate him with joy. . . .[109]

In Aztec poetry, it can be seen that most ordinary ailments and causes of death inspired fear because they led to the mysterious destination of Mictlan. Only the mode of death that assured the recipient of joining the deity was contemplated willingly. This attitude appears in the same poem cited earlier:

> My heart craves death
> by the obsidian edge.
> Only this my heart craves:
> death in war.

The Medical Establishment

Rather than list different types of healers, we will delineate some general principles of organization that underlay the healing professions. In the etiology of disease, there was no clear separation between natural and supernatural forces. Consequently, health care providers cannot be divided along these lines. The causes of illness lay on a continuum between the purely natural and the purely supernatural poles. The same cure might involve empirical, magical, and religious elements. Some useful distinctions depend on the source of the authority to cure, the source of diagnostic and therapeutic knowledge, and the difference between "true" and "false" doctors.

Humphrey Osmond cites T. T. Paterson's definition of "Aesculapian authority," which is the authority possessed by doctors. This consists of a combination of three types of authority—sapiential, moral, and charismatic. Sapiential authority is the right to be heard, which derives from knowledge or expertise. Moral authority is the right to control and direct, which derives from uprightness and goodness as it is judged according to the ethos of the enterprise. The moral authority of doctors, expressed in the Hippocractic oath, stems from their doing what is expected of them as physicians and from their concern for the good of the patient. Charismatic authority is the right to control and direct, and it derives from God-given grace.[110] This element reflects the unity of religion and medicine that exists in many parts of the world and that certainly existed in Aztec medicine. Osmond claims that in Western culture the charismatic element has to do with the possibility of death and the fact that there are too many known and unknown factors in illness for medicine to rest entirely on sapiential authority. Osmond worries that physicians and health-related personnel today attain adulthood without being exposed to life-threatening illness and death in their own homes. They have not learned the role of the sick person and cannot fully place themselves in the sick person's position. The "sick role" has four essential aspects: (1) depending on the nature and severity of the illness, sick persons are exempted from some or all of their normal responsibilities; (2) they cannot help being ill and cannot get well by an act of decision or will; (3) they are expected to want to get well as soon as possible; and (4) they are expected to seek appropriate help, usually from a physician. The failure of either the patient or the physician to understand and act out the appropriate role will hinder the healing process.[111]

Charismatic authority was very important among the Aztecs since much of the medical tradition was derived from shamanism. The shaman was a link to the supernatural and also a healer. The complex Aztec religious system was linked to the elaborate (and sometimes personal) manifestations of nature. Such a philosophy viewed the cosmos as a sign of living powers. The use of hallucinogens in the diagnosis of disease is a direct link to shamanism. Osmond's concern for a shared ethos between patient and doctor through shared experience of illness would be a minor problem in Aztec culture. Many types of Aztec healers received their charismatic authority by virtue of the fact that their vocation was signaled by a bout of severe illness, a birth defect, or some life-threatening event (such as "a narrow miss by lightning").

Anzures y Bolanos describes the basis on which the Aztecs divided doctors into two classes: the goddess Toci was the patroness of doctors, surgeons, phlebotomists, midwives, aborters, diviners, and those who extract harmful objects from the body; Tezcatlipoca was the patron of the *nanahualtin*, necromancers, and magicians, who could cause harm and illness. The distinction rested on whether the knowledge possessed by the person was used to cure a patient or to cause illness and harm.[112] This distinction between "good" and "bad" doctors has also been explored by León Portilla.[113] Since a "good doctor" *(qualli ticitl)* is also a "wise man" *(tlamatini)*, it is necessary to list some of his characteristics according to Fr. Bernardino de Sahagún's informants. The word *tlamatini* is derived from the verb *mati* ("to know") and means "he who knows things." Such a man teaches truth but also teaches people to be prudent and cautious and to have self-knowledge. He also teaches morality:

The wise man: a light, a torch, a stout torch that
does not smoke.

. . . .

He himself is writing and wisdom
The wise man is careful (like the physician) and
preserves tradition

. . . .

Teacher of the truth, he never ceases to admonish.
He makes wise the countenances of others; to them he
gives a personality;
he leads them to develop it.

. . . .

He puts a mirror before others; he makes them prudent,
cautious; he causes a face (a personality) to appear in
them.

. . . .

Thanks to him people humanize their will and receive
a strict education
He comforts the heart, he comforts the people
he helps, gives remedies, heals everyone.[114]

León Portilla summarizes a long discussion of the above passage as follows:

It might be noted that the Nahuatl philosopher was symbolically described putting together the most meaningful aspects of his intrinsic nature: he throws light upon reality; he is a concentrated vision of the world; "his are the illustrated manuscripts"; "he himself is writing and wisdom"; He also appears in his relationship with other men. He is a teacher *(temachtiani)*, "the road"; "his is the handed-down wisdom"; "he is the teacher of the truth and he does not cease to admonish"; moreover, he performs the duties of a psychologist *(teixcuitiani)*, through whom "the faces of others look wise"; "he opens their ears

... and is master of teachers." That he also functions as a moralist *(tetezca-huiani)* becomes evident in these words: "He puts a mirror before others, he makes them prudent, cautious." Immediately after this, his interest in examining the physical world is discussed: *"cemahuactlahuiani,"* "he attends to things, he applies his light to the world." One single sentence shows him to be a metaphysician, for he studies that which escapes our finite comprehension—"the region of the dead," the hereafter. Finally, as though in summation of his qualities and in explanation of his principal goal, we are told that "thanks to him people humanize their will and receive a strict education."[115]

León Portilla points out that the Aztecs distinguished the "good" physician as one who derived knowledge from observation and experience and the "bad" physician as one whose knowledge was based on magic and superstition. However, as Anzures shows, "good" doctors also included those who use mixed therapies and psycho-religious techniques, such as the ones listed under the patronage of Toci. Here the distinction between empirical and supernatural knowledge is not as sharp as León Portilla would have it. The key distinction is not possession of sapiental authority, since both types of doctors possessed more knowledge than the layperson, but rather the moral authority of the physician. "Good" doctors had moral authority because they performed their duties in an ethical fashion and with the best interests of the patient in mind. The "bad" doctors may have had knowledge, even empirical knowledge, but lacked moral authority because they intended to harm rather than cure. This distinction is more useful than one that tries to dichotomize solely on the basis of natural versus supernatural cures. In describing the goals of Aztec education, León Portilla points out that wisdom, as an ideal of Aztec education, implied purity of heart,[116] as shown in the description of the qualities required for those who would be elected high priest:

> Even if he were poor and lowly,
> even if his mother and father were the poorest of the poor . . .
> His lineage was not considered,
> only his way of life mattered . . .
> The purity of his heart,
> his good and humane heart . . .
> His stout heart . . .
> it was said that he had God in his heart,
> that he was wise in the things of God.[117]

The description of the characteristics of the "good" and the "bad" doctor in the *Florentine Codex* is as follows:

> The true doctor *(qualli ticitl)*.
> He is a wise man *(tlamatini)*;
> he imparts life.
> A tried specialist,

he has worked with herbs, stones, trees and roots.
His remedies have been tested;
he examines, he experiments,
he alleviates sickness.
He massages aches and sets broken bones.
He administers purges and potions;
he bleeds his patients;
he cuts and he sews the wound;
he brings about reactions;
he stanches the bleeding with ashes.
The false physician.
He ridicules and deceives the people;
he brings on indigestion;
he makes illness worse;
his medicines are fatal.
He has dark secrets he will not reveal;
he is a sorcerer *(nahualli)* and a witch *(tlapouhqui)*;
he is familiar with the noxious herbs and possesses
their
seeds,
he practices divination with knotted ropes.
He makes sickness worse;
his herbs and seeds poison and his cures kill.[118]

León Portilla enumerates the qualities of the good physician thus:

> The true physician is a tlamatini, or wise man, who has learned his profession
> by practising it—*tlaiximatini,* which means literally, "he who has firsthand
> knowledge *(imatini)* of the character or nature *(ix)* of things *(tla)*." . . . He pro-
> ceeds by a "scientific" method, studying the effects of his medicines and test-
> ing their curative powers before applying them. Finally, he restores health by
> setting broken bones, massaging, administering purges, bleeding, performing
> surgery, and inducing beneficial reactions in his patients. The standards which
> the good Nahuatl physicians had to meet were not very different from our
> own.[119]

In fact, the Aztecs did possess much valid empirical information and
could claim sapiential authority. They had excellent empirical knowledge
of the pharmacological properties of plants, and this was based on
lengthy observation and practice.[120] One factor contributing to this success
may have been the opportunities for research and the facilities established
by emperors starting as early as the 1460s. In that time Motecuhzoma I
established a botanical garden in Huaxtepec, which, by the time of the
conquest, was seven miles in circumference and contained several thousand species. Other gardens, established at Tenochtitlan, Chapultepec,
Tetzcotzinco, and Itztapalapa, were available to doctors for mixing prescriptions and for experimenting with new drugs.[121] The efficacy of Aztec

wound treatments has been validated,[122] as well as their accurate knowledge of the physiological activities of plants.[123] Their extensive ethnobo-
tanical knowledge and accurate taxonomy indicates that herbals may
have existed and were taught in school, although no genuine pre-Columbian herbal has survived.[124]

Further evidence for this empirical approach to health was the
advanced state of public health and personal hygiene; standards were
much higher than those of contemporaneous Europe. Tenochtitlan in the
sixteenth century was a city of approximately 300,000 inhabitants. Its
public water supply provided pure spring water in aqueducts running
from Chapultepec and Coyoacan. Fresh water was piped to all palaces
and to public outlets and fountains. At this time reliable municipal water
supplies were almost nonexistent in Europe; the usual source of water was
a river running through the city, which itself became a source of disease
since it also served as a sewer.[125]

Personal cleanliness and hygiene were highly prized. The Spanish
conquerors were amazed at the amount of bathing done by the people,
since in Europe bathing was not considered to be healthy. Motecuhzoma
bathed twice daily, and everyone bathed often. The *temazcalli*, or steam
bath, was used frequently—particularly by pregnant women, both for
hygiene and well-being, as well as for ritual purification. The midwife
would enter the sweat bath with the gravid woman, providing massage
and manipulating the child for easier delivery.[126] These hygienic conditions during childbirth may have helped to reduce the incidence of puer-
peral fever. Further evidences of the preoccupation with hygiene are prescriptions in native sources for deodorants, dentifrices, and breath
sweeteners. The city was kept very clean. Garbage was picked up and
dumped at the edge of the city. The upkeep of the streets was organized
in each quarter of the city under the general supervision of the Uey Calp-
ixque. The streets were swept daily, and night soil and urine were collected and removed.[127]

Sapiential authority required a good deal of training. Doctors went to
school for many years in the *calmecac*, the school wherein priests and
scribes were also trained. A lengthy apprenticeship was available to
obtain herbal and other types of knowledge. This description of modern
herbalists would apply equally well to the Aztecs:

> We often think that the village herbalist is an untrained charlatan working in
> the realm of magic that in no way relates to science. In the same vein, we also
> confuse the educational attainments of the practitioner with the therapy—
> M.D.'s and Ph.D.'s do scientific things, while the "uneducated" do magical
> things. Yet in Western cultures, mental illness was thought to be caused by
> witches only a century ago. In other words, it is not difficult to mix a bit of
> illogic, fantasy, and a placebo with the healing science, and at times it may be
> beneficial. Many people are unaware that much time and effort are expended

before an individual is recognized as an herbalist or witch doctor (comparable in indigenous medicines to our pharmacist or psychiatrist), for he must train for many years often under several instructors, in one region and then in another, to learn the use of herbs in several localities, the methods of preparation, and how the materials are related to various spiritual rites.[128]

Empirical knowledge was one, but not the sole source of medical authority. Charismatic or god-given authority was an authority that could be obtained in several ways: (1) A doctor could be divinely predestined in a medical career because of his or her birthday. Doctors and midwives were born on a day 1-House or on a particular day sign ruled by Mictlantecuhtli;[129] while *nanahualtin*, classified as "bad doctors," were born on 1-Rain or 1-Wind.[130] (2) Evidence for predestination could be present at birth, regardless of the date. For example, those who were destined to become *nahualli* would emerge and return to the womb four times before they were finally born.[131] Those who were born lame, cross-eyed, or with other birth defects were destined to be healers because they had received this grace from God in their mother's womb.[132] (3) There are also cases of illness vocation in which the ability to cure was revealed to the participant during a life-threatening illness.[133] This type of selection, a direct shamanic remnant, continues to be important in present-day Mesoamerica. One of the symbols of being a *granicero*, a person capable of stopping hail as well as of healing people, is having been "touched by lightning" in order to be reborn in a new status.[134] Since religion and curing were inextricably mixed, charismatic authority was an important component of the healer's authority.

Moral authority, not the amount or source of knowledge, was the key distinguishing factor between "good" and "bad" doctors. The important point was the intent of the practitioner in the use of the knowledge or the charismatic power either to cure or to harm. We see in the description of the qualities of the doctor that the "bad" doctor had sapiential knowledge but was lacking in moral authority. Persons with charismatic authority could also be distinguished by their ethical or unethical intent. The *nanahualtin* were predestined to be so by birth and were capable of voluntarily sending their *ihiyotl*, in the form of an animal, to harm other people and to make them ill. Their patron god was Tezcatlipoca, and thus they come under the rubric of "bad" doctors. But even in this case, it was possible to have a "good" *nahualli*, as can be seen from this description of them in the *Florentine Codex:*

The Sorcerer *(naoalli)*

The sorcerer [is] a wise man, a counselor, a person of
trust—serious, respected, revered, dignified,
unreviled, not subject to insults.

The good sorcerer [is] a caretaker, a man of
discretion, a guardian. Astute, he is keen, careful,
helpful; he never harms anyone.

The bad sorcerer [is] a doer [of evil], an enchanter.
He bewitches women; he deranges, deludes people; he
casts spells over them; he charms them; he causes them
to be possessed. He deceives people; he confounds
them.[135]

Conclusion

Aztec religion was inextricably intertwined with medicine. From a very
early age, origin myths and religious beliefs inculcated the primary ethical
duty and principal goal in life: to serve one's group or state and accept
suffering or inequity in the distribution of goods. The body was hostage
to the performance of duty and to communal expectations; the gods punished the body with disease or death for transgressions against the rigid
moral order. Thus, supernaturally ordained illnesses reinforced the *status
quo* and the secular legal system. In the order of creation, differences in
individual physiology reflected moral status or hierarchical rank. Social
stability, a prime goal of Aztec society, was supported by the view that
the ruling class was physically, as well as morally, superior to the commoners. Transgressors of the moral code became physically altered
through their evildoing and emitted noxious forces that could harm and
sicken those around them.

Doctors possessed charismatic or moral authority as well as sapiential
authority derived from empirical study. The Aztec penchant for duality
and opposition held that there were "good" and "bad" physicians and
other medical practitioners. Moral authority distinguished the "good"
doctors whose intent was to benefit their patients. Cultivating this moral
authority was a key goal of Aztec education.

Modern Mesoamerica has creatively synthesized both Catholic and
pre-Hispanic beliefs. Contemporary Mesoamerican folk medicine can best
be understood by recognizing the continued presence of many Aztec
beliefs about health and illness. This description of the original concepts
in Mesoamerica aims to serve as a benchmark for those who wish to
untangle the twisted skein of contemporary Mesoamerican medical practice and belief.

Notes

1. Richard E. W. Adams, *Prehistoric Mesoamerica* (Boston, 1977), pp. 5, 12.
2. L. Marie Musgrave-Portilla, "The Nahualli or Transforming Wizard in
   Pre- and Postconquest Mesoamerica," *Journal of Latin American Lore* 8,
   no. 1 (1982):3–63.

3. Alfonso Caso, "Religion o Religiones Mesoamericanas?" *Verhandlungen des XXXIII internationalen Amerikanisten kongresses, 1968,* vol. 3 (Stuttgart-Munich, 1971), pp. 189–200.
4. Michael D. Coe, "Religion and the Rise of Mesoamerican States" in *The Transition to Statehood in the New World,* eds. Grant D. Jones and Robert R. Kautz (Cambridge, England, 1981), pp. 157–171.
5. Henry B. Nicholson, "Religion in Pre-Hispanic Central Mexico," in *Handbook of Middle American Indians,* vol. 10, eds. Gordon F. Eckholm and Ignacio Bernal (Austin, TX, 1971), p. 396.
6. Bernard R. Ortiz de Montellano, "Empirical Aztec Medicine," *Science* 188 (1975):215–220; same author, "The Rational Causes of Illnesses among the Aztecs," *Actes du xlii Congrès international des américanistes, 1976,* vol. 6 (Paris, 1979), pp. 287–289; J. R. Davidson and Bernard R. Ortiz de Montellano, "The Antibacterial Properties of an Aztec Wound Remedy," *Journal of Ethnopharmacology* 8 (1983):149–161.
7. Musgrave-Portilla, "The Nahualli."
8. Peter T. Furst, *Hallucinogens and Culture* (San Francisco, 1976), pp. 4, 57–86.
9. Nicholson, "Religion in Pre-Hispanic Mexico," pp. 398–402.
10. John Eric Sidney Thompson, *The Rise and Fall of Maya Civilization* (Norman, OK, 1966), pp. 277–278.
11. Nicholson, "Religion in Pre-Hispanic Mexico," p. 402.
12. Alfredo López Austin, *Cuerpo humano e ideología,* 2 vols. (Mexico City, 1980), p. 402.
13. W. Lehman, ed. and trans., *Die geschichte der königreiche von Culhuacan und Mexico* (Stuttgart, 1938), pp. 330–338; Nicholson, "Religion in Pre-Hispanic Mexico," p. 400.
14. Miguel León Portilla, *Aztec Thought and Culture,* trans. Jack E. Davis (Norman, OK, 1963), p. 111.
15. Davíd Carrasco, *Quetzalcoatl and the Irony of Empire: Myths and Prophecies in the Aztec Tradition* (Chicago, 1982), pp. 70–72.
16. Mircea Eliade, *The Myth of the Eternal Return* (New York, 1965), pp. 12–17.
17. Eduardo Matos Moctezuma, "El templo mayor de Tenochtitlan: Economia e ideologia," *Boletin de antropologia americana sobretiros* 1 (1980):179–189.
18. Fr. Bernardino de Sahagún, *Florentine Codex: General History of the Things of New Spain,* eds. and trans. Charles E. Dibble and Arthur J. O. Anderson (Salt Lake City, 1950–1969), bk. 3, pp. 1–5.
19. Matos Moctezuma, "El tempo mayor de Tenochtitlan."
20. López Austin, *Cuerpo humano e ideología,* pp. 171–174, 396–399.
21. Thompson, *Maya Civilization,* p. 177.
22. López Austin, *Cuerpo humano e ideología,* p. 173.
23. Ibid., p. 9.
24. Ibid., p. 398.
25. Nicholson, *Religion in Pre-Hispanic Mexico,* pp. 408–430.
26. Sahagún, *Florentine Codex,* bk. 1, p. 31.
27. Ibid., p. 39.
28. Ibid., p. 45.
29. Alfredo López Austin, "Ideas etiologicas en la medicina Nahuatl," *Anuario indigenista* 30 (1971):255–275.
30. Fr. Bernardino de Sahagún, *Historia general de las cosas de Nueve España,* (Mexico City, 1956), vol. 1, p. 277.
31. Sahagún, *Florentine Codex,* bk. 2, p. 58.

32. Sahagún, *Historia general*, vol. 1, pp. 72–75.
33. Wigberto Jiménez Moreno, "Religion o religiones mesoamericanas?" *Verhandlungen des XXXIIII internationalen Amerikanisten kongresses, 1968*, vol. 3 (Stuttgart-Munich, 1971), pp. 201–206 (my translation).
34. Coe, "Religion and Mesoamerican States," p. 183; Carrasco, "Quetzal-coatl," pp. 151, 161.
35. López Austin, *Cuerpo humano e ideologia*, p. 272.
36. Miguel León Portilla, *Pre-Columbian Literatures of Mexico* (Norman, OK, 1969), pp. 87–88.
37. Alfonso Caso, *The Aztecs: People of the Sun* (Norman, OK, 1958), pp. 58–65.
38. Nancy K. Rhoden and John D. Arras, "Withholding Treatment from Baby Doe: From Discrimination to Child Abuse," *Milbank Memorial Fund Quarterly* 63, no. 1 (1985):18–51.
39. Jacques Soustelle, *The Daily Life of the Aztecs*, trans. Patrick O'Brian (Stanford, CA, 1970), p. 157.
40. Cited in R. Gordon Wasson, *The Wondrous Mushroom: Mycolatry in Meso-america* (New York, 1980), p. xiv.
41. López Austin, *Cuerpo humano e ideologia*, pp. 408, 411.
42. Wasson, *The Wondrous Mushroom*; Peter T. Furst, *Hallucinogens and Culture* (San Francisco, 1976).
43. López Austin, *Cuerpo humano e ideologia*, p. 412.
44. Alfredo López Austin, "Almas y experiencia entre los antiguos Nahuas," *Boletin de la sociedad Mexicana de historia y filosofia de la medicina* 6, no. 45 (1983):223–234.
45. Sahagún, *Florentine Codex*, bk. 4, p. 55.
46. Ibid., p. 73.
47. Ibid., p. 83.
48. Soustelle, *Daily Life of the Aztecs*, p. 165.
49. Sahagún, *Florentine Codex*, bk. 4, p. 25.
50. López Austin, *Cuerpo humano e ideologia*, pp. 228–233, 254.
51. Sahagún, *Florentine Codex*, bk. 4, p. 184.
52. Calixta Guiteras Holmes, *Los peligros del alma: Vision del mundo de un Tzotzil* (Mexico City, 1965), p. 248.
53. López Austin, *Cuerpo humano e ideologia*, pp. 244–245, 354.
54. Ibid., p. 243.
55. Ibid., pp. 224, 332.
56. Friar Alonso de Molina, *Vocabulario en lengua Castellana y Mexicana y Mexicana y Castellana* (1571), facsimile ed. (Mexico City, 1970).
57. H. Ruiz de Alarcón, "Tratado de supersticiones y costumbres gentílicas que oy viuen entre los indios naturales de esta Nueve España," in *Tratado de las idolatrías, hechicerías y otras costumbres gentílicas de las razas aborígenes de México (1629)*, ed. Francisco del Paso y Troncoso (Mexico City, 1953), p. 137.
58. Angel Ma. Garibay, "Paralipomenos de Sahagun," *Tlalocon* 2 (1943):235–254.
59. George M. Foster, "Relationship between Spanish and Spanish-American Folk Medicine," *Journal of American Folklore* 66 (1953):201–217.
60. Bernard R. Ortiz de Montellano, "*Caida de Mollera*: Aztec Sources for a Mesoamerican Disease of Alleged Spanish Origin," *Ethnohistory* 34 (1987):381–399.
61. Bernard R. Ortiz de Montellano, "Las Yerbas de Tlaloc," *Estudios de cultura Nahuatl* 14 (1981):287–314.
62. Ibid.

63. William Madsen, "Hot and Cold in the Universe of San Francisco Tecospa," *Journal of American Folklore* 68 (1955):123–138.
64. C. Viesca Trevino, personal communication, 1981.
65. López Austin, *Cuerpo humano e ideologia*, p. 256.
66. Antonio García de Léon, *Pajapan: Un dialecto Mexicano del Golfo* (Mexico City, 1976), p. 32; Evon Z. Vogt, "H?iloletic: The Organization and Function of Shamanism in Zinacantan," in *Summa antropologica en homenaje a Roberto J. Weitlaner*, ed. Antonio Pompa y Pompa (Mexico City, 1966), pp. 359–369.
67. Alfredo López Austin, "Sahagun's Work and the Medicine of the Ancient Nahuas: Possibilities for Study," in *Sixteenth Century Mexico: The Work of Sahagun*, ed. M. S. Edmonson (Albuquerque, NM, 1974), p. 220.
68. Sahagún, *Florentine Codex*, pp. 129–130, 155, 165, 181.
69. Ortiz de Montellano, "The Rational Causes of Illnesses among the Aztecs."
70. López Austin, *Cuerpo humano e ideologia*, pp. 389, 407.
71. Ortiz de Montellano, "The Rational Causes of Illnesses among the Aztecs."
72. León Portilla, *Aztec Thought and Culture*, pp. 149–150.
73. López Austin, *Cuerpo humano e ideologia*, p. 256.
74. López Austin, "Sahagun's Work and the Medicine of the Ancient Nahuas."
75. López Austin, *Cuerpo humano e ideologia*, pp. 212, 257–260.
76. Ibid., pp. 245, 357.
77. Sahagún, *Florentine Codex*, bk. 6, p. 97.
78. Alarcón, "Tratado de supersticiones," pp. 110–112.
79. J. de la Serna, *Manual de ministros de indias* (Mexico City, 1953), p. 250.
80. López Austin, *Cuerpo humano e ideologia*, p. 344.
81. Sahagún, *Florentine Codex*, bk. 4, pp. 190–192.
82. Luis A. Vargas, "Las relaciones interpersonales y la enfermedad en la época prehispánica," *Actes du xlii congreès international des Américanistes, 1976*, vol. 6 (Paris, 1979), pp. 341–347.
83. Alarcón, "Tratado de supersticiones," pp. 112–115.
84. López Austin, *Cuerpo humano e ideologia*, pp. 294, 299.
85. Léon Portilla, *Aztec Thought and Culture*, pp. 73–79.
86. Sahagún, *Florentine Codex*, bk. 6, p. 93.
87. Ibid., p. 168.
88. Sahagún, *Florentine Codex*, bk. 3, p. 41.
89. León Portilla, *Aztec Thought and Culture*, p. 72.
90. López Austin, *Cuerpo humano e ideologia*, pp. 277–280.
91. Ibid., pp. 201–206.
92. Adrian Recinos, trans., *Popol Vuh*, eds. Delia Goetz and Sylvanus G. Morley (Norman, OK, 1950), pp. 167–169.
93. Sahagún, *Florentine Codex*, bk. 6, p. 101.
94. Ibid., p. 125.
95. Pedro Carrasco, "Una cuenta ritual entre los Zapotecos del Sur," in *Homenaje a Dr. Alfonso Caso* (Mexico City, 1951), p. 95.
96. López Austin, *Cuerpo humano e ideologia*, pp. 333–335.
97. Ibid., pp. 345, 348.
98. R. Moreno, "Las Ahuianime," *Historia nueva* 1 (1969):3–31.
99. Fr. Bartolomé de las Casas, *Apologetica historia sumaria*, ed. Edmundo O'Gorman (Mexico City, 1967), vol. 2, p. 387.
100. Seymour D. Levine et al., "The Mexican Plant Zoapatle (*Montanoa*

tomentosa) in Reproductive Medicine, " *Journal of Reproductive Medicine* 26 (October 1981):524–528.

101. Sahagún, *Florentine Codex*, bk. 6, p. 160.
102. López Austin, *Cuerpo humano e ideologia*, p. 217.
103. Ibid., pp. 344–345.
104. Noemi Quezada, "Metodos anticonceptivos y abortivos tradicionales," *Anales de antropologia* 12 (1975):223–242.
105. Sahagún, *Florentine Codex*, bk. 11, p. 24.
106. Noemi Quezada, *Amor y magia amorosa entre los Aztecas* (Mexico City, 1975), pp. 100–106.
107. López Austin, *Cuerpo humano e ideologia*, p. 347.
108. León Portilla, *Pre-Columbian Literatures*, p. 85.
109. Ibid., p. 86.
110. Humphrey Osmond, "God and the Doctor," *New England Journal of Medicine* 302 (March 1980):555–558.
111. Talcott Parsons, "Definitions of Health and Illness in the Light of American Values and Social Structure," in *Patients, Physicians and Illness: Source Book in Behavioral Science and Medicine*, ed. E. Gartley Jaco (New York, 1958), pp. 165–187.
112. Maria del Carmen Anzures y Bolanos, *La medicina tradicional en Mexico* (Mexico City, 1983), pp. 45–47.
113. León Portilla, *Aztec Thought and Culture*, pp. 3–27.
114. Ibid., p. 10.
115. Ibid., pp. 15–16.
116. Ibid., pp. 142, 147.
117. Sahagún, *Florentine Codex*, bk. 3, p. 67.
118. León Portilla, *Aztec Thought and Culture*, pp. 26–27.
119. Ibid., p. 27.
120. E. del Pozo, "La farmacologia indigena," in *Libellus de medicinalibus indorum herbis*, ed. M. de la Cruz (Mexico City, 1964), p. 338.
121. Bernard R. Ortiz de Montellano, "Curanderos: Spanish Shamans or Aztec Scientists?" *Grito del Sol*, 1, no. 2 (1976):21–28.
122. Davidson and Ortiz de Montellano, "Aztez Wound Remedy."
123. Ortiz de Montellano, "Empirical Aztec Medicine."
124. Bernard R. Ortiz de Montellano, "Una clasificacion botanica entre los Nahoas?" in *Estado actual del conocimiento en plantas medicinales Mexicanas*, ed. X. Lozoya (Mexico City, 1976).
125. Ortiz de Montellano, "Curanderos."
126. Sahagún, *Florentine Codex*, bk. 6, p. 155.
127. Ortiz de Montellano, "Curanderos."
128. Walter H. Lewis and Memory P. F. Elvin-Lewis, *Medical Botany: Plants Affecting Man's Health* (New York, 1977), p. 3.
129. Sahagún, *Florentine Codex*, bk. 4, pp. 41–42; Serna, *Manual de ministros de indias*, p. 167.
130. Sahagún, *Florentine Codex*, bk. 4, pp. 93, 101.
131. Angel Ma. Garibay, "Paralipómenos de Sahagún," *Tlalocan* 2, no. 3 (1947):235–254.
132. Serna, *Manual de ministros de indias*, pp. 240–242.
133. Ibid., pp. 86–87, 242.
134. Carmen Cook de Leonard, "Roberto Weitlaner y los graniceros," in *Summa antropologica en homenaje a Roberto J. Weitlaner*, ed. Antonio Pompa y Pompa (Mexico City, 1966), pp. 290–298.
135. Sahagún, *Florentine Codex*, bk. 10, p. 31.

CHAPTER 15

Religious

Foundations

of Health and

Medical Power

in South America

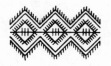

LAWRENCE E. SULLIVAN

In January 1986 Brazil's president, Jose Sarney, provoked a storm of controversy concerning indigenous medicine. On Tuesday, January 21, Sarney pleaded with a healer from an unnamed Amazon tribe to save the life of Augusto Ruschi, a seventy-year-old ecologist whom many Brazilians revere as a national hero. Ten years earlier, it was believed, a dendrobata frog had poisoned Ruschi with fatal venom. Summoned by the president of the Republic, an Amazon Indian healer named Raoni rushed to the bedside with his medicines and his apprentice, a younger colleague named Sapaim.

Raoni and Sapaim brought their patient to a wooded park in Rio de Janeiro. Raoni inserted the ceremonial lip-plug that lends the tones of his voice an extraordinary power. Healer and apprentice decorated the upper parts of their bodies with stripes of dark paint. For more than an hour they smoked vision-inducing cigars, bathed their patient in tobacco smoke, and washed him with *atorokon*, a potion prepared from forest plants. The treatment sessions were closed to the press. Only selected friends and relatives attended. They reported later that Raoni and Sapaim massaged the entire body of their patient and then extracted pasty substances from inside of him. The healer held out the substances for all the observers to see. Raoni rubbed his hands together to make the substances disappear. Over the course of the treatments the pathogenic extractions gradually changed color, from green to white to black, as the poison diminished.

After six sessions Raoni pronounced the patient cured. Ruschi agreed with this assessment and pointed to the fact that he no longer suffered nosebleeds and that the tenor of his dreams had changed so that he now saw beautiful things when he slept. The professional medical community of Rio reacted negatively and strongly. Prominent doctors condemned the treatments as "mere quackery." They suggested that Ruschi's medical problems stemmed not from frog poison but from deterioration of his liver due to the harmful side effects of modern medicines used to combat malaria. Others hypothesized that the dose of venom Ruschi had absorbed was small enough so that he could recover. Flavio Martino, a toxicologist from a Rio medical foundation, summarized the conventional view: "Even if there was some poison and the Indians took it out of Ruschi, he would continue in a critical state because of his liver." He added, "I do not believe in a cure."[1]

The newspapers of any city in the modern world contain reports of this sort. On the one hand the stories testify, usually in condescending tones, to the persistence of indigenous medical systems and to their undiminished value for some modern practitioners and patients. On the other hand, they often depict the exasperation of health care professionals trained to fight disease by eradicating ignorance concerning illness and well-being. Trained to interpret "folk" practices as obstacles to optimal health, institutionally schooled practitioners educate the community against the heresies that impede the progress and triumph of "modern" medicine.

Disease and cure always confront realities that are *other* than ordinary: realities that are strange, unsuspected, unseen, or unfamiliar. Medicine and strangeness are related, although where that strangeness is located and what its symptoms mean depend on a culture's history. The experiential encounter with a mode of being foreign to one's normal state (and symbolically present under the signs of poison, virus, invasive pathogen, agent of physical injury, chemical imbalance, or traumatic event) makes sickness a condition definable as out of the ordinary. Once the extraordinary and alien character of affliction is recognized, the afflicted may be excused from normal work, behavior, and culpability. A patient is "sick" and no longer responsible for his or her abnormal state; an alien condition has forcibly intervened.[2] Indigenous medical practices in South America reflect the relationship of disease to the supernatural order. The goal of individual or cosmic life and the nature of the human constitution are religious concepts. These and other fundamental ideas lead cultures toward distinct evaluations of health and sickness. The incident involving President Sarney, ecologist Ruschi, healer Raoni, and toxicologist Martino shows how therapy can proceed from vastly different appraisals of the nature of reality—political, cosmic, supernatural, or chemical.

This essay does not aim to resolve the tensions that arise from conflicts of meaning. Rather, it scans only one side of the issue—the local logics of some South American medical systems.[3] Religious imagery provides the context for understanding these practices and warrants their tenacious existence at the heart of vital cultures. Religion is not held separate from cultural or individual life in South American societies. Insofar as existence is authentic, it is a religious situation, a life that keeps in touch with what is sacred.

Medicine lies at the heart of the religious evaluation of existence. Religion and medicine are symbolic strands forming a single fiber that binds together the framework of meaning. Medicines such as plants, animal products, crystals, paints, or songs bear special relationship to sacred realities. A supernatural being first gave them to humankind, or a holy place produced them, or the ritual process of preparation consecrated them. The category of medicine includes people, dreams, concrete objects, sounds, and times. In general, medicine should be seen as a mode of being, a condition that fills an entity with sacred power or manifests an extraordinary relationship to supernatural realities. That is why, among the many other purposes it serves, medicine deals effectively with powers of affliction. In an exemplary way, the human body and its outward signs, especially the symptoms of sickness and cure as well as the symbolic trappings of medical practice, manifest realities on which the creativity and degeneracy of culture are founded.

Wellness and Illness

South America contains some 1,500 distinct language groups.[4] One could say that there are hundreds of separate medical traditions.[5] Rather than attempt an impossible historical treatment of any or all traditions, the following pages offer a reflection on the evidence that exists as a whole, with an eye toward the religiousness of health and medicine. What are the religious values that underlie and coincide with the *intentions* of indigenous medicine? No essay that scribes this wide a compass can dwell at length on the particularities of distinct traditions. At this stage, South American medical systems cannot be subjected to exhaustive, seamless, and smooth description. Not only is our general knowledge of South American medicine incomplete and inconclusive, but the interpretation of any single culture's medical practice must remain as open as the good practitioner's search for powers of cure.[6]

In general, the elimination of organic disorder is not the only goal of the most powerful medicine. "Health" and "sickness" are comprehensive modes of being that transcend the individual organism. The states of wellness and illness encompass relations with all manner of cosmic beings: the creator, mythic heroes who invented culture, monsters left over from earlier worlds, and potent spiritual aspects of sun, moon, stars, rains, plants, earth, or human society.

THE CENTER AS MEDICAL RESOURCE AND HEALTH HAZARD

Medicine manages communication among all significant realms of being in the cosmos that impinge on the body. The reason for this is religious: through ritual, humans situate themselves at the center of the world. Several examples make clear how this fundamental belief finds multiple and creative expression in the religious traditions of South America.

The Inca capital of Cuzco, the ritual heart of a sixteenth-century empire that stretched across 3,000 miles of mountains and coast, was the navel of an immense feline body and the center of the five divisions of the earth. The contemporary Andean village of Misminay near Cuzco is constructed directly beneath the Milky Way and exactly in the middle of the four solstitial points on the intercardinal horizons, the outermost reaches of the rising and setting sun during its yearly travels. The roundhouse of the Yekuana people from the Orinoco area of Venezuela is a miniature image of the world, located at the world's center. The entire community lives there. The same is true of the *malocas* (longhouses) of Tukano-speaking peoples of the Vaupés River area of southern Columbia and northeastern Brazil. The Campa people of eastern Peru live halfway between "upstream" and "downstream," the two directions that contain the outermost markers of the world's boundaries. The dance and ritual plazas at the center of villages among the Apinayé, Boróro, and Kayapó peoples from the southern branches of the Amazon in Brazil are set in the middle of the four cardinal points at the midpoint between the places where the sun sets and rises. Many South American peoples locate their living space, especially their ritual sites, in the center of vertical space. The Kogi of Colombia, for example, picture the universe as having nine layers; they inhabit the middle one.

In medical practice throughout South America the healer's rattle figures prominently. This powerful instrument is often a centering device. Its sound marks the world's center. Rattles of many Guaraní-speaking peoples in Paraguay, for example, contain noisemaking seeds. These were the same fruit seeds spit out by a hero who had scaled an enormous tree during the primordial flood. The pits fell to the soil with a *ping* as they struck the dry ground at the foot of the cosmic tree, the first and central patch of earth to emerge after the Deluge. The sounds of the seeds still mark the sacred center and the hopes of salvation from destruction. The Kari'ña healers of Venezuela carve designs in their medicinal rattles. The cross-hatching and holes describe how the rattle marks the intersection of the four cardinal directions, the place where all spirits come together to feed on tobacco smoke when summoned by the rattle's sound.

Living at the center of the world is a religious posture, for the center itself is a symbolic construction based on the recognition of sacred powers.[7] This religious stance offers South American peoples access to powerful realities; here they can traffic with all manner of beings both helpful and harmful. By assuming its proper place in the world, therefore, human existence becomes "medically" hazardous. Maintenance of health and the restoration of a condition of well-being become the first responsibilities of cultures making the religious choice to live in contact with the full range of powerful beings. Myths often report that heroic forerunners of culture made this decision for human beings toward the beginning of time. These heroes, such as Kuai among the Baniwa of the upper Rio Negro of Brazil or the first *xon* (healer) of the Selk'nam of Tierra del Fuego, serve as models of medical practice. The same beings who created the conditions of culture also provided medicine. Medical powers redress the disorders occasioned by the spiritual hazards associated with the foundations of culture: food, sex, hunting, agriculture, social existence, crafts, and so on. The imagined causes of disease (through breach of food restrictions, incest, improper behavior during hunting or farming, harmful intentions of a neighbor or in-law) remain closely bound to religious symbols that reveal the meaning of fundamental realities of culture and cosmos.[8]

To extract from South American medicines a unique source of wellness would be a futile gesture. In general, these cultures show little interest in isolating a single force responsible for wellness, nor do they seek a single cause of illness, whether that explanation be theological, psychological, or technico-chemical. They prefer to explore the nature of a *complex movement* of forces at work in this world. Wellness reveals itself in the following symbolic complexes: the fullness of time, the wholeness of space, the soundness of tone, and the indivisibility of formless conditions (such as sleep, darkness, invisibility, breath, silence or total noise, and the emotional plenitude of the community during ritual).

THE FULLNESS OF TIME

To capture the sense of wellness manifest in the images of fullness of time, it is essential to emphasize that, in most South American accounts, human beings appear rather late on the cosmic scene. In many cases, whole worlds existed and disappeared before the creation of the world containing human life as it is now known. Universal flood, fire, or petrification destroyed the first worlds. Each of these failed primordia contained the germ of its own destruction, for each was built on a single temporal principle. For example, the Desana people of southern Colombia say that the sun and moon followed the same course at the beginning of time. Many other cultures describe how solar and lunar time were identical before tragic events caused their separation into separate periodicities (day versus night, lunar versus solar months and years). In the Desana case, the tragedy was the incestuous union of the Sun with his daughter: his light penetrated her eye and inseminated her. Many peoples living in the Amazon hold to another image of the uniqueness of primordial time. In the beginning, conditions were such that one could paddle a given distance upstream or downstream in the same amount of time.[9]

A primordial world founded on only one temporal principle cannot contain change (and containing change is a prerequisite for bodies that experience the changes manifest as sickness and cure). The only change in the primordial world could be a total one: destruction. Peoples in the Andes, for example, report the existence of several ages in succession. Each one was destroyed for reasons intrinsic to its own temporal character. In some accounts, the first world was consumed by fire. An unbroken rainy season governed the second world. It was destroyed by flood.[10]

Although the disintegration of those first worlds was due, ironically, to their unchanging mode of being, their appearance and demise continue to affect human history. The present world is an accommodation of such primordial realities as light, darkness, water, unique sound, and stone to a kind of temporality which did not exist in the first epochs: alternation and periodicity. The present world in which humans live contains the effective signs of both primordial light and darkness because it subjects these primordial realities to periodic time. Light shines during the day, and darkness reigns at night. There is accommodation of the periodicity of the moon to the sun and to the stars. There is alternation between the rainy and dry seasons. The Inca calendar, for example, contained units that combined solar, lunar, and sidereal time into one-, eight-, and sixteen-year megacycles, among other units, and coordinated these with the growth cycles of animals, plants, and humans.[11]

Indeed, this is the cosmos, the human world, which enjoys the appearance of all these temporalities. The fullness of time (as opposed to the absoluteness of any single kind of time) is a cosmic ritual that carefully orchestrates and controls the intercalation of multiple modes of time. Each temporal mode, on its own, has proven itself destructive in the past and shows itself as sickening in the present. When all modes are taken together, however, they constitute a generativity characteristic of this world. The human being shares this periodic and reproductive nature. The temporal complexity of the human constitution is demonstrated during therapeutic dances when the movements of separate limbs exhibit the ability to embody complex polyrhythms in a simultaneous event. Human beings show themselves to be amalgams of times in other ways as well. The substances of breath, bone, and blood, for example, each manifest a separate kind of temporal rhythm or pulse. There are souls that govern the beating heart, the vital respiration, and nocturnal dreams, and each has its history: according to the Sanemá-Yanoama of the Brazil-Venezuelan border, for instance, the various souls and physical substances of the human constitution emerge from separate periods of mythical history, bone being the most ancient and blood the most recent.[12] That is why each substance in the human constitution brings a different kind of temporality to the ensemble that composes human experience. Should the multiplicity of times threaten to collapse into a single dimension, the life of this world would also be threatened. That is why eclipses so often signal the onset of an annihilating epidemic. The Guayakí of Paraguay, for example, contend that a primordial jaguar of celestial blue color devours the sun or the moon during eclipses; they drive him away with furious noise. The jaguar's partial success brings disease. If he ever devoured the moon or sun completely, the world would end either in the rotting darkness of total night or in the conflagration of total day.[13] The loss of multiple times is also the reason why the cessation of breath, the diminution of pulse, the irregularity of excretions, or the absence of the soul from the body are temporal signs that spell possible disintegration of health. Well-being is a temporally complex and dynamic state of being. The fullness of time preserves itself at the cost of any single kind of temporality. Wellness includes the periodic limits of its component parts: the "death" of the sun each evening, the end of night with the dawn, the end of the dry season, the curtailment of the wet season, the disappearance of the moon each month. The temporal limits of human components must also contribute to the complex movements of well-being: the end of sleep for work is as important to individual and communal health as the termination of work in order to rest and dream, the end of each exhalation and inhalation, the loss of blood in menses, the confinement during the menstrual period or during initiatory seclusion, the closing of ritual periods open to transcendent forces, the decomposition of flesh at death, the pounding and consumption of cremated bones, the termination of the postmortem soul's presence on earth.[14] In order to have good health, it is essential that every appearance of life make its proper disappearance and yield to the periodic time governing the well-being of this world. These intermittent and multiple "deaths" of specific time lines are an integral part of the continuing fullness of time characteristic of this world. This explains why sickness, as a symbolic emblem of death, is an integral part of this world and why healers themselves sometimes reenact the disappearance or "death" of primordial forms through ecstasy or possession. Wellness and illness are part of the complex temporal process—the only kind of time that has, thus far, managed to sustain itself in the cosmos.

THE WHOLENESS OF SPACE

Just as the temporal mode of these primordial worlds was ill adapted to change, the spatial stage, too, of the first primordia was univalent. Each world was a space of its own kind, uninterrupted by the kinds of space that existed elsewhere or would exist later in time. These singular spatial conditions failed to sustain themselves and fell apart. In the beginning of creation, for example, the Yanomamö universe existed on a single plane, but, under its own weight, parts of it crumbled and fell to become other levels of the extant universe. The same thing happened to the griddle-sky of the first Barasana (northwest Amazon) world. It sank to become the earth; a new space, a new sky, was set in place of the first one. The creator Romi Kumu had to set up several more griddles because the first and unique one fell. The Wayãpi report that, in the beginning, the sky and earth were one place, until a team of dancing architects in the shape of birds raised the heavenly vault on high.[15] For many South American peoples, different spatial worlds now exist above and below the earth and are peopled with various sorts of beings. The first spatial worlds of mythic beings, univalent and unreplicable, contrast with the presently known universe of human residence, which consists of many different cosmic regions, each with its own quality of space and conditions of being.

This level of the universe may itself consist of a variety of ontological econiches (places where diverse kinds of beings thrive in surroundings that are in keeping with their character of being): the forest, the world of water creatures, the garden, mountains, the world inside plants, the worlds at the four cardinal points. These spaces are fragments from failed creations. The body itself is an arrangement of spatial entities, such as hair, bone, orifices, fluids, and shadows—the residue of dramatic episodes in long-gone spatial worlds.

The success of the present cosmos and of human physiology is due to their coordinated arrangement. In spatial terms, well-being is driven by an aesthetic principle demanding that everything create a place proper to its mode of being. The human occupies a privileged place in this spatially complicated scheme. Through myth cultures learn the meaning of all modes of being because myth reveals the significance of spatial symbolism. That is, myth illustrates how the myriad spaces of this world form part of a history of sacred realities.

Because human knowledge is rooted in the meaning of symbols, and because symbolic existence is the profoundly human mode of experience, humans are in the central position to practice medicine; that is, they create the *beauty* that displays the dynamic arrangement of forces in the cosmic process. In fact, healers are often at home in the plastic and performing arts. In the course of their general practice they must often be craftspeople, potters, weavers, set designers, songsters, and pictorial or instrumental artists. Their healing performances embody local canons of style and grace. What we might call objects of art, especially ritual artifacts, play a large role in maintaining health and preventing or dispelling sickness. Above all, beauty appears in the rites that maintain the community's contact with sources of well-being in good times and that restore the sick to health in times of crisis. In fact, the healing rites that humans perform reconstitute the wholeness of the universe in which spirits, heroes, colors, directions, and bodies achieve a regenerative arrangement. The cadenza at the closing of many healing songs and prayers is a petition that beauty—an effective arrangement of what is powerful and real—surround the patient.[16] Well-being is that state where the universe takes its proper order around and within the human being. Since that proper order is a religious perception, sickness and cure are deeply religious affairs. The proper arrangement of the cosmos, itself a symbolic construction dependent on the appearance of sacred beings apparent in the human imagination, affects the well-being of the patient. The social universe of the patient is likewise depicted in spatial terms. Relatives and ritual friends take specified places during healing seances.[17]

In the view of South American medicine, pathogens may exist prior to the creation of the state of wellness brought about by cultural heroes. Some pathogens may be fragments of ancient epochs destroyed by fire, flood, or petrification. According to Baniwa accounts, for example, a cosmic fire destroyed a previous world. The fire was set beneath a tree on which hung the body of Kuai, a great mythic hero. As he burned, fluids streamed from his body orifices. Those liquids are now the poisons of the world. His singed body-hair became disease-bearing splinters. To this day, the ashes found at the center of the world, where he burned, have a deadly power.[18] When bone-splinters, spirit-darts, thorns, spiders, hairs, or ancient stones from previous epochs lodge in the sufferer, they disrupt healthy relations within the space of the body and within the space of the community. Knowledge of the past events related in myth helps one to recognize displacements of this kind for what they are and empowers the healer to place the pathogenic fragments of past worlds once again in their proper perspective.[19]

Medicine is, in spatial terms, restorative. However, it does not restore the cosmogonic orders of the first ages of the world. Instead, its restoration is actually a re-creation, as is all aesthetic order. Medical practice produces new forms of beauty by extending into new circumstances the aesthetic principles sketched out roughly by the transforming heroes of the culture whose exploits are recounted in myth. In particular, the actions of the divine twins found throughout South America provide a stimulating example for medical practitioners. They revived one another after near fatal exploits and, in some cases, avenged their mother's murder or even raised her from the dead before ascending into heaven. They also wrought havoc on the primordial world, especially by slaying the mythic jaguar who presided over it.[20] As medical models, the twins and other mythic healers bequeath to contemporary practitioners the power over life and death, but they do not prescribe detailed treatments for every case. Those remain the province of the physician.

The portrayal of wellness in images of time and space points out how diagnosis and cure are "historical" endeavors. When healers retrieve lost souls or expel possessing spirits, they resituate elements that have strayed from their proper temporal mode or spatial locus. They thereby reintegrate the patient in his or her proper set of spatiotemporal relations. In this respect, cure overlaps the fundamental religious act of orientation—assuming one's proper posture toward sacred powers by discerning them in the symbolic structures of the world.

Since the focus of diagnosis and cure falls on discovering the *meaning* of temporal and spatial dislocations, we may say that curing is a careful exercise in historical interpretation. The Canelos Quichua healer, for example, seeks out not only the patient's immediate case history but also the spiritual history of elements comprising the patient's personality—elements acquired at conception, at birth, at naming-ceremonies, at first-food rites, and at initiation.[21] In order to uncover this spiritual history a healer induces vision, hallucination, trance, stupor, or the delirium of exhaustion in order to visit other spatial realms and primordial times.[22] The examination may reach back through generations of the dead, movements of villages, mythical epochs. It recollects the qualities of lineages in the patient's descent (or in that of his associates and enemies), the moral actions of neighbors and relatives, and whatever is known of ancient pathogenic elements and powers.[23]

This historical vision of wellness and illness views degenerative processes as coextensive with the cosmos. Degeneration and consumption are conditions that human beings share with other beings including spirits (such as the Yanoami *hekula*) who consume offerings of food, tobacco, or fermented liquids and monsters (such as the Andean Pishtaco or Naqaq and the Cubeo Abahuwa) who devour fat or flesh.[24] However, medicine appears to be a human possibility not available to all other modes of being. Humans remain practitioners of medicine even if all other modes of being benefit from it. Medicine begins with the heroes who established the conditions of human culture. Wellness, as it is known in the present epoch, is not usually the work of the Supreme Being but of a culture hero who brings to society both medicine (an empowering relationship to sacred power) and an order more dynamic than the one established by the creator.

The human body is a space with a history. Corporeality, a condition that embodies transformative powers, is a state that humans share with animals. For that reason, the meaning and origin of the body-space and its temporal functions (eating, menstruating, defecating, vomiting, urinating, passing gas, emitting semen, expressing milk) are often revealed in myths that tell of the division between animal species and humans. The distinction between animal and human bodies often originated during the first drinking festival or at the time of the flood or fire, the great divide between epochs. The various species and races scampered into different habitats, shouting different sounds of panic. This accounts for the different geographic locations and languages of birds, animals, and humans. In many cases, the water monster who caused the flood was slain and the mythic beings bathed in its blood or feces. The streaks of blood, stains from excrement, or scars from the cosmic fire explain the distinctive body marks of animals and the ceremonial decorations of humans.[25]

The multiplicity of body forms is often associated with the universal destruction by flood or fire that fractured the first uniprincipled creations. In the case of the Incas of the Andes and the Toba peoples of the Gran Chaco area of Argentina, distinct species emerged from separate holes in the ground after the cosmic fire. That is, the multiplicity of body-space arrangements accompanied the multiplicity of "universes" and epochs generated in the processes of disintegration, fragmentation, and regeneration.

In terms of the wholeness of space, wellness consists in discovering one's proper place in the universe and in taking up this place in such a way as to effect and extend meaningful order in the cosmos. Knowledge of myth is essential to the process. For this reason myth is also essential to those who wish to understand how South American medicine works and what it tries to achieve. For South American healers the knowledge of myth is experiential. Medical specialists not only hear about the first times and places, but they often have intimate acquaintance with these symbolic realities. They journey to mythical realms or traffic with beings and spirit helpers who come from there.

THE SOUNDNESS OF TONE

One can hardly overstate the power of song, especially rhythmic ceremonial chant, in South American medicine. Sound is one of the great manifestations of being; it reveals the significance of each entity, for each species possesses sounds unique to it. The entire creation, to its farthest reaches, forms a symphony of sounds, ritually empowered and orchestrated by a fathomable movement of sacred forces. South American mythic traditions explain the reason for sound's effectiveness.

Creation itself may result from sound. The supreme being of the Avá-Chiripá of Paraguay, for instance, called beings and worlds into existence with his creative word. Today every human being possesses a soul element consisting of an eternal divine word. The Wakuenai of the northwest Amazon describe a different use of creative sound. The Wakuenai world was created from a small lump, such as a pebble or the excrement of a hero. Mythic figures of the day, probably a female band led by Amaru, the formless spirit of water, played sacred flutes over the tiny mass until it opened and grew to the size of the earth. During boys' initiation, the Wakuenai now reproduce the same sounds with those flutes in order to "open" the boys and make them grow into young men.[26] For the Kari'ña of Venezuela, every sound creates a species. This is why each species of animals makes its own sound or possesses its own language. Furthermore, every species of sound creates a *tamu*, a bodily form in which the sound appears on occasion. The state of the body and the structure of the sound are bound together. Some cultures report that Earth once spoke to humans and animals at the beginning of creation. According to the Campa of eastern Peru, Earth spoke infrequently and slowly, using a limited scale of tones. She ceased speaking after she became fed up with the rotting flesh of cadavers buried in her.

The tones and melodies of medical incantations are often human imitations or rearrangements of sounds that originally belonged to other species of being. During rituals, performers compose the sounds into a whole just as healing practitioners recompose the sick person with ritual sound. The Ayoreo of the northern Chaco Boreal sing medical myth-chants called *kucáde kíke uháidie*, the "cyclical vestiges of things." The incantations have healing properties. Each myth-song consists of two parts: a narrative *(eró)* and a sacred song that is called *saúde* if used to cure illness, *paragapidí* if used to prevent illness. The "cyclical vestiges of things" are acoustic fragments of sacred beings who have withdrawn from this world. When mythic beings disintegrated at the time of creation, their spirits departed on high, their forms changed into the creatures and shapes of the earth, and whatever was left became healing songs. The myth-chants make present once again the full manifestation of powers that were active during the primordium. Performing them allows the physician to transform the patient's soul and body just as transformation of sacred beings occasioned the first performance of the sounds.[27]

According to some Guaraní-speaking people, it is tiny fruits and seeds inside the medicine rattle that utter the sharp sounds it makes. These fruits have power to speak healing sounds because they come from a tree located in the Land Without Evil, a place where no disease exists. Ecstatic dancers may be transported there in their living bodies while they sing and shake rattles. The Land Without Evil is not a postmortem world. The power of sounds, when coupled with the light body-weight of the dancers, who have fasted and observed a vegetarian diet as well as weight-dissolving moral commands, sweeps the dancers across the primeval sea without necessitating their dying.

The sounds of the Guaraní rattle proved effective in the beginning of time. Kuarahy, the sun and the first medicine man, was a divine twin. His father was the creator Nanderú Guazú. When the creator withdrew from the earth after the creative episode, Kuarahy chanted to the accompaniment of his rattle until his father transported him into the celestial realm. The powerful apparel and rattles of contemporary healers are modeled on those of Kuarahy.[28] Among the Warao the songs of medical practitioners were originally sung by flowers in another time and place. These flowers had special colors coordinated with their sex and song. They adorned the houses of deities dwelling at the cardinal points of heaven. The divine residences were constructed of tobacco smoke, which is the living-space or embodiment of supernatural beings. Humans learned the healing songs when they overheard mythical birds (of the same color and sex as the primordial flowers) singing the songs at dawn and at sunset during the seasons of the year that threaten the health of children. The female bird sings her song to protect young male children. The male bird, as he rises into the sky, sings a chant that protects the growth of girls. The birds are, in fact, starry constellations of the night sky of certain seasons. Medical songs possess power because they manifest the same movement of forces that orders the universe: colors, flowers, supernatural spaces and beings, birds, seasons, stars, male and female children. The healer's ritual performance of songs orchestrates all of these realities into a powerful harmony of life forces, which compose their well-being.[29]

In some South American societies, song composes one element of the mature human soul. Sought during initiation, it becomes part of one's mature spirit when provided during an adolescent's initiatory vision. Well-being is impossible without a song of one's own. In the Gran Chaco area, for example, youths quest for songs during dreams.[30] The song is unique to the individual. A person runs the risk of death if he or she should sing the song-element of another's personality. Equipped with this power, the growing person uses the song for protection, cure, and acquisition of greater knowledge—in the form of song as well. Among the Shipibo of eastern Peru, the soul (*kayá*) makes the sound of a flute when it enters or leaves the body at night. All during the soul's nocturnal journey, the flute sounds to prevent the sickness that would occur if the soul became lost in an eternal dream.[31]

As in the case of the well-being manifest in the images of time and space, wellness expressed as sound cannot be a homeostatic condition. Sound is dynamic and requires constant transition from one state of being to another.[32] Myths underline the fact that sound always accompanies change. This is true of the great number of sounds that we have no chance to examine here but that have medical value: names used to order the individual and society in healthy ways or to expel evil beings from the living-space of the body or communal residence; ritual weeping that plays a prominent role in many South American societies as they cope with the changes wrought by sickness, initiation, or death; or stylized racket needed to make the transition into a healthy new year.[33] The incessant transitions between states of wellness and illness fill the world with the sounds of preventive and critical care.

THE INDIVISIBILITY OF UNCONSCIOUS CONDITIONS AND FORMLESS STATES

Some elemental conditions of wellness are indivisible: darkness, invisibility, air, emotional plenitude. These modes of being manifest a power that is irreducible to conscious states of articulation; that is, they are internally indivisible. They comprise part of a larger world of significance that cannot be factored into historical (in this case, individual) and nonhistorical components. For example, the dynamics of wellness embed themselves in the forces of sleep that blur the distinctions between life and death; they embed themselves in the forces of darkness and invisibility that erase the visual distinctions between separable forms. The Waiwai perform important healing ceremonies at night because snakes make the transition from water to earth under cover of darkness. Moving from one medium to another, the snakes (emblems of physical rejuvenation) assume the forms of supernatural animals and mythic beings who attended the first feast, when beings took on their specific incarnate form with all its capacities and vulnerabilities.[34] Many South American peoples hold that darkness, as a form of supernatural seclusion, allows beings to shed their skin like crabs or snakes; or darkness helps one to dissolve like a larva in a cocoon. In the undifferentiated darkness, the larval chaos of the cocoon or of the earth-buried seed, one transcends the distinctions between forms. In ritual seclusion and hidden from the ordinary gaze, one passes from child to mature woman; or from sick patient to healthy person. One emerges reconstituted from the chrysalis of darkness.[35] Since unconscious conditions are revealed as meaningful, they become strong images of the indivisibility of meaning itself, which underlies all movement of forces. Among the Guayakí, for example, pregnant women have special healing power that comes from their fetal children. In the darkness of the womb, the unborn child lives the undifferentiated experience of the divine twins before the end of the mythic age. The baby dwells in primal darkness, experiences the meaning of all things, recognizes the significance of symptoms, divines the disease, and prescribes a therapy that the mother communicates to the patient.[36]

Sleep is another instance in which indivisible conditions affect wellness. A medical practitioner must often "conquer" sleep. He or she not only masters the physical demand for sleep through extended nocturnal vigil, but also overcomes the apparent meaninglessness of sleep. Ultimately, some practitioners penetrate the meaning of sleep to such an extent that it becomes the foundation of their therapeutic training and practice.

Among the Chiripá, for instance, the period of apprenticeship takes place mainly while the trainee sleeps. A medicine man who, before dying, chose the candidate as heir to his knowledge appears to the novice in his dreams and instructs him in the medical arts. Throughout the medical career, sleep continues to be the cornerstone of continuing education, diagnosis, and cure. After many years, sleep gradually offers access to the knowledge of other dead shamans dwelling in the Land of the Dead. In turn, they introduce the sleeping physician to their helper-spirits. Finally, one of these spirits may conduct the sleeper to the very realm of the Sun, the model medicine man.[37]

To become powerful and effective, Chiripá healers must learn to integrate the experience of sleep into everyday existence. Wellness consists in respecting the indivisibility of the sleep state by allowing it to carry through into the waking state. The Chiripá distinguish four grades of healers, based on the degree to which they can dramatically represent the powers of their sleep while awake. The most powerful medical practitioners most effectively reactualize the life encountered in their dreams by singing the songs revealed by the dead during their sleep. Only the healer who can reactualize in the day and for the public what his own solitary soul encounters during sleep at night has the power to heal. He has penetrated the mystery of consciousness and its forces; he transmutes sleep and inertness into control of the powers of reality.[38] In fact, public and collective life are "real" and "powerful" only to the extent to which a medical practitioner can make them like his dream.

Night, the period when most humans and animals sleep, is frequently the "daylight" of awakened supernatural beings. Consequently, for the sake of general well-being, it becomes imperative to draw the actions and intentions of more powerful supernatural beings into the relatively pallid "daylight" of less powerful human consciousness. In short, night and sleep for some South American cultures are more "real" than day and wakefulness. For the sake of wellness the former must be seen as the pillars of the latter. For the Goajiro, for example, humans see in the light and with their eyes only approximations of the true realities created by the supreme being in his dream. The extraordinary power of night chants

and cures, and the popularity of sleep therapies that practitioners undertake on behalf of their clients take root in this vision of the movement of
forces manifest in formless states.

Passages

Many South American societies divide up the human life cycle by celebrating key moments of transition, such as conception, birth, puberty,
marriage, parenthood, ritual sponsorship (or "godparenthood"), and
death. The rites of passage *create* the states of being into which one
passes; they are not superfluous celebrations of changes that would happen without them. One could say that rituals of transition force the
changes they signify. A discussion of several of these passages follows:
conception, birth, initiation, and death—and the end of the world, which
is a transition of cosmic proportions.

CONCEPTION

Human conception usually requires intercourse. Many South American languages assign a dynamic role to women in sexual relations leading
to conception. The womb sucks the seed out of the penis and transforms
it, just as the medicine man's mouth sucks pathogens out of the body and
changes them. Conversely, the penis blows semen into the womb in the
same way that ancestors or the creator himself blew breath through
ancestral flutes to inseminate the first fruits with sound.

Conception results not only from the sexual performance of parents
(for not every act of sex results in conception) but from other conscious
acts as well. The symbolic causes of successful conception include acts of
dancing, singing, decoration, fasting, hunting, gardening, and eating in a
proper manner. The health and destiny of the new child depend on the
significant acts of others, especially the prospective parents. An individual
does not fashion his or her own signifiers. Conception among the Baniwa,
for example, requires the deposit of male blood (*lirana* or *likai*, "sperm")
from the father into the mother's womb. However, this is not sufficient in
itself. Yaperikuli, "Our Father" the creator and supreme being, produces
the child's soul, bones, and organs. He inserts them into the uterus. Conception reenacts the mythic event when Yaperikuli's "knowledge"
impregnated Amaru, the primordial water serpent, to provoke the first act
of conception. In the same way, human knowledge, a spiritual awakening
through intimate contact with the sacred, is a prerequisite of proper conception. That is why fathers must be properly initiated. Baniwa initiation
opens the male sexual orifice when the young man comes to "know"
Kuai, the culture hero/ancestor/flute (he is all three at once). Kuai is the

fruit of the union between Yaperikuli's thought and Amaru's form. Contact with Kuai at male initiation (when the sound of Kuai's flutes enters the cuts in the boy's skin) causes the boy to become open (*kewiken*, to menstruate) and makes him capable of conceiving an authentically human child.[39]

Most South American peoples recognize that conception is more than a physical process. It is the outcome of powerful spiritual processes. According to the Tapirapé of Brazil, conception occurs when the soul of a child enters the woman's womb and decides to stay. But the spirit child has a choice; it is the offspring of primordial and supernatural animals, fish, or thunder. A healer (*panché*) transports the child-soul to the desirous womb. If it decides to stay, the father should ejaculate more semen into the woman's womb to build up the flesh of the child. For that reason, the Tapirapé say that a child can have several fathers.[40]

BIRTH

Birth rituals are usually very simple. This fact is ironic, since the process of conception, gestation, and birth becomes a model for elaborate cultural metaphors of initiatory rebirth at other points in the life cycle. Birth becomes an exemplary moment, no matter how plain, because something is appearing for the first time.[41]

The midwife is often more than a physical nurse. She is a spiritual functionary.[42] Among the Apinayé, for example, grandmothers act as midwives. They maintain ritual ties throughout life with the grandchildren they deliver. They rearrange the body-space of the newborn by painting it with rubber pigment and decorating it with ornamental bones, seeds, and wood-bits. These dressings ward off harm and instigate growth. The Apinayé give birth to children in a conical hut of palm leaves. Ritual seclusion is a common feature of rites of transition throughout South America. Also typical are restrictions on eating and behavior. In the case of the Apinayé, parents refrain from cutting their hair or painting their bodies. They also watch their diets in prescribed ways. The father goes out on a ritual hunt, first for an ostrich, and then for a deer. Sound is a key factor in the hunt. (In other societies, such as the Kari'ña, the father actually hunts down a sound, which he captures (imitates) ventriloquially and places in the child's voice.) In the Apinayé instance, attendants smear red *urucu* (*Bixaorellana*, a shrub whose seeds yield a dye used as body paint) on the baby to keep it from crying while the father kills the game.[43]

The child's posture at birth can be important. In the Afro-Brazilian religious traditions practiced in the city of Bahia, the moment of birth affects the individual's destiny. The details of birth shape one's *ase*, a mystical force that fills the cosmos. Girls born in a particular posture, for example, come under the patronage of the deity named Ìyá Mapo to whom offerings are made to prevent the girl from becoming a lesbian.[44]

Rituals of birth frequently prescribe the first acts of a new child. The newborn is made to act just as did the first human beings at the time of their appearance on earth. The Aché of Paraguay, for example, make the child repeat the first act of standing upright. The Aché rite of birth includes two moments, *waa*, "a falling" from the womb to the earth; and *upi*, "a lifting up" by the *upiaregi*, "she who lifts up" (a ritual parent). This is what the first humans did when they emerged from the earth, and these acts distinguish humans from animals.[45]

In other cultures, the child is massaged, washed, wrapped in special clothes, and placed in contact with the sacred earth, or it has its head molded to conform to sacred models. Disposal of the placenta often requires special care. The Kaingáng place it in a basket and affix it to the bed of a stream. Some Quechua-speakers burn it in a bundle of clean white woolen cloth. Manipulation of the placenta can sometimes cause infertility and is used as a means of birth control.[46] The precarious state of the neonatal soul often leads to infant mortality. Through their actions, parents, relatives, and neighbors help protect and stabilize the constitution of the newborn so that its soul does not become lost. Foods, heat, and liquids are presented in controlled ways. Chanting and lullabyes help the newborn negotiate the transitions from waking to sleep and from day to night.

INITIATION

Initiation is often the most significant event of an individual's life and the most dramatic spectacle in cultural life. For this reason, South American initiatory scenarios are well reported and known. Initiation awakens one to symbolic realities; it places sacred realities at the disposal of human understanding for the first time. Learning the meaning of the sacred through a mature encounter with its symbolic expressions lies at the heart of human culture. Novices learn that humans are the beings who apprehend their world in symbolic terms.

Women's initiation in South America highlights the ways in which the female body serves as an instrument for transforming not only individuals but humanity itself. The aim is to construct a perfect container, often on the model of the goddess or supernatural heroine who sealed herself in a container or a gourd during the Deluge. Perhaps this is why women's initiation is so frequently performed in association with a large drinking bout. By controlling the opening of her eyes, mouth, ears, and vagina the candidate becomes the embodied container of culture and the locus of regenerative life. Many South American myths recount that it was in this way that a heroine saved the very possibilities of culture from destruction and allowed the cosmos to pass through a period of chaos into a state of fertile life. On their bodies, especially their skin, initiated girls bear the cuts of that cosmic battle in the shape of tattoos, bite marks, stamped designs, or ornaments. These signify the punctures cut by body parts (teeth, nails, stingers, or penises) of the monsters that the primordial female subdued. For example, cutting an Akawaio girl's face around the mouth at puberty marks her with the scars of a scorpion's bite, a snake-bite, or the sting of an ant or bee. This readies her for marriage. The scarring occurs at the girl's first menses and is done by an older female relative. The wounds are filled with sweet honey. Even the tongue is scraped and tattooed. From now on the young woman can perform the ceremonial tasks of a mature woman, especially preparing cassava and sweet fermented beverage. She holds the mash in her mouth and her being transforms the beverage into a sweet and powerful drink.[47]

Women's initiations make use of the symbolic strategies of seclusion, hygienic and moral propriety, invisibility, and display. For the Yawalapíti, for example, seclusion is needed to "make" (*um*, "to make" in the sense of "to make a child or a person") a girl. The womb and tomb are similar places where people in transition are symbolically sequestered. During confinement the candidates eat special foods and exaggerate their manners when eating, speaking, bathing, or even touching themselves to scratch their own bodies. The Yawalapíti ritual seclusion is linked directly to death. The demiurge named Kwamuty used such an enclosure when he transformed large logs into the first beings by blowing tobacco smoke over them. However, midway through the process the ritual seclusion was broken and death entered existence. Now Yawalapíti girls, enclosed for initiation, relive that precarious experience on the border of life and death. In their straw enclosure they are covered with tobacco smoke, which symbolizes semen. The act transforms them into full human beings. The girls who come forth from confinement are debutantes in the fullest sense: "these young girls . . . are seen as the first human being: the mother of men."[48]

Male initiation employs many of the strategies found in women's initiation, especially seclusion and physical ordeals such as fasting, vigilance, marathon dancing, or cutting the skin. The origin myths associated with men's initiation frequently describe how male initiatory procedures and paraphernalia (such as musical instruments, masks, or ceremonial clubs) were stolen or forcibly expropriated from women. In fact, men's more violent relationship to reproductive or regenerative processes—including the ceremonial process of reproducing a new generation of mature men—seems to characterize many initiatory ideologies. More than in the case of women, male initiation introduces candidates to participation in the ceremonial, rhetorical, and sociopolitical processes of the public arena, which is frequently a place defined by the official silence of women. Women are absent, for example, from the so-called men's club-houses of Ge societies in central Brazil and from the men's compartment near the front of the *maloca* in the "longhouse" societies of the northwest Amazon.

Men's initiations appear to highlight the violence of change that is a part of symbolic display. Women embody within themselves the powers that threaten them during initiation. Flood waters are consubstantial with the amniotic fluid in her womb; the sheddable skin of mythical snakes becomes the lining of her uterus, which she sloughs off in each menstrual cycle. And the ravaging power of the moon over regenerative life becomes the regular rhythm of her periods. Men, on the other hand, tend not to contain but rather to *instrumentalize* the powers that threaten them in their initiatory seclusion; they employ festival feathers, masks, hair-tubes, penis sheaths, and musical instruments, all of which regularly disappear in the off-season.

Initiation may accompany the assumption of special ritual roles in the public sphere, especially for men. Taught by a master, an educated class, or spirit helpers, the apprentice undergoes a time of training. He not only acquires a fund of information but suffers a change in his psychic and physical constitution. For example, a novice entered the Lóima-yékamuš, the school for apprentice Yamana shamans of Tierra del Fuego, only after showing signs of special sensitivity to the spirit world. He had heard supernatural voices or had seen spirits in his dreams. Under the guidance of an experienced *yékamuš*, a religious specialist, the novice entered seclusion in a special hut made of large logs, and there he suffered extraordinary physical ordeals including immobility, staring at a fixed point for long periods, little sleep, minimal nourishment, and absolute silence. Indeed, the aim of all initiatory trials is to cultivate the spiritual strength necessary to negotiate a constructive relationship with the supernatural powers, especially the spirits of the mythic Yékamuš, who appear in his dreams and deliria. The candidate should aspire to penetrate the supernatural realm of these images in the least amount of time possible. This will make him a powerful healer able to give clear form to the desires and fears that the souls of his future patients may experience. The adventures of the novice's soul have a direct relationship to the condition of his body (as they will to the physical state of his prospective clients). During the six months of confinement and training the novice rubs his cheeks with white clay and yellow wood shavings. The old skin of his face gradually disappears as he grows in wisdom. In its place is a new skin that is softer and shinier. Only experienced healers in states of hallucination can see this finer skin, which is the most beautiful and tender layer. Its appearance, brought on by mystical rubbing that no longer touches the cheeks, signals the end of initiatory confinement and the beginning of medical practice under the watchful eyes of an attending veteran.[49]

The length of initiatory schooling and apprenticeship varies widely.

Generally, training lasts from several months to a couple of years, but longer periods are not unknown. Among the Taulipáng and Arecuna, for example, apprenticeship lasted from ten to twenty years, and, among the Kogi, priests trained for eighteen years. Initiations into various grades of accomplishment and specialization often punctuate training periods that are extremely lengthy.[50]

The appointment of a ritual companion, sponsor, or ceremonial friend is an important feature of initiation. The relationship often remains important in the political and economic life as well as in establishing ritual and matrimonial alliances in the future of the community. Ritual friends may help decorate initiands by making parts of their costume, cutting their hair, or painting their body. In some cases the ritual friend may even undergo the same painful ordeals as the candidate.[51] Some scholars are beginning to view marriage in the context of this large variety of ritual partnerships that come to light during ritual transitions from one state to another.[52] Maturity, brought on at initiation, places adults into more intimate relationships. This occurs not only on the sexual level, to generate more offspring for the community, but also on the intellectual, political, and spiritual planes, in order to produce material abundance, social stability, and religious wisdom for the group. Considering the temporal, spatial, and sonic bases of well-being and illness, it is understandable that these social relations, orchestrated or even generated in ritual, affect individual and communal health.

DEATH

Death is the final transition for human beings because it is an irreversible state. Mythical beings who suffered momentary and reversible deaths may have risen to new life soon afterward. But that is not the case for human beings. Irreversible death defines the meaning of mortal life, human existence. And it marks the definitive limits of human possibilities because it is the ultimate transition. At death one comes up against not only the experience with which life ends *(terminus a quo)* but the condition toward which human life is directed *(terminus ad quem)*.

The signs of death are found in myths of death's origins, the bodily symptoms of death, the symbolic actions of funerals, and the conceptions of postmortem life. Origin myths frequently stress that death entered existence because of a failure to pass a test or undergo an ordeal. In particular, some being at the beginning of time failed to maintain ritual closure. This excessive openness resulted in death. Someone wept or spoke when told to keep silent, or opened a box that should have stayed closed, or peeked when instructed to keep the eyes closed, or had sex (the penetration of the sexual opening and the outpouring of semen) when this was forbidden.

Funeral rites model themselves on the myths of origins of the first death and funeral. Death can bring disease; the presence of the deceased spirit threatens illness or continued death. On the other hand, proper disposal of the dead helps the deceased achieve their postmortem destiny and conduces to communal well-being at every level. A chorus of relatives may imitate the original sound that caused death.[53] They may perform stylized lamentation, ritual weeping, shouting, or ceremonial fury. These imitations of the first death assure that the dying individual succeeds in making the same final transition. Keening can be difficult work but it is required in order to carry the dead through their passage.

Scrutinizing the bodily symptoms of death is an important moral exercise. If the causes of death are apparent, burial proceeds apace. If the reasons for death remain obscure, someone in the community may hold an inquest. The inquest amounts to a communal examination of conscience as well as a review of the individual's immediate and remote life history. Hidden faults should come to light. Illnesses of unknown origin, such as epidemic diseases brought by foreign invaders, prove especially difficult to reckon with. Their meaning cannot easily be appraised, since they bear no relationship to the sacred as it has revealed itself in the mythic history. Death is not generic. Each death manifests its peculiar meaning through its unique circumstances. This meaning affects the entire community and even the cosmos. Every effort is made to bring that significance to light.

Games, such as blindman's buff and games of chance, as well as competitive contests, such as log races, athletic matches, or musical competitions, are a common feature of funerals.[54] Perhaps the widespread Brazilian practice of relay races, in which runners carry heavy logs, was "a way of practicing bringing home the fallen warrior to his matrilineal family. The training has later become a pure ceremony, a sport."[55] We need not accept this historical explanation to connect competitive spectacles to death. Games contest the powers of death and highlight the way in which the ambiguity of death calls for a fitting symbolic response. By forming dance teams or competing antiphonal choirs, cultures recognize the ambivalence of sacred powers manifest in death and resolve that ambivalence in a responsible and creative way. Death is a struggle with forces that are obscure, opaque, and invisible. Contests bring the opposing powers in that struggle to light in a public arena and celebrate them as elements of regenerative life.

Because they take on a thoroughly spiritual existence the dead are treated with fearful respect, an ambivalence appropriate to sacred beings. After the death of a mate the Kaingáng spouse, for example, sleeps with his or her arms wrapped around the stems of a large fern, just as they clung to their spouse at night. This same plant enwreathes the cremated bones of the deceased, and is also used to ferment beer. The fern becomes an ambiguous marker of both death and the festive life that ferments after liquidation, for the plant is said to frighten away the soul of the deceased.[56]

Regarding the corpse, two sets of acts become especially important. The first is the bundling of the body in a grave, a shroud, mats, animal hide, ferns, or other material. This comprises the last significant ritual enclosure and helps effect the final transmutation of the person. Often the corpse is sealed in finery. Smothered in full ceremonial regalia, the cadaver is set into the ground, immersed in a river, hung in a bundle from a tree, or placed on a platform. Funeral rites multiply the images of enclosure. In the same funeral the body may be painted, wrapped in vines, put in an urn, and placed in a pit. The body openings of the cadaver are sealed shut; the eyes and mouth fixed shut, the ears and nostrils tapped up, the arms and hands wrapped around the torso or head to signal closure.[57]

A second set of funeral acts concerns the consumption of mortal remains. In many instances the earthen grave consumes the dead body or a cremation fire does. Often the corpse is consumed several times over. A primary burial allows the flesh to decompose in the earth or in a mortuary bundle. Then the grave is opened, the wraps undone, and the bones extracted. This secondary burial can also be ceremonious. Mourners scrape the bones free of any remaining flesh, bathe the bones, ornament them with feathers and paint, and replace them in a mortuary urn or install them in a new setting. In some cases the bones are redistributed during the secondary burial so that the integrity of the individual skeleton is no longer recognizable. The Goajiro, for instance, move the bones of the deceased from their individual grave into an enormous urn that contains the bones of the entire matriclan.[58] The deceased merge with the collectivity of the ancestors. Their name no longer bears mention and their individuality dissolves as their supernatural stature increases.

South Americans maintain a variety of ways to dispose of the dead. Important among a number of groups is the consumption of some relic of the dead body by survivors. A small number of peoples appear to have consumed a portion of the flesh of dead enemies as part of a solemn ritual meal. This communion was typically associated with the rites of war as practiced, for example, by the Tupinambá and Carib peoples, largely exterminated by western colonists.[59]

More widespread is the custom of consuming the ashes of deceased relatives in a fermented brew. If the corpse is cremated, some calcinated bones are saved, once the fire has consumed the flesh. If the body was buried, it is exhumed when the flesh has putrified and some bones, often the long bones, are ceremonially cleaned and painted. Then, perhaps after burning, the bones are pounded to a fine powder. Origin myths make clear that bones are the locus of the soul. At the proper time, usually a moment timed with the ripening of forest fruits, a feast is held and the bone powder is placed in a mildly fermenting fruit beverage. Participants commune with the dead by drinking the ashes.

The customs of consuming the flesh of enemies and of imbibing the ashes of relatives are, almost without exception, found quite separately from one another. Groups that practice the one do not usually celebrate the other.[60]

No matter how their remains decompose, the dead make their way to an afterlife. Death is never the end of existence. Irreversible death marks a final transformation to a new and everlasting state. In fact, the personality disintegrates so that various components of an individual take on separate cosmic existences. Sound (such as one's name) may fall absent for a time but then recycle and reappear in the new child of another generation. The power of speech may return to the supreme being whose divine word the speech-soul is (as among the Guaraní speakers), or else it may be kept in the obscurity of a mortuary gourd in the silent form of a darkened dream image, as among the Krahó. Some aspects of the person transmigrate through a series of forms beginning with large animals and finish up as tiny flowers or stones. The forces that account for one's appetite for vegetables may have a different destiny than the appetite for meat.

The road to the afterlife is arduous and marked by ordeals similar to the sort one finds at initiation. The soul undergoes interrogation, is subjected to fire, crosses treacherous passages, risks being devoured by monsters, battles with supernatural birds of prey or with thunder, and so on. The Kamayurá soul, for instance, is sent off with tobacco and song by a ritual specialist and journeys to the Milky Way, where it meets with the same terrible trials as those suffered by the mythical hero Kanaraté. It is slain several times in succession and squeezed through a tiny opening at the western end of the Milky Way, where two predatory birds guard the door to heaven.[61] To overcome such obstacles, the dead are often furnished a guide, a species of ritual companion, to usher them safely into the afterworld. This psychopomp may even be a living healer whose ecstatic experiences have familiarized him or her with the roads to other worlds. In the case of the Kalapalo, however, the guide is a deceased relative who aids the recently dead soul across the slippery, moss-covered log that spans a stream, the final obstacle to the heavenly world.[62]

The circumstances that await the souls of the dead when they finally arrive at their destinations are variable. Some afterlife scenarios are free from care and sickness; food abounds without work. The afterworlds frequently exclude outsiders to one's group, the in-laws or foreigners who bring strife and discord. In some cases, postmortem existence is a ceaseless festival of dancing, singing, and ritual games. The realm to which the dead go is not necessarily a cheery place, for other afterworlds are grim in the extreme. Such is the fate of most Warao, who end up in a smelly and dank underworld, rank with the stench of rotting blood and flesh. The supernatural being named Scarlet Macaw, smoking a cigar and playing a ghoulish bone clarinet, presides over this predatory realm. A nefarious medicine man transports the dead there by carrying them upside down on his back. On their arrival the supernatural bird breaks their necks with his beak and tears off their heads to begin their anti-existence.[63] Death always reduces one to a spiritual existence, and that reduction is evaluated as an ambiguous reward at best. The dead desire offerings, such as food and tobacco, to supplement their impoverishment. In return for these substantial fruits of the periodic world, they send to the living songs and dreams, which are the insubstantial but real tokens of their own, spiritual, sort of existence. These gifts of the dead hold special medicinal power, just as their wrath inflicts sickness, accident, and misfortune.

In general terms, the point to insist on is that death always represents a new beginning, no matter what quality of life ensues in the postmortem world.

THE END OF THE WORLD

One additional passage requires special mention. This is the transition that the entire world undergoes at the end of time. Visions of the end have motivated numerous South American communities, especially since the arrival of the colonists. In search of well-being, visions of the end arose to inspire migrations, pilgrimages, salvific transitions through dance and rite, and millennial revolts. Communities read the realities of their existence—political oppression, physical decimation, social dissolution—as sure signs of the end of the world. In fact, they desire to see that reality end. Led by medical men, or by the sick, they quested for a fuller existence, free of physical and political affliction.[64] Thus, for example, generations of Guaraní people followed healing messiahs who led them toward the Land Without Evil (Ywy Mará Ey), a country free of disease and suffering. There their mother, Nande Cy, has waited for them since the creation of the world.[65]

Fascinating and moving examples of this belief appear throughout the modern history of the continent. South American peoples have always had eschatological imagery. It is an integral part of their mythology; the end of time is set up from the beginning, especially in the myths about primordial destruction. That destruction will occur again to bring in still another age. Although they may seek the goods that modern society offers, millennial movements reject Western values and Christianity in particular. But they do so in subtle and complicated ways, for these movements also embrace Christian beliefs and recast them in their own image. Nevertheless, they refuse to believe that institutional Christianity, the ideological foundation of their oppressors, exhaustively embodies the eschatological realities that the Christian religion promises. Consequently, visions of the end are filled with paradoxes. For example, Wanadi, the supreme being of the Makiritare, is crucified by the Fañuru (Españoles, Spanish) who are led by the cruel Fadre (Padre, Christian priest). Wanadi only pretends to die on the cross but actually his soul dances to heaven, whence it will come again to destroy the world, condemn Christian oppressors, and create a new world for the righteous Makiritare. Wanadi told all this to his twelve disciples before he was captured by his enemies.[66]

The Baniwa messiahs of the 1850s gave evidence of the same complexity. In 1858 Venancio Christo named himself after the Christian messiah but promised that the end of the world could be brought on only by rejecting goods and ideas brought by whites. Venancio Christo made ecstatic journeys to the sky. Another savior, Alexandre Christo, promised that manioc would fall from heaven if only the Baniwa would reject Western ways. Both leaders encouraged the Baniwa to dance ceaselessly in circles so that a conflagration would destroy the world.[67] Everywhere the visionaries of the end encouraged their disciples to do away with the signs of corruption: foreign food, dress, behaviors, authorities, rights to land, and money. They called for a rejection of symbolic life as it stands and denounced the Western view of history in favor of a different evaluation of existence in time. They invoked the end of the world (not without anxiety) in order to prove "history" wrong by ringing in a renewed experience of time, a return to the golden age or paradisal state described in myth or a future utopia depicted in neotraditional imagery.

One of the most dramatic millennial scenarios was led by the sick themselves. This was the Taki Onqoy religious movement that swept through the Andes around 1564. Taki Onqoy means "dancing sickness" or "song-dance of the Pleiades." Taquiongos were messengers seized by the ancient Andean divinities. Celestial gods, associated with stars and Christian saints, swept down from on high and took possession of their victims, forcing them to dance and sing uncontrollably. The seizure spiritually purified the afflicted. The possessed delivered messages from the gods promising that the forces of creation would devastate the world with fever and annihilate the effects of colonial history. Then the ocean would deluge the earth and eliminate all traces of Spanish conquest. The receding tide would reveal a new paradise, free of illness and filled with a new people. The possessed included members of every class and social group of indigenous peoples and more than half their number were women. Expecting an immediate end, they offered their clothes, food, drink, and material items to the divine beings who possessed them. News of them spread like wildfire and their ranks swelled. Their vision helped them diagnose their historical experience, since the conquest could now be seen plainly as a disease whose symptoms had become apparent. The possessed themselves, infested with divine power, carried the possibility of cure—total destruction and creation of a new earth. The swift and punishing campaign led by the Spaniard Cristóbal de Albornoz condemned some 8,000 Indian leaders for their participation in this messianic revival.[68]

PASSAGE AS A MODE OF BEING

The division of the life cycle into a series of temporal units marked off by rites of passage is only a linear arrangement of the human constitution. From the point of view of the fullness of time, a state of well-being, the body and its orifices constitute effective passages for beings of many kinds. Furthermore, the human being is itself a body in passage. The body and its spiritual faculties is an ensemble of transient forces that are sexual, supernatural, nutritive, sonorous, atmospheric, and odoriferous in nature. The human constitution is a simultaneity of passages; cosmic forces course through the body at the same time as the human body passes through the cosmos. The reason for this is essentially religious: the human being and its meaning are understood symbolically. In such a light, the human is "a living cosmos open to all other living cosmoses by which he is surrounded."[69]

Corporeal disorders issue from the complexity of times and spaces of this world as they are embodied in the human being. Unlike the first kinds of beings of the first primordia, the human body experiences many periodicities that, together, comprise the fullness of time. Human nature possesses the capacity to transcend its own mode of being. This valuable talent available to and characteristic of the human spirit is medically dangerous.

Although "passage" is a constant condition of human life, certain key passages are acknowledged as especially important and dangerous. They are accompanied by communal rituals that help the individual effect successful transition from one state of being to another and that protect the health of the individual and collective body by carefully managing the contact achieved with other powers during these times. Under these circumstances, illness, or at least the risk of illness, becomes a sign of a dynamic and maturing human life.

Through the celebrations of an individual's life cycle, the individual's unique historical rhythms leave their stamp on the project of human culture, which orders the cosmos. The body is one of many containers of powers that transform the cosmos: medicine bundles, bark chests, gourds, prophylactic string enclosures, menstrual huts, ceremonial lodges, graves, ritual seclusion screens, and the periphery of the social and cosmic world. This is the best context to understand the body as the locus of processes and passages important to medical practice. For example, the mouth is the locus of transformations effected as speech, singing, eating/fasting, blowing, sucking, devouring, and controlled regurgitation. For the Barasana, for example, the mouth shares in the same powers as a number of other passageways into transformative enclosures: the vagina (for the womb); the men's door (for the communal house); the landing dock (for the village residence space); the Amazon River waters (for the larger Amazon-Vaupés-Pirá-Paraná River area). Ultimately, the mouth (like all its parallel passages) effects transformations from one state to another (e.g., illness to health) because it shares in the power of *the* passageway of all being into the world at the beginning of creation: the Water Door in the east through which passed the great Anaconda whose body was the prime matter of creation. For the Barasana, the human mouth is metonymically related to the passage from nonbeing to being. The penetration of the penis into the vagina is a reenactment of the penetration of the Anaconda into the world. The procession of men playing flutes during the He House (initiatory ceremonies held every few years) is seen in the same light. The file of marching men reactualizes the body of the ancient Anaconda. The pairs of men and flutes are like the paired long bones of the serpent. As they enter the communal house, the *maloca,* they enter the primal universe within which the transformations of human culture (rituals) are carried on. The passing of food, breath, vomit, song, and pathogens back and forth through the mouth of the curer finds its parallel in the gestures and emissions of coitus, as well as in the stylized comings and goings within the communal house. All of these passage events draw their meaning and power from the journey of the primordial Anaconda.[70]

Since wellness is not a static equilibrium but a constant and proper movement of forces, it is imperative that the human person constantly change. The body is a dynamic envelope of physical and spiritual elements or material realities with intrinsically spiritual values acquired through the accumulation of names, ritual privileges, ornaments, animal spirits taken in the hunt, vegetal powers, marriage, and craft specializations. All of these acquisitions signal changes in the body: symbolic wounds, scarifications, body paint designs, coiffure, clothing style, cremation, bone-painting, and consumption of remains.

Normal body growth through the life-cycle passages is the result of ritual processes and the cooperation between human and spiritual forces. In fact, life-passages may be seen as a series of interventions, on the same spectrum as medical-crisis interventions, which transform the human being. In reality, humans (and all creatures of this world) are constantly in a condition of passage. The celebrated rites of passage gather up manifestations of this condition for critical assessment and periodic reflection. Because the body, like the cosmos, is symbolic, it remains "open" and constantly passes from one condition to another and from one meaning to another.

Caring and Curing

Lévi-Strauss . . . suggests that chants are a form of psychological treatment, and refers to them as a "psychological manipulation" of the infected organ. Although this explanation can be sufficiently justified in terms of psychosomatic suggestion in the case of human beings, it is still difficult to explain the cases of cure by chant in the case of animals, where it is unlikely that "suggestion" could be a factor. On more than one occasion I saw a castrated pig, whose wound had become maggoty, cured by chant. As the shaman chanted, the maggots fell off without any sort of powder having been applied. I believe that these phenomena deserve more attention than is usually paid to them without resorting to parapsychological or esoteric explanations. This lack of attention is due to the fact that they cannot be explained by reference to our own system of logical and causal principles although they are part of observed reality.[71]

Care and cure exist on a continuum in South American medicine. The continuum moves from fulfillment of kin and community obligations, through care for members of the group, creatures of the world, and deities or ancestors, to the healing care delivered to the acutely ill by physicians who enjoy a rapport with powerful spirits.

Though less dramatic than the medical specialists, many figures other than the doctor are important in health care: singers, herbalists, informal therapy groups, and dancing or masked societies. Achievement of good community health devolves on parents, ritual friends, sponsors, residence mates, gardeners, artisans, designers of ritual costumes, potters, hunters, cooks, and initiands in periods of transition. Those in charge of the flow of fluids (blood, semen, tears, festival beverage) from or into the body, such as menstruating women, ejaculating men, hunters, potters, or ritual drinkers, must take care to protect the community from the harmful possibilities intrinsic to these periodic exchanges. These acts are ringed round with avoidances, restricted behavior, social constraints, and ritual patterns.

Special responsibilities for public health fall on community leaders and on the heads of households. Among the Canelos Quichua, for instance, a man cannot found a new residential group (*huasi*) until he proves himself capable of handling the spiritual realities encountered in such an endeavor. He enlists the aid of all the spirit helpers he has acquired and proves that their help is adequate to the task of building a new community. In a dramatic hallucinogenic session held in the company of witnesses, the prospective householder must demonstrate his capacity to negotiate with the powers of the spirit world. Only then can he assume the responsibility of leadership for a new social group, for he has proven himself able to overcome the powers of affliction and disorder.[72]

Most ailments are redressed instrumentally and in a quotidian way by herbalists, bone-setters, casual divinations, and neighborly advice. However, as a malady proves intractable, chronically resistant to normal care, life-threatening, or upsetting to optimal relations in the community, it is countered with increasingly more powerful forces. Assembling and arranging powers is the work of ritual; most medical combat is carried on in the ritual theater. The management of this escalation from ordinary care to critical cure falls upon an ad hoc assemblage of blood kin, in-laws, formal ritual friends, loosely affiliated but interested parties, diviners, and experts in diagnosis.

DIAGNOSIS

Illness is often a product of the moral dimension of space or time or sound. These and other signs are symbolic of the movement of cosmic realities that are sometimes personal, usually willful, and always power-ful. The tiniest details of patients' circumstances and of their symptoms are symbolic. They reveal how and why the afflicted have encountered the powers of affliction—whether through their own inadvertence or the malevolence of another. When and where did they fall ill? Where have they been in the past? When were they in that place? With whom? What have they dreamed? Where? When? Their entire network of relations—conscious and unconscious, historical and supernatural—is subjected to a kind of "differential diagnosis." Diagnosticians are often ethicists as well as diviners. They do not simply seek a solution to a problem. They discern how one should behave in the face of a mystery; how one should act toward the powers manifest in space, time, sound, smell, and the social world.[73]

TECHNICIANS OF CURE

In many communities, the diagnostician or diviner refers the patient to other medical specialists. There can be a considerable division of med-ical labor, based not so much on the divisions of the anatomical systems as on the categories of spiritual causes of sickness and kinds of cure. Tech-nicians of cure cover a range of therapies: bleeders, emeticists, washers with solutions of plants (such as the hallucinogenic vine *timbo* which makes a frothy foam), those who bathe patients in smoke or expose them to elements such as water, fire, moonlight, or starlight. Some physicians cover patients with mud; others prescribe travel to a shrine or isolated retreat at a holy place (a sacred mountain, river rapids, oceanside, lake-front, or forest).

SHAMAN AND EXORCIST

A most dramatic therapy is the return of lost souls fetched back from another realm of the universe (the heavens, the forest, the lair of the mas-ter of animals, the land of the dead). The healer himself or herself may retrieve the wayward human spirit that was captured by an enemy or strayed during a dream or during fits of coughing, sneezing, or fainting. In such circumstances the healer undertakes an ecstatic voyage and does battle with the adversary. In many cases, however, the healer enlists the aid of his spirit helpers who fetch the soul for him and deliver it to the operating theater. In any case, the process is a dangerous and life-threatening exercise for the medical practitioner. It requires a special vocation, apprenticeship, and training geared to develop keen knowledge of the spiritual world. The body of the healer is transformed as well. Throughout South America, shamans change their bodies into the forms of supernatural beings, especially primordial jaguars and predatory birds. They become arch-devourers, consumers of the forces of consumption, the powers of affliction.[74] In his function as the master of consumption, the shaman is a master of fire and his lighted cigar is the emblem signaling how fire and consumption link him to the spirit world and to the consumptive powers of disease.[75] The cigar-holder, a forked stick that holds a cigar that is sometimes three or more feet in length, becomes the scaled-down model of the universe and of the realms that the shaman or his spirits visit. In overtly sexual imagery, his cigar penetrates every unexplored plane of the universe, depicted on the crotch of the forked legs of the holder. The sharpened base is set in the middle of the healing arena and marks the center of the world. The shaman's decorative bench, carved in the image of his patron spirits, fulfills the same function (as does his rattle, already mentioned).[76] In service of their desired contact with powers at the outer reaches of the spiritual world and of their wish to heighten their vision of realities only obscurely manifest in the signs of everyday life (including disease symptoms), South American shamans use hallucinogenic plants. This has been true from the most ancient times, as evidenced in burial sites dating from about 650–850 CE. The artifacts surrounding the remains of the medicine man discovered in a Bolivian cave include an entire laboratory of implements used to collect and process hallucinogenic snuff.[77]

Equally dramatic is the opposite practice of the exorcist, who expels the evil spirits of affliction who have invaded the patient. (The two functions, shaman and exorcist, are not mutually exclusive offices.) Although the training of the exorcist may not be as rigorous or lengthy as that of the shaman, previous acquaintance with powers of affliction is required before one may become an accomplished healer. Exorcists may not have suffered the disease of their patients, but they usually have encountered the supernatural beings who possess their sick clients. In that initial confrontation, exorcists learned to recognize the voice (or some other signature) of the pathogenic spirit. That first meeting of the exorcist and spirit of affliction was tantamount to a trial in which the curer practiced the technique needed to expel the spirit. Generally, exorcists establish a dialogue with the sickening being. Through interrogation, it reveals its identity, especially through the sound of its voice or name. These are the sonic structures constitutive of the spirit who hovers formless in the darkness of the body cavity. The songs, names, and babel made by the spirit *are* the manifest expression of the invisible force, just as are the symptoms of disease. Clairvoyance or physical examination through massage helps the curer locate the hidden pathogen. Sounds, in the form of imperatives, curing songs, or curses, cast out the power of primal darkness into the light of day or into the body of another victim (such as an animal familiar, innocent bystander, or unwitting neighbor).[78]

BLOWING AND SUCKING

Blowing and sucking are two principal powers of the flesh. They parallel the acts of soul restoration (an inspirational act) and exorcism (an extractive protocol), respectively. Blowing and sucking appear prominently as transformative processes in myths of creation and in accounts of the first sickness, death, and cure. Fittingly enough, they are rudiments of health practice.

Blowing smoke over the patient is very common.[79] Blowing sound on the sick by whistling or playing a musical instrument over them also conduces to good health. In addition, healers reinstall lost souls by blowing into their patient's mouth, nostrils, or eyes or by whispering the proper sonic structure, especially a name (the phonetic "shape" of the sonic soul), into the sufferer's ear.

Curers who practice massage and suction of the sick body are found throughout South America. Sucking can be a stunning spectacle. Several investigators remark on the violent noise and the aggressive sucking that draws blood from the patient's body. The mouth, throat, and stomach of the sucking healer contain extraordinary powers capable of withstanding the heat and poison of pathogens and even of transforming them into beneficent medicines. The Tapirapé healer of Brazil, for instance, gulps tobacco smoke from his pipe until he is intoxicated. The smoke stimulates the flow of his saliva and makes him nauseous. He sucks back his own vomitus and accumulated spit into his mouth. From time to time during this noisy performance he sucks on the patient's body to extract toxins. Eventually he retches up the entire mess and searches for the intrusive spirit-dart or thorn that caused the sickness. It has been observed that Tapirapé healers gathered in groups to perform sucking cures. On these occasions "the noise of violent vomiting resounded throughout the village."[80]

Confession is a widespread therapy in South America. It also is an extractive or expulsive technique parallel to exorcism, but it employs the symbolism of blowing, because the afflicted themselves use the breath of their speech to cooperate in the expulsion. The Incas had several classes of confessor, including *ichuri* ("grass men"), who advised patients to whisper faults onto a tuft of special grass that the healer pitched into a river before immersing the patient in the water and covering him or her with fine white meal.

Healers offer controlled curative contact with primordial powers. These powers of the creative period offer the possibility of re-creating patients so that they return to the fresh and full state intended at creation. To this end, patients may be placed ceremonially on the soil and raised up again in order to relive the dissolute condition of a buried seed, which then sprouts to new life, or to imitate the emergence of the first people from the womb of the earth. They may be conducted back into their own maternal womb and reintroduced to the powers that fashioned them there. Essentially, this *regressus ad uterum* is an extraordinary exercise of memory, aided by the imagery of myth. Frequently it is the healer, with the help of dream or hallucinogenic plants, who undertakes the journey on behalf of the patient. In trance or deep sleep, the doctor travels back into the womb to encounter the creative forces who once shaped the physical body in primal darkness. Together, the healer and the creative powers remodel the afflicted person so as to overcome their present infirmity.[81]

South Americans knew and practiced abortion and infanticide, but there is little ethnography on the subject. The existing evidence indicates that these practices were deemed reprehensible, even where tolerated. Many reports chronicle the local medical efforts to recall souls of miscarried or stillborn children and, in general, of all the uninitiated who have died. Healers try to effect the reincarnation of spontaneously aborted souls in the forms of animals, plants, or fish. Among the Warao, Akwĕ-Shavante, and Apapocuvá, after miscarriage or still-birth, the medicine man even uses the soul's song and name to call it back into the womb of another woman who may be conceiving a child at that moment.

References to birth control mention imbibing or ingesting contraceptive substances, performing prophylactic acts (such as destroying figurines or jettisoning substances into rivers), bathing in water at inopportune times, or disposing of the placenta in an unprescribed way in order to thwart future fertility. However, "informants" in such cases often claim to be reporting the behaviors of people other than themselves and, consequently, the data take the form of hearsay or even accusations against neighbors. For many peoples, sexual intercourse has a ritual, religious, and magical meaning, and conception often entails divine action. Regulation of fertility was practiced by individuals in accordance with their knowledge of the reproductive processes and supernatural forces, but not as an explicit "social policy" for population control. For these reasons, scientific studies of Indian notions of conception and birth control, studies not grounded in a thorough understanding of religious views, remain incomplete or fail altogether to learn particulars of contraception.[82]

Although there exists a growing statistical literature of demographic studies of birth and fertility rates carried on by national and international agencies, the reports of the native view of these issues consist mainly of asides in narratives written for other purposes. Scattered studies point up ignorance of modern birth control methods and resistance to their introduction. One celebrated case was documented in the film *Blood of the Condor*, set in the Andes of Peru. The movie describes how people of a native community attributed the continued diminution of their numbers, the ruin of their land (through bad weather, infertility, and expropriation) and the infertility of their women to the presence of a family planning clinic in their midst. In fact, the film alleges, their suspicion was well grounded; clinicians were performing sterilizations without obtaining the fully informed consent of their patients. The incident provoked spiritual distress and social unrest in the community. Eventually the clinic was sacked and destroyed by fire.

Systematic efforts toward population control do not preoccupy South American peoples devastated by epidemic diseases, colonial warfare, national policies of dislocation, and extermination of cultural constructs underlying social and economic existence. Accounts of the last living members of evanescing cultures lie in the dusty archives of ethnographic libraries, where demise through sickness and violence is often dismissed as history's inevitable sloughing off of primitive folkways during its progressive march to modernity. Medicine and concepts of health lead the procession while the process of annihilation continues.[83]

STRANGE AILMENTS AND FOREIGN MEDICINE

Medicine is frequently a source of cross-cultural exchange, since the foreign doctor may be the best qualified to treat diseases of foreign origin (arising in the mythical history of a neighboring tribe, for instance). Indigenous peoples seek cure from both local healers and modern hospitals.[84] Each cultural matrix, hailing from different manifestations of primal sacrality, is better equipped to redress the diseases coinvolved with its own history and development. Healers play leading roles in contact with outsiders and in introducing change to their community.

HEALING THE COSMOS

Performances that cure the body often set out to heal the universe in degrees great or small. The sick human body becomes a sacrament for the world,[85] a symbolic complex whose processes effect what they signify: integrity, orientation, dynamism, soundness, relatedness, reflexivity, growth, and degeneration through change. Constituted of cosmic and supernatural elements, the living person is a microcosm. Change (evident in the lifelong wavering between illness and health) recombines these elements and reshuffles the microcosm into a new image of the world, a processual reality in which the patient participates as a reflective overseer.

All of these dynamic transformations are punctuated by intermittent episodes of symbolic death, renewal, and rebirth. The ubiquitous but periodic presence of death in medicine explains why curatives are deadly, why the flesh or bones of healers are often charged with fatal powers of lightning or of the mythic jaguar, and why their bodies often contain deadly poisons in their throats, chests, livers, fluids, or hidden channels of their arms and hands. The Warao healer *(wishiratu)*, for example, embodies in fleshly form the fire of the primordial world. It exists in the forms of deadly poison and sparking crystals of his rattle.[86] Through "death" of the reversible sort present in all aspects of the mortal condition, the healer regenerates life. Human life shares in the periodic nature of *this* world (for there have been other, less successful, worlds). The relationship between the processes of the human body and those of the world is not one of detached analogy. Human wellness and illness are not only metaphors that describe the state of the world. The human state of being partakes of the world's condition and is a metonymic extension or culmination of the cosmic condition. Cosmos and body share in the same movements of the same sustaining forces. They are part of one another's transitory existence.

Curative acts may be directed to beings located within the suffering person. The intentions of such homeotherapy may, for example, have the desperately ill patient dancing feverishly to quicken the recuperative powers within. This course is frequently taken when the therapeutic goal is to jog the patient's memory, so that sacred beings of the mythic period reappear there. Their epiphany, their very presence in the images of memory or delirium, is salutary. On the other hand, the patient may remain passive while forces are brought to bear upon him or her from without. In such allotherapeutic circumstances, it may be the medical practitioner who undergoes sleep therapy on behalf of the client or who ingests the powerful medicines (tobacco, hallucinogenic *banisteriopsis caapi*) needed to cure the patient. Either choice for the direction of therapy implies knowledge of the whole world of significant powers of order and disorder, cure and affliction, wellness and illness. In the first place, *realities* must *appear*—either in memory, vision, dream, or in the staged communal enactment of the sacred events in which powerful beings first appeared. In the second place, the practitioner must discern, in the patient's wider case history, patterns of symptoms that include misfortune: bad luck in hunting, broken tools, poor agricultural yield, disruptive personal relationships. Thirdly, the healer must possess a repertoire of appropriate curing techniques. Healing technology is only one more form of knowledge relating to the sacred and affecting health. This knowledge is essentially historical, in the wide sense. Knowledge of past events reveals to the medical practitioner the true meaning of illness, wellness, and the powers of cure. These past events are recounted in myths that describe the failed beginnings of the cosmos, the origin of pathogens, and the possibilities of therapeutic re-creation.

Although not every South American culture includes all medical options mentioned in the above discussion, each one provides the sick a range of possible therapies that equals the broad spectrum of sacred realities appearing in its religiously complex world.

Ethics and Justice

An examination of the processes of moral discernment in South American cultures underscores the degree to which concepts and definitions of ethics are wedded to Western intellectual history.[87] If we employ these terms in this study we need to know better what ethics and justice really mean as *cultural* realities in the West. How are *ethics practiced* in a clinical or social setting? Ethical conflicts, as they are adjudicated in the modern medical forum, often flow from ritualized or procedural performances, such as family councils (presided over by physicians or pastors), staff or floor meetings, so-called death-boards, organ-bank policy committees, particular service policy committees, the courts, and so on. Presided over by attending physicians or even the chief of staff, hospital policy and decisions on critical care may be hammered out in adversarial proceedings—a performative genre to which physicians are acculturated in medical school and in which nurses and other health care staff are only now gaining some voice. The performative nature of these contests needs to come more to the foreground of our attention lest we think of ethics as a coldly reasoned set of deductions from abstract premises and try to compare that notion with South American practices.

The concept and images of justice should likewise be better located in the cultural setting from which they arise. For example, the image of a lottery lies at the foundation of John Rawls's influential study *A Theory of Justice*. He uses the lottery as a metaphor. However, drawing lots is an ancient and widespread ritual practice used to divine the principles of distributive justice (as in the ancient Greek concept of *moira*, "a share," "one's lot"),[88] and casting lots (or votes) is a divinatory procedure whose process and outcome, as in the case of democratic elections, exercise the meaning, and determine the fate, of the community.

Theories of economic justice seldom seem to take account of the full range of symbolic values of money and the cultural significance of exchange.[89] The meaning of justice that we use to probe ideas from South American societies should not derive only from the solitary visions of professional ethicists, economists, political theorists, or scholars ritually secluded in the isolation of their studies (a valuable cultural exercise)[90] but should also reflect the meaning of justice embodied in general cultural praxis. More attention could be given the performed manifestations of justice and ethics in the ritual proceedings of courts, corporate board-rooms, and stockholders' policy meetings.[91] Otherwise, whenever talk of ethics or justice arises, we might continue to appeal to only one style of intellectual exercise, used to establish duties, principles, or rules for adjudicating conflict in ways that are "purely rational," in the narrowest sense of the term reason.[92] The moral life of South American peoples paled under the ethical beacon of the Enlightenment and appeared to be amoral, unaffected by ethical conflict, or thoughtlessly repetitious of mythic models. Or, using the theory of the Noble Savage as a lens, South American forms of rationality appeared distorted and romantically portrayed, as if they were latent neo-Kantian moralists hobbled only by poor, mythical (nonrational) axioms. In short, it is still said that native South Americans (and others called "primitive peoples") observe simple mores and customs but do not exercise moral judgments that resolve ethical conflicts. These assumptions are wide of the mark. The following paragraphs outline several bases for moral discernment in South America.

AUTHORITIES

Moral conflict often prompts an appeal to authority, in the person of an individual respected for wisdom and moral character. These individuals need not be persons with politically significant statuses and roles. However, insoluble conflict is frequently brought to legitimate authorities, such as a village headman, a council of elders, assembly of blood kin forming the core of a residence group or phratry, and so on. This is what the native chronicler Philipe Guaman Poma de Ayala did between 1584 and 1614. His book, *El primer nueva corónica y buen gobierno,* is less a narrative history than a letter of appeal to the sacred power of the imperial Inca, now embodied in the king of Spain. Guaman Poma makes clear that the very act of writing, the act of creating visible, legible signs of the abomination and injustice of the present age, should provoke the king to a messianic act of justice—the destruction of the current world order and the installation of a new age with equitable relations. The Inca (manifest after Atahuallpa's bloody death in the person of the king of Spain) was not just "an historical personality but a metaphysical principle capable of resolving order."[93] The Inca was the linchpin in the dynamic structures composing the just order (the dynamic movement of spatial and temporal forces, as described in myth). The distribution of legitimate authorities on every social plane stood for the coordinated jurisdictions of space in the impeccable order of the cosmos. Moral order was one with cosmic geography and with the social network of relations linked to it in the four

quarters and in the moieties (the division of the Inca empire into two ritual halves). Propriety in land, hygiene, manners, ritual acts, marriage, and
social hierarchies reflected the order of the stars, the altitude of residence
space, and the individual's distance from the capital.

Inca authority exercised moral judgment by virtue of its proximity to
sacred being and its embodiment of spatial and temporal principles (lineage, age, moment in a temporal cycle, relation to social space). For
instance, the Incas maintained a complex calendar with four seasons of
three months' duration. The seasons were ranked hierarchically. The
king's feast followed the March equinox, the queen's preceded the September equinox; the solstice ceremonies honored the sun, a male emblem;
the equinoctial rites revered waters associated with female entities. During these ceremonies that punctuated the seasons, the rank order of
sacred sites (corresponding to the temporal cycles of stars and planets)
was adjusted. These adjustments were also moral adjudications that
affected the right relations among individuals and between peoples and
the cosmos. At the time, new alignments shifted the assignments of property, tribute, labor, leadership, and guilt for every community in the
empire and for Cuzco in particular. Relations had to change over time
because the spaces and times of this world are constantly in flux. Viracocha created the world in its spatial and temporal complexity and he-she
is manifest in its signs:

> O Virachoca, Lord of the world,
> Whether you are male or female,
> you are for certain the one
> who reigns over heat and creation,
> the one who can work charms with his saliva.
> Where are you?
> I wish you were not concealed from these your sons!
> . . . .
> Where is your mighty tribunal?
> . . . .
> You created us and gave us a soul.
> Watch over us that we may live in health and peace.
> . . . .
> [G]ive us long-lasting life,
> and accept our offering,
> O Creator.[94]

The creator Viracocha had a temporal constitution linked to his-her
creation: the body of Earth (Pachamama, World Mother) opened periodically, in accordance with agricultural rhythms and ritual schedules. The
capital and its sanctuaries formed a microcosm of cosmic reality. Its order
reflected that of the starry heavens and was made evident on a human

scale in architecture, woven textiles, and social order. The landscape of Cuzco changed like a kaleidoscope over the course of solar, lunar, and sidereal years. This desired dynamism created moral uncertainty. Nevertheless, myth provided principles to discern, in symbolic structures of the land, one's moral obligations to neighbors and gods, ancestors and progeny. The Incas seasonally adjusted their alignment to the shifting realities of the cosmos by reassessing the spatial locations of their shrines and by rotating the responsibilities and locations of representatives from local groups. These realignments were essential to dispelling disease from humans, animals, and crops.[95]

DIVINATION

In the face of moral uncertainty or conflicting moral demands, people may turn to a diviner. On the level of day-to-day action, divination clarifies that which is morally binding and uncovers those persons or realities that furtively, or even unintentionally, disrupt the moral order. Since moral breach creates medical and cosmic consequences, misfortune often stirs one to ask advice of a diviner who can disclose the "causes" of disorder. The diviner seeks these "causes" not in the competing premises and deductions of the epistemological realm but in the relations that appear disordered, when compared to those that "ought" to obtain, as revealed in myth and precedent history. South American diviners practice a variety of techniques, including the reading of the innards of animal parts, the movements of flames, casts of leaves, kernels of maize, colored objects, the twinklings of stars, movements of constellations, and so on. Second opinions are commonly sought, especially when misfortune continues. Many forms of divination, such as coca-leaf divination in the Andes or the reading of the movements of lice near a fire among the Kaingáng, are simple and inexpensive. They are consulted frequently and casually. Others can be more expensive and complicated.[96]

Divination guides moral action, an advisory power that depends on the ability to clarify the links between client, community, and cosmic powers. Divination is itself a ritual, even if, at times, the performance is highly informal. Further remedial rites are often prescribed by the diviner to reconstitute right relations symbolically and to redress moral breach. Emphasis falls on *how one experiences* the world (an effective mode of action), not on an examination of the processes of *how one knows* (i.e., on the mode of moral discourse that assures certainty).

Divination constructs an argument of images. The imaginal order of cosmology, which underlies the divinatory system, recontextualizes and clarifies uncertainties in the moral realm. This appears to be an example of what James W. Fernandez calls "edification by puzzlement": "a devaluation or a rejection of language-based thought and the discursive reason that lies in it and that has been the intellectual power tool of modern technical-rational man."[97] The diviner resituates the client's dilemma within the wholesome symbolic structures of moral language. The problem is not dismantled but set in increasingly more comprehensive perspectives until a higher principle is discovered that enlightens the conflict. The mesa, or divining board, of a healer from northern Peru, for example, incorporates all the significant structures of the universe. Its three fields correspond to the cosmic zones (Pachas) of space-time. Objects on it represent the forces at work in the world, and their arrangement embodies the powerful relations impinging on the patient. Intercardinal axes divide the board into the four quarters of the earth. A crucifix at the intersection marks the center of the world and the place where one can pass from one zone to another. Along the northern border of the board are twelve vertical columns that coordinate the twelve hours of the day, twelve hours of the night, and twelve months of the year with the twelve apostles (including a length of hallucinogenic cactus called San Pedro) and with the movements of the stars. The mesa contains many other references to the coordinates of space and time. These multiple layers of space and time are essential to divination and to the successive recontextualization of the client's difficulties. When he activates the power of his board, the diviner sets the world in spin. He manages the patient's experience of the cosmos and discerns what actions are necessary to effect that experience in a proper and moral way.[98]

Borrowing an explanation offered by Fernandez in another context and rephrasing it to fit this case: the mesa does not operate so differently from discovery procedures used in science, procedures that "take things apparently incoherent and inconsistent and show them to be instances of a more general principle. The important difference is that [the mesa diviner] only suggests and does not aim to discover and state those principles in so many verifiable and refutable words. Rather than struggling relentlessly to deprive puzzles of their mystery, [he] works with puzzles."[99]

SACRIFICE AND ORDEAL

The practice and ideology of sacrifice may prove to be a resource from which to extract a society's principles of distributive justice. Mythic sacrifices become models for the establishment of political hierarchies. We saw above, for example, that, in the beginning of time, the supernatural Anaconda came through the Water-Door in the East and entered what was to become the Amazonian universe, and swam upstream until it reached the center of the earth, where the Barasana now live. At that point, the Anaconda split into pieces, and its dismembered portions, especially the long bones, were arrayed along the river in rank order from head to tail. Each one of these portions represents a settlement of Barasana-speakers, who think of their villages as siblings descended from the single body of their supernatural ancestor. They keep sacred flutes, which are replicas of those first bones. When they assemble for their fruit festivals, they bring the bone flutes. The ranks and files of the musical parade at the feast carefully respect and reinforce the hierarchical order of the ranked sibs and the distribution of ritual goods among them. The form of the procession reconstitutes the body of the Anaconda, and reenacts its journey into the universe and the sacrificial disintegration that brought life to the world. The relationship of the parts of the dismembered body becomes the model for the relationship among generations, men and women, work roles, village alliances, and ritual roles among festival participants.[100]

The actual practice of sacrifice also sets up an ideal hierarchy of resources and distribution. The public distribution of portions of sacrificed animals and offerings (through fire, disposal, or communion among social actors) outlines an ideal distributive order against which one may measure contradictions in theory and fact.[101] Nowhere is this more apparent than in the dramatic sacrifices of a human victim, as reported among the Tupinambá, Carib, Incas, and others. The fact that victims were drawn from areas that were systematically rotated reveals a patterned order of relations among these areas and provides an opportunity for examining the moral logic of the political economy. In the case of the Incas, for instance, "the children sent from the outlying lands to imperial temples for sacrifice were part of the tribute the provinces were forced to pay."[102] Similar light comes from scrutinizing the sacrifice of young men as warriors in battles for the sake of virtues sacred to a culture (although these sacrifices never occurred on the same scale as modern Western civilizations). The details of these sacrifices, as well as those executed by shamans through supernatural means, are the economic, political, and military expression of justice, freedom, power, or other virtue apparent in the imagination.

Sacrifices need not be literal. They include mock combats, ritual battles, or contests, and they are important because virtues (especially fairness, justice, equality, humility, asymmetry, overlordship, and distributive power) show their mettle and disclose their structure in the course of trial. For that reason, South American cultures make wide use of staged combat and ritual ordeal. The above section on passages called attention to the ordeals inflicted during initiation. These mark moments of transition from one state to another, one condition of being to another, or one level of the cosmos to another. Some ordeals render the initiand partly "senseless," because they suppress or restrict the use of one of the senses. In her initiatory seclusion, for example, a Guayakí girl keeps her eyes closed even when eating food. "She must not only keep herself hidden [*kaku*, invisible], but must even avoid turning her face toward others, especially toward men who are neither her father nor her male ritual sponsor,"[103] lest she place them in a state of *bayja* (vulnerability to super-natural forces that kill men or make them ill).

Ordeals highlight divisions between qualities of existence: between femininity and masculinity, youth and age, in-groups and out-groups, this world and afterlife, humans and supernaturals. Ordeals are a species of apportionment or allotment. They separate and order realities into hier-archies and systems. Ordeals reveal, reinforce, or reforge the cosmic and social orders. This is because they simulate the conditions of the first sep-aration, especially the Great Divides—the destructions of flood, fire, and dismemberment (or cutting) that detached this existence from the pri-mordial one. The Akwẽ-Shavante ceremonies of immersion in water, for example, last some three weeks and derive their significance from the myths in which heroes, tossing in the floodwaters that deluged the earth, refused to come to land. Instead, they created things in the water, includ-ing women of a marriageable degree of social distance.[104]

Ordeals of the dead provide another resource for studying religious evaluations of distributive justice. The personality undergoes a sacrificial episode, and its elements are made sacred as the personality disintegrates into its component parts. Soul elements journey to different cosmic realms, flesh disappears into the earth (or into fire or the liquid of putre-faction), the spiritual and material elements of bone seek their destiny.[105] As they make their way to their respective afterworlds, the elements of human beings suffer trials and, in some cases, face judgment in formal tribunals.[106] The images of trial and the criteria of judgment offer a basis for understanding the principles of justice at work in a culture. This cosmic redistribution of the person introduces us to the widest possible economy of human life and furnishes evidence of its distributive logic, processual order, and conceptual clarity.

According to many South American peoples, ordeals and sacrifice reveal the orders, just or unjust, of existence, because life in this world is a sacrificial (Latin *sacer facere*, to make sacred) mode of being. That is, human existence is one that is constantly passing from one state to another, through its encounters with sacred realities in the myriad guises of their symbolic expressions. This is the context in which to appreciate the widespread South American judgments that sickness is an ordeal, a sacrificial (sacralizing) condition, that ritual combats (tugs of war, dance teams) and competitive sports epitomize a culture's perception of justice and fair play, and that tests of strength stimulate good health for the com-munity and the cosmos.

PARLIAMENTARY PROCEDURE

Forensic debate is another ritual procedure for adjudicating ethical conflict. In South America a large number of groups carry on a tradition known as ceremonial speech, a judicial institution. During a formal exchange of words, two speakers, representing the two sides of the issue, confront one another. Procedures are highly structured and stylized. Among the Ranqueles, for instance, there are two distinct forms of this ritual speech. Full participation is given by a chorus of "backbenchers," who interject their disagreement or approval. The orator for one side enumerates the reasons why his group's position is the more acceptable. In rapid monotones, the advocate pleads his case in prescribed formulas and in rhymed chant. The speaker finishes each brief argument with a rhetorical question to which his group answers in the affirmative. After the first oratorical round, the speaker rests while the second speaker launches immediately into an even longer enumeration of arguments for the other side. The goal is to arrive at consensus and contractual agreement. Throughout the South American continent such solemn dialogues are notoriously long-winded. Said one observer of the Ranqueles' performance, "It lasted long enough to annoy a saint."[107] Among the Waiwai, sessions have lasted twenty-six hours without any break. "During this time the two chanting persons did not eat or move at all."[108]

In some societies the respondent repeats his adversary's claim, shouting each syllable back to the main speaker as soon as he utters it, or else the respondent barks "yes" after every syllable or phrase from his opponent's mouth. The performance makes public the combativeness needed to sustain human culture in a world of paradox and contradiction. This same performative genre is often used to recount myths (as among the Kalapalo), intone healing chants, greet strangers, and contract marriage. This form of combative speech "de-emphasizes the boundaries between individuals, perhaps more so than any other speech event. . . . the speaker attempts to create or enhance certain images in the mind of the listener, images that will, with skill, begin to approximate his own very closely."[109] In fact, parliamentary procedure often imitates the dialogue of mythical beings during key events. For instance, Trio debaters sit on special benches to present their arguments for judgment. The stools imitate the mythical ones carved in stone during an incident involving the origin of human death. In the ancient times of the creative period, a Trio man was commanded to answer only to the voice of stones while he wandered, but when he heard a tree fall for the first time, he mistook it for the voice of a stone calling out to him, and he answered it. Instead of living eternally, like the stone, "the Trio have been like trees or wood (same word for both, *wewe*) both in terms of softness and ephemerality. People, i.e., the Trio, die like trees."[110] Because of its association with mortality and transition, Trio ceremonial dialogue has pressing urgency and deadly effect. Elsewhere, adjudicatory speech imitates the dialogue between the mythical twins, the sun and moon, or the sky and earth, whose creative words brought the world, with its good and bad points, into existence.[111]

Moral suasion is efficacious in a deep sense. It not only coerces others to agree and binds them to a decision (and thereby makes visible a hierarchy of powers relevant to the study of local concepts of justice), but it *creates* consensus, a *new* condition that mediates between two incompatible choices.

Prospects

In order to give as broad a picture as possible, this essay has presented a panoramic overview of South American cultures in a way that risks effacing important and creative differences among them. Such a seamless presentation must be no more than a prelude to particularity. Scrutiny of the moral life of specific South American peoples, via such works as those mentioned in the notes, not only calls attention to modes of moral reflection that have been overlooked until now but forces us to reconsider the *way* we undergo and think about moral experience itself. Among these South Americans, awareness of ties between the good life and well-being is as vivid as their perception of the mutual influence of cosmic order, social life, individual experience, and religious imagination on one another. Across these many realms, the moral tone of well-being blossoms in color, sounds forth in music, takes shape in space, and dances through time. To experience the plenitude that signals well-being, individuals center themselves on powerful realities revealed in myth. Traffic with these forces affords an experience of the fullness of time, the wholeness of space, and the soundness of tone that primordial existence signifies, but such a religious stance exacts its price. A life of passage, which opens the symbolic universe to other dimensions, is medically hazardous. Sickness announces the presence of realities more powerful than human life and presages a period of discernment, contact, and negotiation with powers that intrude upon the course of human history. This reflective process gleans new knowledge of the world and its spirituality. The Spanish conquest has installed tragedy and disease, death and critical reflection on an unprecedented scale. For many South American groups, the only solution for such unparalleled injustice—suffered at the hands of Western cultures that have pushed to new heights the vocabulary of social ethics, the inventory of technical medicines, and the catalog of epistemological categories that continues to strip South American concepts of any creative role in wider human history—lies in an unprecedented passage of the entire cosmos into a truly new world.

Notes

     1. *The Japan Times*, 27 January 1986, p. 5.
     2. Allan Young, "Some Implications of Medical Beliefs and Practice for

Social Anthropology," *American Anthropologist* 78, no. 1 (1976):5–24. The notion of pathogenic invasion cuts across the spectrum of disease and the range of South American cultures. For an example, see G. J. E. Salazar Escobar and M. Chuy, "Beliefs regarding the Etiology and Treatment of Infantile Diarrhea in Lima, Peru," *Social Science and Medicine* 17, no. 17 (1983):1257–1269, which describes invasion of the body by "cold."

3. This essay passes over two possible approaches to the topic that are amply illustrated in the references. The first approach would inventory types of disease, types of cure, types of healer, and so on. By contrast, I wish to reflect on sickness and cure as religious situations. The second would present several extended cases. However, much interesting material pertinent to our themes would fall by the wayside if coverage were limited to only a few cases.

Regarding the logic of medical systems, which are patterned on a mythical view of the cosmos within which one is sick and cured, see A. T. Delgado Sobrinha, "A lógica simbolica na medicina popular," *Perspectivas* 6 (1983):27–36.

4. Arthur P. Sorenson, "South American Linguistics at the Turn of the Seventies," in *Peoples and Cultures of Native South America*, ed. Daniel R. Gross (New York, 1973).

5. Irwin Press, "Problems in the Definition and Classification of Medical Systems," *Social Sciences Medical Bulletin* 14 (1980):45–57; Juan Somolinos Plaencia, "Medical History in Latin America," *Clio Medica* 15, nos. 3–4 (April 1981): 233–247.

6. The open-endedness demanded by cultural creativity is usually expressed as a scientific problem: "The degree of systematicity present in modes of medical treatment is problematic and culturally variable, and is often 'etic' imputation or projection of the anthropologist onto his or her field material" (Peter Worsley, Sir James George Frazer Memorial Lecture, 1981). Scientists of culture find it difficult to accommodate the expectations of their forms of knowledge to the creativity of religious life, especially as evidenced in the changing variety of myth and rite. Religion-based medicine is another instance of the difficulty.

7. See Mircea Eliade, *The Sacred and the Profane* (New York, 1957), which develops this interpretation of the sacredness of the center as a religious structure of human consciousness.

8. See Christian Scharfetter, "Psychiatrie der Chaco-Indianer Südamerikas," *Curare* 7, no. 3 (1984):189–194; Scharfetter illustrates how illness, including acute and chronic psychosis, manifests what Scharfetter calls a transcendent power or hierophany.

9. On the Desana, see Gerardo Reichel-Dolmatoff, *An Amazonian Cosmos: The Sexual and Religious Symbolism of the Tukano Indians* (Chicago, 1971). For myths of travel upstream and downstream (and their association with the times of sun, moon, and stars as well as with the proper distance of relationships in marriage, alliances, and economic activities), see Claude Lévi-Strauss, *Introduction to a Science of Mythology*, vol. 3: *The Origin of Table Manners* (New York, 1978).

10. See the many myths, spanning three centuries of reports, in Franklin Pease G. Y., *El dios creador andino* (Lima, 1973).

11. R. T. Zuidema, "The Inca Calendar," in *Native American Astronomy*, ed. Anthony F. Aveni (Austin, TX, 1977), pp. 219–259.

12. Daniel de Barandiarán, *Introducción a la cosmovisión de los indios ye'kuana-makiritare* (Caracas, 1979).

13. Pierre Clastres, *Chronique des indiens Guayaki* (Paris, 1972).

14. For a discussion of the ways in which funeral practices, especially drinking the bone ash of dead relatives in fermented brew, affect health, see Otto Zerries, "El endocanibalismo en la América del Sur," *Revista do Museu Paulista* 12 (1960):125–175; also Otto Zerries, "Krankheitsdämonen und Hilfsgeister des Medizinmännes in Südamerika," *Proceedings of the International Congress of Americanists* 30 (1955):162–178. On dreams as a form of primordial temporality that must be entered but also exited from time to time in order to maintain optimal health, see Miguel Alberto Bartolomé, "Orekuera royhendu (Lo que escuchamos en sueños): Shamanismo y religión entre los Ava-Katu-Ete del Paraguay," *Instituto indigenista interamericano de antropología social* 17 (1977):41–58.

15. On the Yanomamö, see Napoleon Chagnon, *Yanomanö: The Fierce People* (New York, 1968). For Barasana creation accounts see the appendixes in Stephen Hugh-Jones, *The Palm and the Pleiades: Initiation and Cosmology in Northwest Amazonia* (Cambridge, England, 1979); for the Wayãpi accounts see Françoise Grenand, *Et l'homme devient jaguar: Univers imaginaire et quotidien des indiens Wayãpi de Guyane* (Paris, 1982).

16. See Terence S. Turner, "Black Bracelets" (unpublished), which offers an analysis of the concept of beauty among the Northern Kayapó of the Xingu River area of Brazil.

17. For an example of the careful spatial arrangement of objects and persons who symbolize modes of power in healing rites, see Douglas Sharon, *Wizard of the Four Winds: A Shaman's Story* (New York, 1978). The four winds of the title are the four cardinal directions as well as the four sides of the healer's *mesa*, a cloth or board on which the healer constructs a microcosm of universal space. Eduardo Calderon, the Peruvian healer whom Sharon interviews, is employed as an artist, restoring the fine art unearthed in archaeological ruins.

18. See Wilhelm Saake, "Die Juriparilegende bei den Baniwa des Rio Issana," *Proceedings of the International Congress of Americanists* (1958):271–279; also Robin M. Wright, "History and Religion of the Baniwa Peoples of the Upper Rio Negro Valley," 2 vols. (Ph.D. diss., Stanford University, 1981).

19. See Norman O. Whitten, *Sacha Runa: Ethnicity and Adaptation of Ecuadorian Jungle Quichua* (Urbana, IL, 1976), which graphically describes the extraction of pathogenic spirit-darts and provides accounts of their mythic history as told by the Canelos Quichua of Ecuador. Whitten also shows how sickness due to the upset of spatial well-being reflects not only the relations within cosmic space and within the sick body but also the ailing relationships among individuals and groups in the social space of the community and its neighbors.

20. For a summary of the myths of divine twins see Alfred Métraux, "Twin Heroes in South American Mythology," *Journal of American Folklore* 59, no. 232 (1945):114–123. More lengthy and varied myths of divine twins can be found in the series Folk Literature of South American Peoples, edited and indexed by Johannes Wilbert and Karin Simoneau and published by the University of California Latin American Studies Center. For a discussion of the Quechua Indian concept of *ticci muyu capac*, the endless cycle of creativity, see Rodolfo Kusch, *America profunda* (Buenos Aires, 1962), which demonstrates how rituals that imitate the creative acts of mythic beings actually impose on contemporary humans the obligation to be creative.

21. Whitten, *Sacha Runa*, passim; Mario Califano, "El concepto de enferme-dad y muerte entre los Mataco Constaneros," *Scripta ethnológica* (Buenos Aires) 2, pt. 2 (1974):33–73.

22. The importance of vision in healing is explored in Marlene Dobkin de Rios, "The Vidente Phenomenon in Third World Traditional Healing: An Amazonian Example," *Medical Anthropology* 8, no. 1 (1984):60–70. For a different approach, one that investigates the organic response of the autonomic nervous system to vision-inducing mescaline, see Donald Jor-alemon, "The Role of Hallucinogenic Drugs and Sensory Stimuli in Peruvian Ritual Healing," *Culture, Medicine and Psychiatry* 8, no. 4 (1984):399–430.

23. See Kenneth Kensinger, "Cashinahua Medicine and Medicine Men," in *Native South Americans: Ethnology of the Least Known Continent*, ed. Patri-cia J. Lyon (Boston, 1974), pp. 283–288; the author shows how compli-cated the process can be when he presents the eight categories of *hekula*, spirits who can cure or kill the Yanoami. These spirits undergo a series of deaths and transformations during which they transmigrate through a succession of different existences including human, animal, and plant form.

24. The Cubeo live in the Northwest Amazon area; see Irving Goldman, *The Cubeo: Indians of the Northwest Amazon*, 2nd ed. (Urbana, IL, 1979).

25. See, for example, Neils Fock, *Waiwai: Religion and Society of an Amazon-ian Tribe*, Nationalmuseets skrifter, Etnografisk raekke, vol. 8 (Copen-hagen, 1963); also Christine Hugh-Jones, *From the Milk River: Spatial and Temporal Processes in Northwest Amazonia* (Cambridge, England, 1979).

26. Jonathan Hill, "Wakuenai Society: A Processual Structural Analysis of Indigenous Cultural Life in the Upper Rio Negro (Guainía) Region of Venezuela" (Ph.D. diss., University of Indiana, 1983); see also Hill, "Kamayura Flute Music," *Ethnomusicology* 23, no. 3 (1979):417–432.

27. Marcelo Bórmida, "Ayoreo Myths," *Latin American Indian Literatures* 2, no. 1 (Spring 1978):1–13 (especially p. 2); Lucien Sebag, "Le chaminisme ayoreo," pts. 1, 2, *L'homme* (Paris) 5 (January–March, April–June 1965):732, 92–122; Otto Zerries, "Die Ayoré in Ostbolivien," *Wiener völkerkundlische Mitteilungen* 3, no. 2 (1955):218–223; Ulf Lind, *Die Med-izin der Ayoré-Indianer* (Bonn, 1974).

28. Bartolomé, "Shamanism among the Avá-Chiripá," in *Spirits, Shamans, and Stars: Perspectives from South America*, eds. David L. Browman and Ronald A. Schwarz (The Hague, 1979), pp. 95–148.

29. Johannes Wilbert, "Eschatology in a Participatory Universe," in *Death and the After-Life in Pre-Colombian America*, ed. Elizabeth P. Benson (Washington, DC, 1975), pp. 163–189.

30. Alfred Métraux, *Religions et magies indiennes d'Amérique du Sud* (Paris, 1967), pp. 105ff.

31. Peter G. Roe, *The Cosmic Zygote: Cosmology in the Amazon Basin* (New Brunswick, NJ, 1982), p. 115.

32. Anthony Seeger, "What Can We Learn When They Sing? Vocal Genres of the Suya Indians of Central Brazil," *Ethnomusicology* 23, no. 3 (Sep-tember 1979):373–394.

33. On names, see David Maybury-Lewis, "Name, Person and Ideology," in *Naming Systems*, ed. Elisabeth Tooker (Washington, DC, 1984), pp. 1–10, which deals especially with Ge-speaking peoples of the southern Ama-zon; also J. Christopher Crocker, "Selves and Alters among the Eastern Bororo," in *Dialectical Societies*, ed. David Maybury-Lewis (Cambridge,

MA, 1979), pp. 249–300. On ritual weeping see Charles Wagley, *Welcome of Tears* (New York, 1978); Wagley explores this subject among the Tapirapé people of Brazil. On the powers of performed din see Lawrence E. Sullivan, *Icanchu's Drum* (New York, 1988).

34. Fock, *Waiwai*, passim.

35. See Bruce Lincoln, *Emerging from the Chrysalis: Studies in Rituals of Women's Initiation* (Cambridge, MA, 1981), pp. 50–70, for an examination of this symbolism among the Tukuna of the northwest Amazon region.

36. Clastres, *Chronique*, p. 183.

37. Bartolomé, "Shamanism," pp. 97ff. Regarding healers who are assisted by the spirits of the dead, see also A. Pollak-Eltz, "Magische Operationen und ihre Wirkung in Venezuela," *Ethnomedizin* 7 (1981–1982):117–126.

38. Bartolomé, ibid. Darkness often has a medical origin, escaping from a gourd of medicines kept by a mythic healer. In the case of the Makiritare of the Orinoco River region of Venezuela, darkness escaped from a medicine pouch at the beginning of time. It was a healing element, but one intended for containment. The creator divinity would put his head in the pouch in order to dream the dead back to life; see Marc de Civrieux, *Watunna: An Orinoco Creation Cycle*, ed. and trans. David M. Guss (San Francisco, 1980), pp. 23–27. Among the Guajiro darkness was a necessary precondition for creation of the world. It surrounded the creator Apusunai and allowed him to dream. Creatures are the dream images of the creator, who is immersed in primal darkness. Michel Perrin, *Le chemin des indiens morts: Mythes et symboles guajiro* (Paris, 1976).

39. Wright, *History and Religion of the Baniwa*, p. 386.

40. Wagley, *Welcome of Tears*, pp. 134–135.

41. As is true for all topics treated in the present essay, stunning differences in birthing practice and belief exist among South American peoples. An article that underlines the need to keep in mind even intracultural variation of childbirth techniques is Ruthbeth D. Finerman's study, "Pregnancy and Childbirth in Saraguro: Implications for Health Care Delivery in Southern Ecuador," *Medical Anthropology* 6, no. 4 (1982):269–278.

42. The absence of a spirituality of obstetrics in so-called Western medicine may largely account for the avoidance of hospitals during pregnancy and delivery. A study of 727 households in four Indian societies of Ecuador, for example, determined that hospital care, though readily accessible, was rarely sought and that only 15 percent of even severe pregnancy complaints were presented to modern health services for care. See B. Blessin and A. Kroeger, "Quantitative Daten zur Schwangerschaft und Geburt in vier Indianergesellschaften Ecuadors," in *Die Geburt aus ethnomedizinischer Sicht*, eds. W. Schiefenhovel and D. Sich, special supplement no. 1, *Curare* 6 (1983):210–216. Other studies that illustrate and analyze resistance to seeking biomedical health care at modern hospitals or clinics include Ruthbeth D. Finerman, "Experience and Expectation: Conflict and Change in Traditional Family Health Care among the Quichua of Saraguro," *Social Science and Medicine* 17, no. 17 (1983):1291–1298, and, in the same volume of the same journal, Judith Davidson, "The Survival of Traditional Medicine in a Peruvian Barriada," pp. 1271–1280.

43. Curt Nimuendajú, *The Apinayé*, Anthropological Series, no. 8 (Washington, DC, 1939), p. 100.

44. Waldeloir Rego, "Mitos e ritos africanos da Bahia," in Hector Carybé,

Iconografia dos deuses africanos no candomblé da Bahia (Sao Paulo, 1980), pages unnumbered. For further consideration of the notions of well-being, illness, and therapy in Afro-Brazilian traditions, see H. H. Figge, "Funktionen der Therapieversuche in der brasilianischen Umbanda," *Curare* 3, no. 3 (1980):159–164; O. M. Ravagnani, "Diagnóstico popular e incidéncia de doenças e males tratados pela fitoterapía tradicional," *Perspectivas* 5 (1982): 39–52; A.T. Delgado Sobrinha, "A Umbanda em Araraquara: Uma contribuição para o estudo da psicoterapía religiosa," *Perspectivas* 6 (1983):37–48.

45. Clastres, *Chronique*, pp. 14–15.

46. On the Kaingáng see Jules Henry, *Jungle People: A Kaingang Tribe of the Highlands of Brazil* (1941: New York, 1964), p. 194. On burning the placenta among some Quechua-speakers, see Abel Adrián Ambía and Rodolfo Sánchez Garrafa, *Amaru: Mito; Realidad del hombre* (Lima, 1970), p. 18; on birth control through cooling the placenta and ovaries see Susan C. Bourque and Kay Barbara Warren, *Women of the Andes: Patriarchy and Social Change in Two Peruvian Towns* (Ann Arbor, MI, 1981), p. 89.

47. Audrey J. Butt, "The Mazaruni Scorpion," *Timehri* (1957):40–54.

48. Eduardo Viveiros de Castro, "A Fabricação do corpo na sociedade xinguana," *Boletim do Museu Nacional* (Rio de Janeiro), n.s. antropologia, no. 32 (May 1979):40–49; see especially p. 42.

49. Martin Gusinde, "In der Medizinmannschule der Yamana-Feuerlander," *Ciba Zeitschrift* 4, no. 38 (October 1936):1307–1310.

50. Alfred Métraux, "Religion and Shamanism," *Handbook of South American Indians* 5 (Washington, DC, 1949), p. 590; Gerardo Reichel-Domatoff, "Training for the Priesthood among the Kogi of Columbia," in *Enculturation in Latin America: An Anthology*, UCLA Latin American Studies, vol. 37, ed. Johannes Wilbert (Los Angeles, 1976), pp. 265–288.

51. See Roberto Da Matta, *A Divided World: Apinayé Social Structure* (Cambridge, MA, 1982), which analyzes the Apinayé system of ritual friendship; also Maria Manuela Carneiro da Cunha, "Amigos, formais e pessoa: De companheiros, espelhos e identidades," *Boletim do Museu Nacional*, n.s. antropologia, no. 32 (May 1979):31–39, which examines the Krahó system; Jacques M. Chevalier, *Civilization and the Stolen Gift: Capital, Kin, and Cult in Eastern Peru* (Toronto, 1982), pp. 114, 198f., 204, 212; also see Stefano Varese, *La sal de los cerros: Notas etnográficas e históricas sobre los Campa de la selva del Perú* (Lima, 1968), pp. 22, 107, for a discussion of the ayompari/niompari *relationship of ritual trading partners.*

52. P. G. Rivière, "Marriage: A Reassessment," in *Rethinking Kinship and Marriage*, ASA Monograph, no. 11, ed. R. Needham (London, 1971), pp. 57–74: see also Stephen Hugh-Jones, *The Palm and the Pleiades: Initiation and Cosmology in Northwest Amazon* (Cambridge, England, 1979), p. 13.

53. On death originating from inopportune noise see *Folk Literature of the Mataco Indians*, UCLA Latin American Studies, vol. 52, eds. Johannes Wilbert and Karin Simoneau (Los Angeles, 1982), pp. 79, 89, 90.

54. Rafael Karsten, "Zeremoniell Spiele unter den Indianern Südamerikas," *Acta Academiae Aboensis Humaniora* (Abo) 1, no. 4 (1920):92–94; Otto Zerries, "Algunas noticias etnológicas acerca de los indígenas Puinave," *Boletin indigenista venezolano* 9, no. 1 (1964):29–36; on funeral games, see R. Hartmann and U. Oberem, "Beiträge zum 'Huairu-Spiel,'" *Zeitschrift für Ethnologie* 93, no. 2 (1968):240–259.

55. This hypothesis of Curt Nimendajú was reported by Carl Gustav Izikowitz in "Rhythmical Aspects of Canella Life," *Proceedings of the 31st International Congress of Americanists* (Sao Paolo, 1955), pp. 195–209.

56. Henry, *Jungle People*, p. 184.

57. Pedro Agostinho, *Kwaríp:* Mito e ritual no Alto Xingu (Salvador, Brazil, 1974).

58. On secondary burial of bones among the Boróro, see Renate Brigitte Viertler, "A noção de pessoa entre os Boróro," *Boletim do Museu Nacional*, n.s. antropologia, no. 32 (May 1979):27. The Goajiro burial of bones in the collective urn is described in Michel Perrin, *Le chemin des indiens morts: Mythes et symboles Goajiro* (Paris, 1976), p. 186.

59. Neil Whitehead, "Carib Cannibalism: The Historical Evidence," *Journal de la Société des américanistes de Paris* 70 (1984):69–88; Alfred Métraux, *Religions et magies indiennes d'Amérique du Sud* (Paris, 1967), pp. 43–78 ("L'anthropophagie rituelle des Tupinambá"); also Theodor Koch-Grünberg, "Die Anthropophagie der südamerikanischen Indianer," *Internationales Archiv für Ethnographie* (Leiden) 12 (1899):78–110.

60. See Otto Zerries, "El endocannibalismo en la América del Sur," *Revista do Museu Paulista*, n.s., vol. 12 (1960):125–175, which inventories some thirty-three groups that imbibe ashes of the dead. Detailed descriptions of the rite, as practiced among the Yanomamö of Venezuela, can be found in Hans Becher, "Bericht über eine Forschungsreise nach Nordbrasilien in das Gebiet der Flusse Demini und Araca," *Zeitschrift für Ethnologie* 82, no. 1 (1957):115–116, and in Daniel de Barandiarán, "Vida y muerte entre los indios Sanemá-Yanoama," *Antropológica* (Caracas), no. 21 (December 1967):3–65.

61. Orlando Villas Boas and Claudio Villas Boas, *Xingu: The Indians, Their Myths* (New York, 1973), pp. 213–225.

62. Ellen B. Basso, *The Kalapalo Indians of Central Brazil* (New York, 1973), p. 57.

63. Wilbert, "Eschatology in a Participatory Universe," p. 173.

64. For an overview of eschatological movements in South America, see Alicia M. Barabás, "Movimientos étnicos religiosos y seculares en América Latina: Una aproximación a la construcción de la utopía índia," *América* indígena 46, no. 3 (July–Sept. 1986):495–529; also Egon Schaden, "Le messianisme en Amérique de Sud," in *Histoire des religions*, vol. 3, ed. Henri-Charles Puech (Paris, 1976), pp. 1051–1109. One of the most stirring accounts of an eschatological movement in South America is the historical novel by Mario Vargas Llosa, *The War of the End of the World* (New York, 1984), which conveys the ferment, the mixture of hope and despair, that accompanied the eschatological movement in Canudos, Brazil, at the turn of the century.

65. Egon Schaden, "Der Paradiesmythos im Leben der Guaraní-Indianer," *Proceedings of the 30th International Congress of Americanists* (London, 1952), pp. 179–186.

66. Civrieux, *Watunna*, pp. 161ff.

67. Robin M. Wright and Jonathan D. Hill, "History, Ritual, and Myth: Nineteenth Century Millenarian Movements in the Northwest Amazon," *Ethnohistory* 33, no. 1 (1986), pp. 31–54.

68. On the Taki Onqoy and other eschatological movements in Peru, see Steve J. Stern, *Peru's Indian Peoples and the Challenge of Spanish Conquest: Huamanga to 1640* (Madison, WI, 1982); also Nathan Wachtel, *Vision of*

the Vanquished: The Spanish Conquest of Peru through Indian Eyes (New York, 1977).

69. Mircea Eliade, *Patterns in Comparative Religion* (New York, 1958), p. 455.
70. Hugh-Jones, *From the Milk River*, passim.
71. Bartolomé, "Shamanism among the Avá-Chiripá," p. 134.
72. Whitten, *Sacha Runa*, pp. 65ff.
73. See Joseph Bastien, *Mountain of the Condor: Metaphor and Ritual in an Andean Ayllu* (Saint Paul, 1978), which shows how this process works in the case of divination with coca leaves. For discussion of the diviner's mesa, see Douglas Sharon, *Wizard of the Four Winds*, passim; Ana Maria Mariscotti de Görlitz, *Pachamama santa tierra* (Berlin, 1978), passim; Billie Jean Isbell, *To Defend Ourselves: Ecology and Ritual in an Andean Village* (Austin TX, 1978), p. 160. Divinatory items (leaves, power objects, the mesa) are creatively rearranged to fit the personal circumstances of the patient, who is in turn rearranged through ritual to obtain healthier relationships with mysterious powers. For other perspectives on the relationship of medical imagery and the social world see also Irwin Press, "The Urban Curandero," *American Anthropologist* 73 (1971):741–756; Mark Munzel, *Medizinmannwesen und Geistervorstellungen bei den Kamayurá (Alto Xingu-Brasilien)* (Wiesbaden, 1971); also Leon Cádogan, *Apuntes de medicina popular guairena* (Asunción, 1967).
74. G. Reichel-Dolmatoff, *The Shaman and the Jaguar: A Study of Narcotic Drugs among the Indians of Colombia* (Philadelphia, 1975); Alfred Métraux, *Religions et magies*, pp. 79–176.
75. Jürgen Riester, "Medizinmänner und Zauberer der Chiquitano-Indianer," *Zeitschrift für Ethnologie* 96, no. 2 (1971):250–265.
76. Günther Hartmann, "Zigarrenhälter Nordwest-Brasiliens," *Festschrift Otto Zerries*, special supplement no. 1, *Ethnologische Zeitschrift Zürich* (1974):177–189; Otto Zerries, "Tierbank und Geistersitz in Südamerika," *Ethnologische Zeitschrift Zürich* 1 (1970):47ff.
77. S. Henry Wassén, "A Medicine Man's Implements and Plants in a Tiahuanacoid Tomb in Highland Bolivia," *Etnologiska studier* (Göteborg) 32 (1972):8–114; see especially pp. 13f.
78. Examples and suggestions may be found in J. W. Helbig, *Religion und Medizinmannwesen bei den Cuna*, Münchner Beiträge zur Amerikanistik, vol. 5 (Munich, 1982); Franz Xaver Faust, *Medizinische Anschauungen und Praktiken der Landbevölkerung im andien Columbien*, Münchner Beiträge zur Amerikanistik, vol. 10 (Munich, 1983); Moisé S. Bertoni, *La civilización guarani*, vol. 3; *Etnografía, conocimientos: La higiene guarani y su importancia científica y práctica; La medicina guarani, conocimientos científicos* (Asunción, 1983); Angelina Pollak-Eltz, *Folk-Medicine in Venezuela* (Vienna, 1982).
79. Audrey J. Butt, "Ritual Blowing: *Taling*—A Causation and Cure of Illness among the Akawaio," *Man* (London) 62 (April 1956):49–55.
80. Wagley, *Welcome*, p. 191.
81. Claude Lévi-Strauss, "The Effectiveness of Symbols," *Structural Anthropology* (New York, 1963), pp. 186–205, offers a brief but lucid depiction of this process at work in difficult childbirth and makes suggestive remarks about its relationship to modern psychotherapy. The author further assesses the connection between the uses of mythic imagery among South American people and in Euro-American psychoanalysis in *La potière jalouse* (Paris, 1985), wherein he talks about the image of the

"shrink" and the custom of shrinking trophy heads among the Jivaro peoples of Ecuador.

82. The point that studies of contraception have failed because of their lack of grounding in the religious cosmology of the people under study is argued in S. H. Wassén and H. Krumbach, "Indianische Kontrazeption," *Ethnología americana* 18, no. 2 (1981):1013–1016.

83. Walter Dostal, ed., *The Situation of the Indian in South America: Contributions to the Study of Inter-Ethnic Conflict in the Non-Andean Regions of South America* (Geneva, 1972).

84. See D. Pedersen and C. Colima, "Traditional Medicine in Ecuador: The Structure of the Non-Formal Health Systems," *Social Science and Medicine* 17, no 17 (1983):1249–1255, which shows how traditional and Western medicine can be combined in the health care of four villages. See also A. B. Colson and C. De Armellada, "An Amerindian Derivation for Latin American Creole Illnesses and Their Treatment," *Social Science and Medicine* 17, no. 17 (1983):1229–1248, which stresses that local religious and conceptual structures serve as bases for selecting new information from incoming medical systems and adapt themselves to new health needs; the same case is made in S. M. S. Carvalho, "Reflexoes sobre 'pensamento tradicional' e 'pensamento selvagem,'" *Perspectivas* 6 (1983):19–26; also in James W. Larrick, James A. Yost, Jon Kapalan, Garland King, and John Mayhall, "Patterns of Health and Disease among the Waorani Indians of Eastern Ecuador," *Medical Anthropology* 3, no. 2 (1979):147–189. On the role of the healer in cultural exchange, see Miguel A. Bartolomé, "El shaman guaraní como agente inter-cultural," *Sociedad Argentina de anthropología* (Buenos Aires), n.s., 5, no. 2 (1971):107–114.

85. The global reach of the sickness experience is true also in cases of what might appear to be idiosyncratic neurotic episodes. See, for instance, Michel Tousignant, "*Pena* in the Ecuadorian Sierra: A Psychoanthropological Analysis of Sadness," *Culture, Medicine and Psychiatry* 8, no. 4 (1984):381–398.

86. J. Wilbert, "The Calabash of the Ruffled Feathers," *Artscanada* 30, nos. 5–6 (December 1973–January 1974):90–93.

87. "Is anything we say about morality in general inevitably tainted by our own moral traditions and perspectives?" This is the question that opens a fascinating review of recent works in comparative religious ethics, namely: John P. Reeder, Jr., "Moralities and Cosmogonies," *Religious Studies Review* 13, no. 3 (1987):223–229.

88. Arthur Adkins, "Cosmogony and Order in Ancient Greece," in *Cosmogony and Ethical Order: New Studies in Comparative Ethics,* eds. Frank Reynolds and Robin Lovin (Chicago, 1985), pp. 39–66.

89. The point is made in Steven Lukes, "Marxism, Morality and Justice," in *Marx and Marxism,* Royal Institute of Philosophy Lecture Series, no. 14, ed. G. H. R. Parkinson (Cambridge, England, 1982), pp. 177–205; the same point is made in a different manner in David Tracy, "Religion and Human Rights in the Public Realm," *Daedalus* 112 (1983):237–254.

90. A good example is Owen J. Flanagan, "Quinean Ethics," *Ethics* 93 (1982):56–74.

91. See, for example, Richard Fenn, *Liturgies and Trials* (New York, 1982), as well as the works of Michel Foucault and Erving Goffman. In regard to the rituals of the workplace and monetary exchange, as they reflect

historical concepts of justice, see Michael Taussig, *The Devil and Commodity Fetishism in South America* (Chapel Hill, NC, 1980).

92. This narrow construction of a single band of moral reasoning (as opposed to the broad spectrum of forms of rationality) has come under attack in Richard Rorty, *Philosophy and the Mirror of Nature* (Princeton, 1979); also in Jeffrey Stout, *The Flight from Authority* (Notre Dame, IN, 1984). It has long been questioned in cultural studies, for there is need to get beyond the narrow construction of reasoning and principles of adjudication found in such works as David Little and Sumner B. Twiss, *Comparative Religious Ethics: A New Method* (San Francisco, 1978); also Ronald Green, *Religious Reason* (New York, 1978); and Tom Beauchamp, and James F. Childress, *Principles of Biomedical Ethics* (New York, 1983).

93. Juan M. Ossio, "Guaman Poma: Nueva crónica o carta al rey: Un intento de aproximación a las categorías del pensamiento del mundo andino," in *Ideologiá mesiánica del mundo andino*, ed. Juan Ossio (Lima, 1973), pp. 155–213; see especially p. 157.

94. Quoted from Philip Means, *Ancient Civilizations of the Andes* (New York, 1931), pp. 437ff.

95. I have presented a lengthy treatment of the spatial, temporal, and ritual bases of Andean ethics in "Above, Below and Far Away: Andean Cosmogony and Ethical Order," in *Cosmogony and Ethical Order: New Studies in Comparative Ethics*, eds. Robin W. Lovin and Frank E. Reynolds (Chicago, 1985), pp. 98–130. Grasping the local logic of Inca moral reasoning (or that of any other South American culture) requires the kind of running start provided in that article.

96. Afro-Brazilian tradition has adapted the complex form of Yoruba divination that combines casts of shells with enigmatic poems. Linking these symbolic forms to the destiny of an individual and his or her immediate symptoms is left to the discretion of accomplished diviners. See William Bascom, *Sixteen Cowries* (Bloomington, IN, 1980).

97. Fernandez, *Bwiti: An Ethnography of the Religious Imagination in West Africa* (Princeton, 1982), pp. 569–570.

98. Sharon, *Wizard*, pp. 64–65, 72, 106–107.

99. Fernandez, *Bwiti*, pp. 571–572.

100. Hugh-Jones, *The Palm and the Pleiades*, passim.

101. In regard to the connections among sacrifice, ritual distribution of portions, and hierarchies of social value, see the stimulating discussions in *Divisione delle carni: Dinamica sociale e organizzazione del cosmo*, special issue, *L'uomo* (Rome) 9, nos. 1, 2 (1985).

102. Alfred Métraux, *History of the Incas* (New York, 1969), p. 140; Whitehead draws the same conclusion in regard to Carib sacrifice; Florestan Fernandes, "La guerre et le sacrifice humain chez les Tupinambá, *Journal de la société américaniste* 41 (1952):139–220, comes to similar conclusions in regard to the Tupinambá.

103. Clastres, *Chronique*, p. 135.

104. David Maybury-Lewis, *Akwe-Shavante Society* (Oxford, 1967), pp. 248–249.

105. José María Cruxent, "Indios guaika: La incineración de cadáveres," *Boletin indigenista venezolano* 1, no. 1 (1953):149–151.

106. See Chagnon, *The Yąnomamö*, p. 48, which describes how the dead are separated by a supernatural judge. The Goajiro and Warao must be able to name animals and plants that no longer bear their familiar form. Only

their initiatory acquaintance with the esoteric names of the items in question allows them to proceed along the path to their destiny. Otherwise (if their memory fails them or if they failed to learn thoroughly the hidden meanings of symbolic orders during life), they become monsters who live "neither here nor there."

107. Mansilla, *Excursion*, p. 182.
108. Fock, *Waiwai*, p. 216.
109. Basso, "A 'Musical View of the Universe': Kalapalo Myth and Ritual as Religious Performance," *Journal of American Folklore* 94, no. 373 (1981):283.
110. Peter Rivière, *Marriage among the Trio* (Oxford, 1969), p. 262–263; see also Peter Rivière, "The Political Structure of the Trio as Manifested in a System of Ceremonial Dialogue," in *The Translation of Culture*, ed. T. O. Beidelman (London, 1971), pp. 293–311.
111. For example, see Roberto Cortez, "Dialogo cerimonial e dialogo mitologico entre os Tiriyo," *Boletim do Museu Goeldi* (Belém, Brazil), n.s., no. 61 (November 1975):1–25.

A Guide to

Further Reading

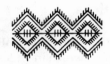

Buddhist Traditions

A slightly dated but still solid introduction to the various aspects of Buddhism is provided by Edward Conze in *Buddhism, Its Essence and Development* (New York, 1951). As Arthur Waley says in the preface, this book is "comprehensive, easy and readable." A handy (only 243 pages), well-balanced historical study of the rich and complex Buddhist development is found in Richard H. Robinson and W. L. Johnson, *The Buddhist Religion: A Historical Introduction* (Encino, CA, 1977).

A clear and competent exposition of Buddhist philosophy, especially that of the Mahāyāna tradition, is given by Junjiro Takakusu in *The Essentials of Buddhist Philosophy* (Honolulu, 1947). For over half a century Edward J. Thomas, *The History of Buddhist Thought* (1933; reprint, New York, 1951) has been regarded as a small classic in dealing with the major themes of Buddhist thought in its early as well as later phases. The Ceylonese Bikkhu, Walpola Rahula, author of *What the Buddha Taught* (New York, 1959), was educated at home and in England, and lived in France. According to Paul Demiéville, he is "humanist, rational, Socratic in some respects, Evangelic in others, or again almost scientific." He is certainly well versed in both the Theravāda and Mahāyāna traditions. He is also a genius in presenting difficult subjects simply.

Following E. J. Thomas's insight that the Buddhist movement began "not with a body of doctrine, but with the formation of society bound by certain rules," Joseph M. Kitigawa's *Religions of the East*, rev. ed. (Philadelphia, 1968) emphasizes the importance of the Buddhist "community." Is Buddhism one of the heterodox branches of Hinduism, as many Hindus and some Buddhists as well as certain vocal Western Buddhologists claim, or is it an expression of an autonomous religious experience? Sir Charles Eliot's *Hinduism and Buddhism*, 3 vols. (New York, 1954), is indispensable for answering this question.

Lily de Sylva gathers textual references to and contemporary descriptions of *paritta*, one of the most long-lived of Buddhist healing rites, in *Paritta: The Buddhist Ceremony for Peace and Prosperity in Sri Lanka*, Spolia Zeylanica: Bulletins of the National Museum of Sri Lanka, vol. 36 (Colombo, 1981).

Chinese Buddhist Traditions

The only extended study of the Master of Healing is Raoul Birnbaum, *The Healing Buddha* (Boulder, 1979), which includes translations from Chinese scriptures about this buddha. This work provides a cross-cultural view of the cult of the Master of Healing, emphasizing its scriptural foundations and iconographic manifestations. Further information regarding Chinese traditions can be found in Birnbaum's "Seeking Longevity in Chinese Buddhism: Long Life Deities and Their Symbolism," in *Myth and Symbol in Chinese Traditions*, eds. Norman Girardot and John S. Major, special double issue of *Journal of Chinese Religions* 13–14 (Fall 1985–Fall 1986): 143–176. Paul Demiéville's remarkably comprehensive cross-cultural essay on Buddhist medical theory and healing traditions is available in an English translation by Mark Tatz as *Buddhism and Healing: Demiéville's Article "Byō" from Hōbōgirin* (Lanham, MD, 1985). To examine Chinese medical cosmologies and practices that lie outside a strictly Buddhist perspective, one may begin with Manfred Porkert's excellent study, *The Theoretical Foundations of Chinese Medicine: Systems of Correspondence* (Cambridge, MA, 1974), which contains additional bibliography, and Nathan Sivin's *Traditional Medicine in Contemporary China* (Ann Arbor, 1987).

Contemporary Japanese Traditions

The book from which some of the arguments in Ohnuki-Tierney's article were derived is *Illness and Culture in Contemporary Japan* (Cambridge, England, 1984). It provides a detailed and historically informed account of the cultural practices and cultural meaning of health care in urban Japan. It also offers a comprehensive picture of a pluralistic system of health care, including religious practices, the Chinese-derived Japanese medicine of *kampō*, and biomedical delivery, which, as the author demonstrates, has been thoroughly transformed and has become part of Japanese culture and society. William Caudill, a specialist on Japan with psychiatric training, provides a sensitive account of cultural patternings of day-to-day health care and illness perception through a comparison between Japan and the United States in "The Cultural and Interpersonal Context of Everyday Health and Illness in Japan and America," in *Asian Medical Systems,* ed. C. Leslie (Berkeley, 1976), pp. 159–177.

The Japanese attitude toward cancer illustrates most succinctly how culture patterns the conception and treatment of illness. In "Curable Cancers and Fatal Ulcers," *Social Science and Medicine* 16 (1982):2101–2108, Susan O. Long and B. Long describe their observations of the Japanese attitude toward cancer. A psychotherapy that has developed in Japan and that is deeply embedded in the Japanese conception of human relationships is discussed by Takao Murase in "Naikan Therapy," in *Japanese Culture and Behavior,* ed. T. S. Lebra and W. P. Lebra (Honolulu, 1986), pp. 388–397.

The Ayurvedic Tradition

Jean Filliozat's *Classical Doctrine of Indian Medicine,* trans. Dev Raj Chanana (Delhi, 1964) is an authoritative overview by a trained medical practitioner and South Asianist. It focuses on Vedic pathology, anatomy, and physiology as the background to classical Āyurveda, and it allows for comparative discussions of Avestan, Greek, and Mesopotamian medical theories. *Hindu Medicine,* ed. Ludwig Edelstein (Baltimore, 1948) is a collection of essays from Heinrich Zimmer's lectures at the Johns Hopkins Institute of the History of Medicine in 1940. Although superseded by nearly a half century of studies in Āyurveda, they still reflect the author's perceptive summations of Hindu mythology, philosophy, and symbolism. Twenty essays by historians, anthropologists, sociologists, and others are gathered in *Asian Medical Systems: A Comparative Study,* ed. Charles Leslie (Berkeley, 1976). About half of the book pertains to South Asia, with essays on subjects such as ancient and medieval India (A. L. Basham), the impact of Āyurveda upon Sri Lankan culture and the individual (G. Obeysekere), and medical revivalism in contemporary South Asia (B. Gupta and the editor).

"Ayurveda and the Hindu Philosophical Systems," in *Philosophy East and West* 37 (1987):245–259, by Gerald J. Larson, an expert in South Asian philosophy and religion, presents a concise overview of a natural affinity between the Samkhya and Vaisheshika naturalistic philosophies and Ayurvedic medical practice according to its early literature. Mircea Eliade, *Yoga: Immortality and Freedom* (Princeton, 1969) is a classic study by the foremost historian of religions of the century. This work explores the techniques and symbol systems of yoga in ancient India, classical Hinduism, Tantrism, Buddhism, and Jainism. *Fluid Signs: Being a Person the Tamil Way* (Berkeley, 1984) is an innovative regional study of South India by anthropologist E. Valentine Daniel. He enters the Tamil expressions of region, village, house, and body in order to develop a semiotics of substance, change, and interaction. An overview of Hinduism, its history, interactive worldviews, and dynamics, including the journey of a life-body through stages of existence, is found in David M. Knipe's *Hinduism: Experiments with the Sacred*, forthcoming.

Contemporary Hindu Traditions

A popular account of the traditional system of medicine is given in J. Jolly, *Indian Medicine*, 2nd rev. ed. (Delhi, 1977). *Asian Medical Systems*, ed. Charles Leslie (Berkeley, 1976) presents essays on different aspects of the indigenous medicine of various countries of South and Southeast Asia, as well as Arab and Chinese medicine. Sudhir Kakar, *The Inner World: A Psychoanalytic Study of Childhood and Society in India* (Delhi, 1978) is a psychological analysis of growing up in India and of the belief system in which development takes place.

Sudhir Kakar's study entitled *Shamans, Mystics and Doctors: A Psychological Study of India and Its Healing Traditions* (New York, 1982) is a psychoanalytic interpretation of various Indian traditions of the healing of emotional disorders. Healings by Muslim holy men are the subject of Erna M. Hoch's article "Pir, Faqir and Psychotherapist," *The Human Context* 6 (1974):668–676, where they are seen from the viewpoint of an orthodox Swiss psychiatrist with many years of experience in India. A look at Ayurvedic psychotherapy by the distinguished Sri Lankan anthropologist Gananath Obeyesekere is found in "The Theory and Practice of Psychological Medicine in the Ayurvedic Tradition," *Culture, Medicine and Psychiatry* 1 (1977).

Sinhala Traditions

Both L. R. Amarasingham (Rhodes), "Movement among Healers in Sri Lanka: A Case Study of a Sinhalese Patient," *Culture, Medicine and Psychiatry* 4 (1980):72–92, and L. A. Rhodes, "Time and the Process of Diagnosis in Sinhalese Ritual Treatment," in *South Asian Systems of Healing*, ed. E. Valentine Daniel and Judy Pugh, Contributions to Asian Studies

(Leiden, 1984), deal with actual case studies and the diagnostic procedures in Sinhala medicine and ritual.

An excellent comprehensive study of traditional rituals of exorcism in Sri Lanka, focusing primarily on the aesthetic aspects of ritual drama, is *The Celebration of Demons* (Bloomington, IN, 1981) by Bruce Kapferer. G. Obeyesekere, "The Impact of Ayurvedic Ideas on the Culture and the Individual in Sri Lanka," in *Asian Medical Systems*, ed. Charles Leslie (Berkeley, 1976) focuses primarily on Ayurvedic medicine in Buddhist Sri Lanka and on its integration into popular belief.

Islamic Traditions

Many of the issues touched upon in the two articles on Islam are further developed by Peter Antes in "Islamische Ethik," a chapter in his *Ethik in nichtchristlichen Kulturen* (Stuttgart and Berlin, 1984), 48–81; also by Fazlur Rahman, *Health and Medicine in the Islamic Tradition* (New York, 1987). A general overview of the relation between Islam and medicine is found in R. Alsabah, "Islam and Medicine," *Journal of Arab Affairs* 3, no. 1 (1984):69–83. For reviews of historical practices and attitudes in several Islamic countries see Ševki, *Turkish Medical History* (Istanbul, 1925); Cyril Elgood, *A Medical History of Persia* (reprint, Amsterdam, 1979); E. G. Browne, *Arabian Medicine* (Cambridge, England, 1962); Amin A. Khairallah, *Outline of Arabic Contributions to Medicine* (Beirut, 1946); and L. Leclerc, *Histoire de la médicine arabe*, 2 vols. (London, 1926). An excellent historic sketch of the profession of medicine in Fatimid Egypt is *Medieval Islamic Medicine: Ibn Riḍwān's Treatise "On the Prevention of Bodily Ills in Egypt,"* Arabic text ed. Adil S. Gamal, trans. Michael W. Dols (Berkeley, 1984). This work shows the influence of Hippocratic/Galenic concepts on medieval Islamic medicine. Other works of interest that focus on Islamic medicine of the medieval period include Donald Campbell, *Arabian Medicine and Its Influence on the Middle Ages*, 2 vols. (London, 1926), and Al-Ruhāvī, *Medical Ethics of Medieval Islam*, trans. Martin Levy (Philadelphia, 1967).

Various concepts of disease may be found in the Islamic world, and these have been studied in a variety of ways. For example, see Byron J. Good, "The Heart of What's the Matter: The Semantics of Illness in Iran," *Culture, Medicine and Psychiatry* 1, no. 1 (1977):25–58; and, for a study of the conception of mental illness and the cure of madness, see Michael W. Dols, "Insanity in Byzantine and Islamic Medicine," in *Symposium on Byzantine Medicine*, ed. John Scarborough, Dumbarton Oaks Papers, no. 38 (Washington, DC, 1984). In *Ḥamadsha: A Study in Moroccan Ethnopsychiatry* (Berkeley, 1973), Vincent Crapanzano takes an ethnopsychiatric approach to the study of Sufi therapies of dance, trance, and music. Another approach to curing rites is exemplified in David Howell's "Health Rituals at a Lebanese Shrine," *Middle East Studies* 6 (1970):179– 188.

Akan Traditions

Kofi Appiah-Kubi's study entitled *Man Cures, God Heals: Religion and Medical Practices among the Akans of Ghana* (New York, 1981) is an elaborate work on the healing practices of the Indigenous African Christian churches, stressing the importance of religion in healing. A compilation of articles from all over Africa, emphasizing the spiritual and holistic aspect of African healing, appears in the collected papers of the African Regional Conference on the Churches' Role in Health and Wholeness, sponsored by the Christian Medical Commission of the World Council of Churches, Gaborne, Botswana, October 1979. Pascal J. Imperato, who formerly worked in Mali, examines the beneficial aspects of traditional medicine in *African Folk Medicine* (Baltimore, 1977). P. A. Twumasi's *Medical Systems in Ghana* (Tema, Ghana, 1975) is an examination of the coexistence of the traditional and modern health care systems, suggesting that an integration of the two is possible and desirable.

David Sobel's study *Ways of Health* (New York, 1979) is an excellent book about holistic approaches to health care, both ancient and modern. In *Health and the Developing World* (Ithaca, NY, 1969), John Bryant underscores the health problems of developing nations and offers suggestions for eradicating some of these problems. *The Cultural Crisis of Modern Medicine*, ed. John Ehrenreich (New York, 1978) takes a critical look at the cultural monopoly of health care in Western society and raises questions about the important role of culture in health care in all societies.

Central and Southern African Traditions

The uses and rationales of African medicine and biomedicine in Kongo society are explored in a study by John M. Janzen with William Arkinstall, M.D., *The Quest for Therapy: Medical Pluralism in Lower Zaire* (Berkeley, 1978). In *Lemba 1650–1930: A Drum of Affliction in Africa and the New World* (New York, 1982) Janzen provides an in-depth historical study of a western equatorial cult of affliction that emerged in response to the Great Trade, with exploration of the more general characteristics of African religion and healing.

Harriet Ngubane, *Body and Mind in Zulu Medicine* (New York, 1977) explores Zulu concepts such as balance, pollution, and sorcery in their relation to medicine. Victor Turner analyzes indigenous medical beliefs and practices as found in a series of ritual performances in the life of a single village community in *The Drums of Affliction: Religious Processes among the Ndembu of Zambia* (Oxford, 1968). A health definition that openly recognizes the central role of value-charged ideals and goals in both the culture at large and in health programs is advocated in Janzen's "The Need for a Taxonomy of Health in the Study of African Therapeutics," in *Social Science and Medicine* 15B (1981):185–194.

Haitian Traditions

Alfred Métraux, *Voodoo in Haiti* (New York, 1959) is still the most accurate and complete ethnography on the traditional religion of Haiti. The book is limited in that its author maintains a certain distance from his subject. He focuses his attention on public ceremonies and belief systems. There is little clue in his writings as to the personal or social healing that goes on in Vodou. *Divine Horsemen: The Living Gods of Haiti* (New Paltz, NY, 1983) is a more intuitive, imaginative, and personal book written by dancer and filmmaker Maya Deren. Folklorist Zora Neale Hurston's *Tell My Horse* (Berkeley, 1981) is less rich in basic information than Deren's book but could be described in similar ways. *Life in a Haitian Valley* (Garden City, NY, 1971) by Melville J. Herskovits is a classic study of the Mirebalais Valley. Because Vodou was in decline in the Mirebalais area at the time Herskovits did the study, much of his information about Haitian traditional religion cannot be used for a general understanding of Vodou. Michel S. Laguerre's more recently published *Vodoo Heritage* (Beverly Hills, 1980) is a book that should be used with care; there is valuable information in it about spirits, songs, and rites in the volume, but there is also mistranslation and misinformation. In *The Drum and the Hoe: Life and Lore of the Haitian People* (Berkeley, 1960) Harold Courlander covers some of the same terrain as Laguerre and he does it more responsibly.

Robert Farris Thompson, *Flash of the Spirit: African and Afro-American Art and Philosophy* (New York, 1983) is an invaluable resource for understanding the notions of person, health, and wholeness that underlie all Afro-Caribbean healing systems.

There is little written directly on healing in Haitian Vodou. Erika Bourguignon does use Vodou as one of her case studies in *Possession* (San Francisco, 1976), and the following books contain one or more articles on possession and/or healing in religious systems from other parts of the Caribbean: Vincent Crapanzano and Vivian Garrison, eds., *Case Studies in Spirit Possession* (New York, 1977); Alan Harwood, *RX: Spiritist as Needed: A Study of a Puerto Rican Community Mental Health Resource* (New

York, 1977); and Felicitas D. Goodman, Jeanette H. Henney, and Esther Pressel, *Trance, Healing and Hallucination: Three Field Studies in Religious Experience* (New York, 1974).

Hawaiian Traditions

A broad-ranging account of herbal practitioners, set in a social and religious context, is found in *Kahuna La'au Lapa'au* (The practice of Hawaiian herbal medicine) (Norfolk Island, Australia, 1976), by J. Gutmanis. It details their selection, training, diagnosis, and treatment of illnesses (especially of women and children) and their use of medicinal plants, notebooks, spells, and prayers. *Polynesian Religion* (Honolulu, 1927), by E. S. C. Handy, is a classic comparative study of Polynesian religion and philosophy. *The Polynesian Family System in Ka-'u, Hawai'i* (Wellington, N.Z., 1958), by E. S. C. Handy and M. K. Pukui, is a description of an old-style Hawaiian community by native informants in 1935, covering the physical, legendary, and social setting; the life cycle; psychic relationships; manners and customs; and ecological and historical perspectives.

Fragments of Hawaiian History (Honolulu, 1959) is by the native scholar J. P. Ii (1800–1870), who held important positions in the kingdom from boyhood until retirement. It offers memories of personal experiences of Hawaiian political, social, and religious transition from the time of the ancient taboo system to the constitutional monarchy. *Ka Po'e Kahiko* (The people of old) (Honolulu, 1964) is a description of Hawaiian society, family, aumakuas, spirit world, transfigurations, medical practices, magic, and sorcery by the native scholar S. M. Kamakau. It is based on personal experience and access to firsthand information about the past.

Hawaiian Antiquities (Moolelo Hawaii) (Honolulu, 1951) contains classic ethnography on the old way of life by the native scholar D. Malo (c. 1793–1853), derived from personal experience and information from other native experts. Conversion to Christianity colors his work, and also Kamakau's and Ii's. *Nānā i ke Kumu* (Look to the source) (Honolulu, 1972) by M. K. Pukui, E. W. Haertig, and C. A. Lee is a sourcebook on Hawaiian cultural practices, concepts, and beliefs written to inform the professional staff of today that is serving Hawaiians and part-Hawaiians through the child welfare agency established by Queen Lili'uokalani. A comparative account of South Pacific medical practices and beliefs from modern informants and published works is given in C. D. F. Parsons, *Healing Practices in the South Pacific* (Laie, Hawaii, 1985). Hawaii is not included.

Native North American Traditions

Virgil J. Vogel is the author of *American Indian Medicine* (Norman, OK, 1970), a general, popular introduction to the subject of native North American traditions. Marcelle Bouteiller offers the only analytical treatise on North American Indian shamanism that exists so far in *Chamanisme et guérison magique* (Paris, 1950), 25–162. Åke Hultkrantz, *Conceptions of the Soul among North American Indians*, Ethnographical Museum of Sweden Monograph Series, no. 1 (Stockholm, 1953) is an investigation of the concepts underlying the Indian ideas of disease and shamanism. In *The Religions of the American Indian* (Berkeley and Los Angeles, 1979), the same author discusses medicine men and shamans in chap. 6 and ideas of the afterlife and their connections with soul concepts and shamanism in chap. 9. A detailed study of the occurrence of soul-loss diagnosis in the western part of aboriginal North America is that of William W. Elmendorf, "Soul Loss Illness in Western North America," in *Indian Tribes of Aboriginal America*, ed. Sol Tax (Chicago, 1952), 104–114.

  Yuwipi: Vision and Experience in Oglala Ritual (Lincoln, NE, 1982) by William K. Powers is a well-rounded presentation of an important Lakota Indian medicinal and divinatory ritual. A wealth of materials on Cherokee medicines and their application is found in James Mooney and Frans M. Olbrechts, "The Swimmer Manuscript: Cherokee Sacred Formulas and Medicinal Prescriptions," *Bureau of American Ethnology Bulletin* 99 (Washington, DC, 1932). A well-researched work on shamanic healing among today's Coast Salish Indians is Wolfgang G. Jilek, *Indian Healing: Shamanic Ceremonialism in the Pacific Northwest Today* (Blaine, WA, 1982). Weston La Barre, *The Peyote Cult*, 4th ed. enl. (Hamden, CT, 1975) is the classic work on peyote, the spineless cactus that is taken as a medicine by many Indians.

Mesoamerican Traditions

An excellent short survey of Aztec culture in general is given by Jacques Soustelle in *Daily Life of the Aztecs* (Stanford, CA, 1970). Alfonso Caso, one of the founding scholars of Aztec studies, describes a number of aspects of their religion in *The Aztecs: People of the Sun* (Norman, OK, 1958). Historian of religion Davíd Carrasco provides a provocative study of religion and mythology in central Mexico. His *Quetzalcoatl and the Irony of Empire* (Chicago, 1982) explores the application of anthropology and urban geography to myth. In *Indian Medicine in Highland Guatemala* (Albuquerque, NM, 1987), Sandra Orellana gives a survey of medicine and ideology in the Maya region of Mesoamerica. *The Human Body and Ideology: Concepts of the Ancient Nahuas* (Salt Lake City, 1988), a study by Alfredo López Austin, is an indispensable work for the study of the religion, ideology, and medicine of the Aztecs. This work covers much more and in more detail than was possible to deal with in the present chapter.

South American Traditions

Juan Somolinos Plaencia, "Medical History in Latin America," *Clio Medica* 15, nos. 3–4 (April 1981):233–247, provides bibliography regarding medical ideas and practice (including ethnomedicine) in Latin America. Many articles in the German journals *Ethnomedizin* and *Curare* cover native South American medicine. On ecstatic healers see Peter Furst,"Shamanism: South American Shamanism," in *The Encyclopedia of Religion* (New York, 1987); Gerardo Reichel-Dolmatoff, *The Shaman and the Jaguar: A Study of Narcotic Drugs among the Indians of Colombia* (Philadelphia, 1975); and Mario Califano, "El chamanismo mataco," *Scripta Ethnológica* 3, no. 3 (1976):7–60. Lawrence E. Sullivan, *Icanchu's Drum: An Orientation to Meaning in South American Religions* (New York, 1988) details the vocation of the ecstatic healer (pp. 386–465) as well as the passages of the life cycle (pp. 229–385). Various afflicting and healing spirits are examined by Mario Califano, "El concepto de enfermedad y muerte entre los Mataco-costaneros," *Scripta Ethnológica* (Buenos Aires) 2, no. 2 (1974):32–73; and by Otto Zerries, "Krankheitsdämonen und Hilfsgeister des Medizinmännes in Südamerika," *Proceedings of the International Congress of Americanists* 30 (1955):162–178. An exemplary study of notions of the body is Joseph W. Bastien, "Qollahuaya-Andean Body Concepts: A Topographical-Hydraulic Model of Physiology," *American Anthropologist* 87 (1985):595–611. Irwin Press, "The Urban Curandero," *American Anthropologist* 73 (1971):741–756, presents issues particular to city-dwelling curers.

Index

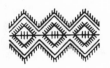